The Chicago Review Press

PHARMACOLOGY MADE EASY
for
NCLEX
PN

Review and Study Guide

Linda Waide, MSN, MEd, RN
and Berta Roland, MSN, RN

Library of Congress Cataloging-in Publication Data is available from the Library of Congress.

© 2001 by Linda Waide and Berta Roland
All rights reserved
This book, or any part thereof, may not be reproduced in any manner without written permission from the publisher.
Published by Chicago Review Press, Incorporated
814 North Franklin Street
Chicago, Illinois 60610

ISBN 1-55652-392-0
Printed in the United States of America

Contents

Acknowledgments

We wish to express our appreciation to the consultants and contributors for their efforts and expertise. It has been very rewarding to associate with such capable and pleasant professionals in the creation of this review and study guide. Because of their valuable assistance, *Pharmacology Made Easy for NCLEX-PN* is now available to help graduates prepare for the PN Licensure Examination.

   We also wish to thank Noreen Pitts for her tireless and tenacious efforts in preparing and preparing and preparing the many revisions that came across her desk for *Pharmacology Made Easy for NCLEX-PN*. She exemplifies professionalism on a daily basis.

Consultants and Contributors

Joanne Brown, MSN, MPH, RN
Health Education and Health Promotion
University of Alabama at Birmingham

Jane Case, MSN, FNP, RN
Vanderbilt University, Nashville, Tennessee

Amy Chrapliwy, MSc, BSN, RN
Director, Faith Wesleyan Child Care Center
Greensboro, North Carolina

Judith Cooper, MSN, RN
CNS—Maternal-Infant Care
Assistant Professor, Troy State University, Troy, Alabama

Mary Ann Dell, EdD, RN
Associate Professor, Troy State University, Troy, Alabama
Coordinator of MSN program at Phoenix City, Alabama

Phyllis Horton, MSN, RN
President of Stellar Systems, Education Consultant
Eden, North Carolina

Joyce Jenkins, MSN, RN
Assistant Professor, CNS—Pediatrics
Troy State University, Troy, Alabama

Margaret Lyles, MSN, RN
Assistant Professor, Adult Health Coordinator
Troy State University, Troy, Alabama

Preface

Mastering pharmacology can be a time-consuming, difficult, and sometimes overwhelming task for graduate nurses preparing for the NCLEX-PN. *Pharmacology Made Easy for NCLEX-PN Review and Study Guide* was created to provide graduates with a quick and efficient way to assure their success. This one-of-a-kind text furnishes the graduate with the knowledge and confidence needed to excel in the classroom and on the pharmacology portion of the NCLEX-PN.

Pharmacology Made Easy for NCLEX-PN prepares the graduate for success on the NCLEX in three important ways.

First, it increases the graduate's knowledge of pharmacology with 15 carefully written practice tests that include answers and rationales for every question, plus a 100-question practice test on an interactive software computer disk, also with answers and rationales. All questions follow the latest NCLEX-PN test plan and format. The answers and rationales given at the end of each practice test are designed to teach the graduate **why** the correct answer is right and **why** the three distractions are incorrect. All phases of Client Need (Health Promotion/Maintenance, Physiological Integrity, Psychosocial Integrity, and Safe, Effective Care Environment) are identified for every question. Graduates can easily trace their competence and success in all of these areas.

Second, *Pharmacology Made Easy for NCLEX-PN* gives each graduate an opportunity to practice and learn test-taking skills and strategies that are vital for success on the NCLEX-PN CAT (Computerized Adaptive Testing). Practicing how to select correct answers using the Critical Thinking Process can improve test scores. Graduates who possess good test-taking skills and are able to apply knowledge correctly are more likely to experience success on the NCLEX-PN.

Third, this review decreases test-taking anxiety for licensure candidates. Many graduates tell us they study for tests but are too anxious to remember the subject matter being tested. By preparing for the NCLEX-PN with the *Pharmacology Made Easy for NCLEX-PN Review and Study Guide*, graduates can feel confident because they have prepared appropriately.

Introduction

The Purpose of Drugs

Drugs are used to treat medical diseases, disorders, and conditions. They are also administered for diagnosis and prevention of diseases and disorders, and to maintain health. In addition to prescribed drugs, "over-the-counter" (OTC) drugs such as aspirin, Tagamet, and Benadryl; various salves, ointments, and solutions; and home remedies such as soda and salt are also used to treat and relieve symptoms.

For nursing purposes, drugs can be defined as agents prescribed by qualified health professionals for the treatment of disorders. Since the early 1900s, many laws have been passed by the U.S. Congress to make drugs safer for use. Drugs are now regulated by the federal government through the Food and Drug Administration (FDA). Prior to FDA control, a retroactive system was employed to assess drugs already on the market. Today we have two broad groupings of drugs defined by the Food and Drug Administration: "over-the-counter" and "prescription."

Persons administering and receiving drugs should be aware that drugs alone cannot cure. They combine with the body's natural defenses to bring recovery and stabilization. Where some drugs are helpful for some individuals, for others they may not be effective. Each of us has our own unique immune system. Drugs that bring astounding relief to some will invariably bring no relief to others.

Medications are classified according to their therapeutic uses. Those that have multiple therapeutic uses, like aspirin, are classified according to their most common usage. Drugs can be toxic to the body. Persons administering and receiving drugs should understand the full consequences of any drug given for a particular condition. Individuals will respond differently to the type of drug and dosage administered. Drug regimens should be established with a health-care provider.

Drug Names

There are three different names for every drug. The chemical name describes the drug in terms of its chemistry. Aspirin's chemical name, for instance, is acetylsalicylic acid. Nurses and other health-care providers usually do not refer to a drug by its chemical name when they are communicating with a client or with each other, partly because it is generally difficult to pronounce.

A drug also has a generic or nonproprietary name and at least one trade or brand name. Each drug has only one generic name, while it can have several trade names. "Aspirin" is the generic name for acetylsalicylic acid. Aspirin's trade names include Bayer Aspirin, Bayer Buffered Aspirin, and many more. Trade names are protected by trademark registration. Even though the generic name can be longer and more difficult to pronounce than a trade name, nurses and other health-care professionals generally prefer to use a drug's generic name.

Routes of Drug Absorption

Drugs can be absorbed into the body by three major routes: the enteral, the parenteral, and the percutaneous.

Enteral Route

Drugs administered by the oral, rectal, and nasogastric routes go directly into the gastrointestinal tract. This is the enteral (intestinal) route. Drugs given via the enteral route have the slowest and least dependable rate of absorption, resulting in a slower onset of drug action. Drugs such as insulin and gentamicin are destroyed by digestive fluids and must not be administered enterally.

The enteral route should not be used if the client is experiencing vomiting, gastrointestinal suctioning (where there is a possibility of aspiration), or if the client is unconscious. The enteral route should not be used if the drug harms or discolors the teeth.

Enteral-route medications can be administered as:

- Capsules
- Elixirs
- Emulsions
- Lozenges
- Suspensions
- Syrups
- Tablets

Parenteral Route

When drugs are given parenterally, they do not go through the gastrointestinal tract. The onset of action is usually more rapid but the effects are of shorter duration. Drugs are administered parenterally when they must be absorbed rapidly and at a steady, controlled rate. The parenteral route of administration is also used when the client is experiencing nausea and vomiting. Several different parenteral routes may be used.

Intradermal (ID) Route
Intradermal injections are administered just below the epidermis into the dermis. The absorption rate is slow. This is the route of choice for:

- Allergy sensitivity
- Desensitization
- Local anesthetics
- Vaccinations
- Intramuscular (IM) Route

Intramuscular injections are carried out by the use of a needle penetrating the dermis and subcutaneous tissue and entering into the muscle tissue. The drug is deposited into the muscle mass. Absorption is more rapid with IM injections due to greater blood supply to the muscles. Injections should be made into healthy tissue with careful placement of the needle so that damage to nerves and blood vessels is avoided.

Intravenous (IV) Route
The intravenous route places the drug directly into the bloodstream. Intravenous administration is the most rapid of all the parenteral routes. Large volumes of drugs can be administered into the vein, usually with little irritation. Most of the time IV medications are given on an intermittent basis, or the drug can be given continuously through an established IV line. The IV route is usually the most comfortable for the client if the drugs are to be given daily for several days.

Subcutaneous (SC) Route
Subcutaneous injections are made into the subcutaneous tissue, the loose connective tissue located between the dermis and the muscle layer. Many drugs cannot be administered by the subcutaneous route because only 2 ml of fluid can be injected into subcutaneous tissue at one time. If circulation is adequate, subcutaneous injections are completely absorbed. Examples of drugs commonly injected subcutaneously are:

- Heparin
- Insulin

Sometimes the terms intralesional (into a lesion), intra-arterial (into an artery), intracardiac (into the heart), intra-articular (into a joint), or intrathecal (within the spinal cord) are used.

Percutaneous Route

Percutaneous administration refers to the application of medication to the skin or mucus membranes. Absorption can be influenced by the drug's concentration, the length of contact with the skin, affected areas, size of affected areas, thickness of the skin, tissue hydration, and how much the skin has been disrupted. The primary advantage of percutaneous administration is localization that reduces systemic side effects. Medications given via the percutaneous route may be difficult to apply, messy, and time-consuming due to the short duration of their action. These drugs require frequent application. Percutaneous administration can be made via:

- Creams
- Inhalants
- Instillations
- Lotions
- Patches
- Powders

Practice Test 1

Anti-Infective Agents

OVERVIEW

Anti-infectives are natural or synthetic compounds that treat, inhibit, and prevent various kinds of infections.

Anti-infectives include:

- Amebicides and antiprotozoals
- Aminoglycosides
- Anthelmintics
- Antifungals
- Antimalarials
- Antituberculars and antileprotics
- Antivirals

- Cephalosporins
- Macrolides
- Penicillins
- Quinolones
- Sulfonamides
- Tetracyclines

AMEBICIDES AND ANTIPROTOZOALS

AMEBICIDES are substances that kill amebas. A person infected with amebas is said to have amebiasis. Amebiasis is caused by the parasite Entamoeba histolytica.

There are two types of amebiasis: intestinal and extraintestinal. The extraintestinal type, such as that found in the liver, is more difficult to treat.

Conditions treated with amebicides include:

- Amebic dysentery
- Amebic hepatitis

ANTIPROTOZOALS are substances that kill protozoa. Protozoa are single-celled parasitic organisms. Protozoal infections are typically spread by the fecal-oral route where food or water are contaminated with cysts or spores. Infections may also occur through the bite of a mosquito or other insect that has previously bitten an infected person.

Conditions treated with antiprotozoals include:

- Sleeping sickness (Trypanosoma gambiense)
- Vaginal infections (Trichomonas vaginalis)

AMINOGLYCOSIDES

Aminoglycosides are chemical compounds found in some anti-infectives. Some of these compounds are derived from microorganisms while others are produced synthetically. Aminoglycosides are effective in treating bacterial infections (especially those caused by gram-negative microorganisms).

Conditions treated with aminoglycosides include:

- Urinary tract infections (UTIs)
- Wound infections
- Septicemia

Aminoglycosides may also be used to decrease the number of normal intestinal flora prior to gastrointestinal surgery.

ANTHELMINTICS

Anthelmintics are substances used to treat people who are infected with worms (helminths). The most common infections are associated with hookworms, pinworms, roundworms, tapeworms, and whipworms.

To determine the treatment of choice, the type of worm must be identified. This is done by examination of stool for the ova (eggs) or the worm itself.

Conditions treated with anthelmintics include:

- Pinworm infection (Enterobius vermicularis)
- Tapeworm infection (Echinococcus granulosus)

ANTIFUNGALS

Antifungal agents hinder or slow the multiplication of fungi (fungistatics) or destroy the fungi (fungicides). Fungal infections are referred to as myotic infections. These infections may be superficial or systemic. Superficial infections would include conditions of the skin and nails. Systemic infections are those occurring inside the body.

Fungi include yeast and molds and are found in the air, soil, and water. Only a few will cause disease.

Conditions treated with antifungals include:

- Histoplasmosis (disease of the lungs)
- Ringworm (skin infection)
- Candidiasis (local and systemic infection)
- Athlete's foot (skin infection)
- Thrush (mouth and throat infection)

ANTIMALARIALS

An antimalarial is prescribed to treat persons with malaria. Malaria is transmitted to humans through the bite of an anopheles mosquito infected with one of the four protozoa that cause malaria (Plasmodium falciparum, Plasmodium malariae, Plasmodium ovale, Plasmodium vivax).

Antimalarial substances are used to suppress (prevent) malaria or to manage (treat) an acute attack of malaria.

Conditions treated with antimalarials include:

- Acute malarial attacks
- Malaria (as suppressive prophylaxis)

ANTITUBERCULARS AND ANTILEPROTICS

ANTITUBERCULARS are used to treat people who have tuberculosis. Tuberculosis is caused by the Mycobacterium tuberculosis bacillus. Treatment of tuberculosis usually includes the administration of two or more antitubercular medications.

Persons receiving two or more medications from the same drug classification are doing so for the drugs' synergistic action (together, the drugs produce a therapeutic effect that neither drug could produce alone).

Conditions treated with antituberculars include:

- Pulmonary tuberculosis (infection of the lung)
- Miliary tuberculosis (tuberculosis infection that spreads throughout the body)
- Open tuberculosis (tuberculosis infection where the bacilli are present in the secretions that leave the body)

ANTILEPROTICS are administered to treat people who have leprosy (Hansen's disease). Leprosy is caused by the microorganism Mycobacterium leprae.

The two main types of leprosy are lepromatous and tuberculoid. Lepromatous leprosy is characterized by skin lesions and involvement of peripheral nerves. Tuberculoid leprosy involves asymmetrical nerve and skin lesions with anesthesia of the skin.

Conditions treated with antileprotics include:

- Lepromatous leprosy
- Tuberculoid leprosy

ANTIVIRALS

Antivirals treat conditions caused by viruses. Antiviral medications are effective only in a small number of very specific infections caused by viruses.

Conditions treated with antivirals include:

- Influenza A (treatment/prevention)
- Retinitis
- Herpes simplex
- Acquired immunodeficiency syndrome (AIDS)

CEPHALOSPORINS

Cephalosporins are structurally related to penicillins. They are used to treat infections where the microorganisms are susceptible. Cephalosporins may also be used when people are found to be allergic to penicillins.

Cephalosporins are separated into first-, second-, and third-generation medications. Generally speaking, the first-generation cephalosporins are more effective in treating gram-positive microorganisms such as streptococci and some strains of staphylococci. The second-generation cephalosporins are effective against the organisms of the first generation and also against Haemophilus influenzae. The third-generation cephalosporins are more effective in treating gram-negative organisms.

Conditions treated with cephalosporins include:

- Urinary tract infections (UTIs)
- Abdominal infections
- Septicemia
- Meningitis
- Osteomyelitis

MACROLIDES

Macrolides are any of a group of antibacterial anti-infectives produced by certain species of streptomyces.

Conditions treated with macrolides include:

- Streptococcus pneumonia
- S. pyogens pharyngitis/tonsillitis
- Haemophilus influenzae

PENICILLINS

Penicillins have antibacterial properties that are used to treat infections that are susceptible to them. It is necessary to perform culture and sensitivity tests to see which penicillin will be most effective in treating a particular infection.

Penicillins may treat infection by actually killing bacteria (bactericidal) or slowing down the multiplication/reproduction of bacteria (bacteriostatic). Occasionally penicillins are used as a prophylaxis (to prevent infection).

Conditions treated with penicillins include:

- Pneumonia
- Otitis media
- Urinary tract infections (UTIs)
- Rheumatic fever
- Syphilis
- Meningitis
- Gonorrhea

QUINOLONES

Quinolones are broad-spectrum anti-infectives that are absorbed rapidly from the gastrointestinal tract. Quinolones have a low incidence of adverse reactions. A subcategory of quinolones is the fluoroquinolones.

Conditions treated with quinolones include:

- Urinary tract infections (UTIs)
- Gonorrhea
- Lower respiratory tract infections
- Skin infections
- Conjunctivitis

SULFONAMIDES

Sulfonamides are not true anti-infectives because they are not synthesized by microorganisms. They are, however, very effective antibacterial agents.

Conditions treated with sulfonamides include:

- Urinary tract infections (UTIs)
- Otitis media
- Streptococcal infection associated with rheumatic fever (as a prophylaxis)

TETRACYCLINES

Tetracyclines are effective against both gram-negative and gram-positive bacteria. Tetracyclines may be used in cases of penicillin allergy. Tetracyclines are very effective when treating conditions caused by rickettsial and mycoplasmic organisms.

Conditions treated with tetracyclines include:

- Urinary tract infections (UTIs)
- Upper respiratory tract infections
- Pneumonia
- Meningitis
- Venereal diseases

Practice Test 1

Questions

1 - 1

A client has been hospitalized with an upper urinary tract infection (UTI). The urine culture is positive for gram-negative bacilli. Intravenous gentamicin (Garamycin) has been prescribed. Which side effects will be monitored during gentamicin therapy?

1. nephrotoxicity
2. neutropenia
3. hematuria
4. gastrointestinal dyspepsia

1 - 2

A client is febrile and complaining of "aching all over." It was determined that the client has Rocky Mountain spotted fever. You anticipate a prescription for:

1. a tetanus vaccine.
2. acetaminophen (Tylenol).
3. diphenhydramine (Benadryl).
4. tetracycline (Tetracap).

1 - 3

A 30-year-old client was diagnosed with varicella (chickenpox). Which of the following medications is most likely to be prescribed?

1. acyclovir (Zovirax)
2. amphotericin B (Fungizone)
3. fluconazole (Diflucan)
4. amoxapine (Asendin)

1 - 4

Diagnostic tests confirm that your client has gonorrhea. Which of these medications is frequently prescribed for the treatment of this condition?

1. neomycin
2. sulfisoxazole
3. streptomycin
4. penicillin

1 - 5

A physician has prescribed pyrantel pamoate (Antiminth) by mouth 11 mg/kg of body weight, as a one-time dosage for a 6-year-old with pinworms. The parents of the child receiving this medication should be taught that this drug may:

1. color the stools bright red.
2. cause perianal pruritus.
3. cause potassium deficit.
4. cause dehydration.

1 - 6

Which of the following drugs will the nurse recognize as a medication commonly used in the treatment of urinary tract infection?

1. metronidazole
2. acetazolamide (Diamox)
3. ciprofloxacin (Cipro)
4. meperidine

1 - 7

Which of the following medications would be administered to a client with Legionnaires' disease?

1. erythromycin, to keep the bacteria from reproducing
2. Adrenalin, to relieve dyspnea
3. rifampin, a bacteriostatic and bactericidal agent
4. aminophylline, to relieve dyspnea

1 - 8

The nurse will administer cefazolin (Kefzol) for a client with pneumonia. Before administering the first dosage, the nurse will determine if:

1. the client is allergic to buttermilk.
2. the client is allergic to penicillin.
3. peak and trough levels have been prescribed.
4. a chest X ray has been taken.

1 - 9

For the past 10 days, your client has received large dosages of the broad-spectrum antibiotic demeclocycline (Declomycin). What can develop if the normal bacterial flora is eliminated?

1. hives
2. high fever
3. immunosuppression
4. superinfection

1 - 1 0

A 6-month-old has been successfully treated for septicemia with gentamicin (Garamycin). This medication was discontinued the day prior to discharge. Discharge teaching should include:

1. Hearing test to be performed at a follow-up visit.
2. Peak and trough blood tests to be drawn on the third day after discharge.
3. Observing for recurrence of symptoms within 7 to 10 days.
4. Giving yogurt or cottage cheese to help replace normal intestinal flora.

1 - 1 1

Hansen's disease (leprosy) is a chronic disease caused by Mycobacterium leprae. The regimen of choice for this disease includes:

1. dapsone and clofazimine (Lamprene).
2. chloramphenicol (Chloromycetin).
3. norfloxacin (Noroxin).
4. pyrazinamide.

1 - 1 2

Your client, a parent of several small children, has been diagnosed with roundworms and is to be treated with pyrantel pamoate (Pin-X). Your teaching plan will take into account that:

1. this medication cannot be used for children.
2. enemas must be administered twice daily after taking this medication.
3. this medication will have to be taken prophylactically for up to 1 year.
4. it is not advisable for infected persons to prepare meals for the family.

1 - 1 3

A client diagnosed with Trichomonas vaginalis is to begin anti-infective chemotherapy. You anticipate a prescription for:

1. penicillin G.
2. ritonavir.
3. Flagyl.
4. gentamicin.

1 - 1 4

A client experiencing an acute respiratory infection has just completed a course of antibiotic therapy. The client is experiencing a low-grade fever and has a coated tongue. Fluconazole (Diflucan) 100 mg intravenously every 12 hours is prescribed. This drug is given for the treatment of:

1. fungal infection.
2. gram-negative infection.
3. drug sensitivity.
4. nosocomial infection.

1 - 1 5

A client experiencing a vaginal infection caused by candida albicans is given a prescription for nystatin (Mycostatin). Into which anti-infective subcategory would you place this medication?

1. antiviral
2. sulfonamide
3. antifungal
4. cephalosporin

1 - 1 6

Which medication would be contraindicated for a client allergic to penicillin?

1. cefoxitin (Mefoxin)
2. trimethoprim sulfamethoxazole (Septra)
3. cefuroxime (Ceftin)
4. ticarcillin (Ticar)

1 - 1 7

A client with pneumonia has been given the first dose of a penicillin (Ampicillin) antibiotic. The client is experiencing a fine rash all over the body. For which medication do you anticipate a prescription?

1. diphenhydramine (Benadryl)
2. ticarcillin (Ticar)
3. cloxacillin (Cloxapen)
4. oxacillin (Bactocill)

1 - 1 8

A client is experiencing a large surface abrasion on the leg. The nurse observes that the leg is swollen and has red streaks. Which of the following medications would be administered?

1. cefazolin (Ancef)
2. heparin (Liquaemin)
3. verapamil (Calan)
4. furosemide (Lasix)

1 - 1 9

You plan to administer the initial intravenous dosage of cefotaxime (Claforan) to a child with meningitis. Your first action will be to:

1. perform a neurological check.
2. assess for signs of superinfection.
3. assess the intravenous insertion site.
4. check for allergy to penicillin.

1 - 2 0

A client has contracted malaria. You will anticipate a prescription for:

1. ampicillin.
2. chloroquine (Aralen).
3. quinidine gluconate (Quinalan).
4. malaria vaccine.

1 - 2 1

A young client diagnosed with syphilis asks you if there is a cure for the disease. You reply:

1. "Syphilis is a viral disease with no known cure."
2. "Only a few antiviral medications are effective in treating syphilis."
3. "Syphilis may be treated effectively with penicillin G."
4. "Azithromycin is the treatment of choice for syphilis."

1 - 2 2

Your client has a fever of 101° F and is complaining of dysuria and urinary frequency and urgency, and is voiding small amounts. It has been determined that the client has a urinary tract infection (UTI). Cefoxitin (Mefoxin) has been prescribed for its:

1. anti-infective effects.
2. antipyretic effects.
3. antifungal effects.
4. analgesic effects.

1-23

A client is to receive tetracycline 250 mg every 6 hours orally to treat leg ulcers secondary to venous insufficiency. For optimum effect, tetracycline should be administered:

1. in orange juice.
2. with milk.
3. 1 hour before meals.
4. with meals.

1-24

Your client is taking zidovudine (AZT) to slow the progression of the human immunodeficiency virus (HIV). You will teach your client that a toxic effect of AZT is:

1. polycythemia.
2. watery diarrhea.
3. weight loss and anorexia.
4. bone marrow suppression.

1-25

Your client is to receive two antitubercular medications (rifampin and isoniazid) for treatment of pulmonary tuberculosis. You understand the purpose for administering these two antitubercular medications simultaneously is for their:

1. prophylactic effect.
2. sedative effect.
3. synergistic effect.
4. absorptive effect.

1-26

A client is experiencing a urinary tract infection and is receiving sulfonamide (Gantrisin). Which action is essential when administering sulfonamide?

1. assessing the client's apical pulse for signs of bradycardia
2. teaching the client to report blurred vision or mydriasis
3. cautioning the client about performing activities that require mental alertness or physical coordination
4. maintaining a fluid intake between 3000 and 4000 ml daily

1 - 2 7

Your client has acquired immunodeficiency syndrome (AIDS). To prevent the development of pneumocystic carinii pneumonia, the physician has prescribed pentamidine isethionate (Pentam 300) aerosol. To administer this medication, you will:

1. mix the contents of 1 vial of the medication in 6 ml of 0.9% NaCl solution.
2. administer the medication using a low-pressure < 20 psi compressor.
3. instruct the client to use the aerosol device until the chamber is empty.
4. position the client in bed at 45 degrees.

1 - 2 8

You are to administer levofloxacin (Levaquin) to a client experiencing pneumonia. Prior to the administration of this medication, you will:

1. auscultate blood pressure.
2. monitor body temperature.
3. obtain a sputum culture.
4. maintain strict NPO status.

1 - 2 9

A client with cancer of the colon is scheduled for surgery and will receive the following preoperative preparation: A saline cathartic, enemas daily times 3, and neomycin sulfate (Neo-Tabs) 1 gm po q 1 hour for 4 doses, then 1 gm po q 4 hours for the balance of the 24-hour preoperative time. You understand the purpose of the neomycin sulfate is to:

1. render the client's urine sterile.
2. reduce the bacterial count of the client's intestine.
3. prevent postoperative pulmonary complications.
4. reduce metastatic spread.

1 - 3 0

Your client has vaginitis caused by the microorganism Trichomonas vaginalis. Four 500-mg tablets of metronidazole (Flagyl) have been prescribed. Which of the following instructions will you give the client regarding the administration of this medication?

1. "Take all 4 tablets at once."
2. "Take 1 tablet a day for 4 days."
3. "You should consume alcohol in moderation while taking this medication."
4. "This medication is for symptomatic relief only. There is no cure for this infection."

Practice Test 1

Answers, Rationales, and Explanations

1 - 1

(1) **Effects of nephrotoxicity will be monitored during gentamicin (Garamycin) therapy. Nephrotoxicity (a toxic condition that may damage kidney tissues) is the most frequent and serious effect of gentamicin.**

2. Neutropenia (an abnormally small number of neutrophils in the blood) is not a known side effect of gentamicin therapy.

3. Hematuria may occur as a consequence of the upper urinary tract infection, but not as a side effect of gentamicin therapy.

4. Gastrointestinal dyspepsia is not a known side effect of gentamicin therapy.

Pregnancy Category: D

Client Need: Physiological Integrity

1 - 2

(4) **A prescription for tetracycline (Tetracap) will be anticipated. Rocky Mountain spotted fever is a rickettsial infection carried by ticks. It is potentially fatal. Tetracycline is an antibiotic frequently prescribed for rickettsial diseases.**

1. There is no indication that a tetanus vaccine is needed. A tetanus vaccine is usually given for cuts and puncture wounds that expose clients to the toxins of tetanus bacilli, Clostridium tetani.

2. Acetaminophen (Tylenol) may be an effective comfort measure but would not arrest the disease.

3. Diphenhydramine (Benadryl) is an antihistamine and would have no impact on rickettsial infection.

Pregnancy Category: D

Client Need: Health Promotion/Maintenance

1 - 3

(1) **Acyclovir (Zovirax) is the most likely medication to be prescribed for clients with varicella (chickenpox). Acyclovir (Zovirax) is an antiviral agent and a miscellaneous anti-infective medication. It may inhibit the replication of some viruses such as varicella.**

2. Amphotericin B (Fungizone) is an antifungal and has no impact on viruses; e.g., chickenpox.

3. Fluconazole (Diflucan) is an antifungal and has no impact on viruses; e.g., chickenpox.

4. Amoxapine (Asendin) is a tricyclic antidepressant and has no impact on viruses; e.g., chickenpox.

Pregnancy Category: C

Client Need: Health Promotion/Maintenance

1 - 4

③ **Streptomycin is the drug of choice for the treatment of gonorrhea because of the likelihood of coexisting chlamydial infections. Chlamydia is resistant to penicillin, and 45% of clients with chlamydia also have gonorrhea.**

1. Neomycin is not used in the treatment of gonorrhea because the gonococcus is resistant to this medication.
2. Sulfisoxazole (Gantrisin) is an anti-infective frequently prescribed in the treatment of urinary tract infections and has no impact on gonorrhea.
4. Penicillin for many years was prescribed for the treatment of gonorrhea. However, the gonococcus has become resistant to penicillin, and streptomycin has become the drug of choice.

Pregnancy Category: C
Client Need: Health Promotion/Maintenance

1 - 5

① **The parents of children receiving pyrantel pamoate (Antiminth) should be taught that it colors stools bright red. Antiminth is an anthelmintic that paralyzes and kills worms. Enterobiasis (pinworm) is the most common helminth (parasitic worm) in the United States. Mature worms live in the intestine. The female migrates to the perianal area to deposit ova. Infection and reinfection is not uncommon in children where poor hygiene and hand-to-mouth activity occurs. The medication may cause vomiting, and parents should be taught that the vomitus may also be bright red. Other adverse parameters include gastrointestinal distress, headache, drowsiness, dizziness, and skin rash.**

2. Perianal pruritus is caused by the female worm crawling out of the anus to deposit ova, not by the medication.
3. Potassium is not affected by pyrantel pamoate.
4. Pyrantel pamoate may cause nausea, vomiting, and diarrhea. However, dehydration is not associated with administration of the drug.

Pregnancy Category: C
Client Need: Physiological Integrity

1 - 6

③ **Ciprofloxacin (Cipro) is effective therapy for urinary tract infections. Cipro is an anti-infective. It is administered on an empty stomach at least 1 hour before or 2 hours after meals with a full glass of water.**

1. Metronidazole (Flagyl) is an anti-infective frequently prescribed for gynecological, not urinary tract, infections.
2. Acetazolamide (Diamox) is an antiglaucoma agent that lowers intraocular pressure.
4. Meperidine (Demerol) is an opioid analgesic used in the management of moderate to severe pain.

Pregnancy Category: C
Client Need: Physiological Integrity

1 - 7

① **Erythromycin is the drug of choice for the treatment of Legionnaires' disease because it is bacteriostatic (keeps the bacterium Legionella pneumophila from reproducing).**

2 and 4. Adrenalin and aminophylline relieve dyspnea caused by bronchoconstriction by relaxing the smooth muscles of the bronchial tree. However, they have no direct impact on Legionnaires' disease.

3.   Rifampin may be added to the treatment of Legionnaires' disease in severe cases, but should never be given alone because of the chance that resistant organisms may develop during monotherapy. It is a bactericide (an agent that kills bacteria but may not kill their spores).

Pregnancy Category: B

Client Need: Physiological Integrity

1 - 8

② **The client should be assessed for an allergy to penicillin. Cefazolin (Kefzol) is a first-generation cephalosporin. There can be a cross-allergy between penicillins and cephalosporins.**

1.   Yogurt and buttermilk are useful for intestinal flora replacement, but allergies to yogurt or buttermilk do not affect drug use.

3.   Peak and trough levels are appropriate with aminoglycosides, not first-generation cephalosporins such as Kefzol.

4.   Blood and other cultures should be completed before beginning antibiotics, but not necessarily a chest X ray.

Pregnancy Category: B

Client Need: Safe, Effective Care Environment

1 - 9

④ **Superinfection can occur when normal bacterial flora are eliminated. Demeclocycline (Declomycin), a tetracycline, is thought to exert a bacteriostatic effect. A client can develop a superinfection after prolonged use of broad-spectrum antibiotics. When a superinfection occurs, normal bacterial flora are eliminated, allowing disease-producing microorganisms to multiply.**

1.   Hives are produced when there is an allergic reaction to an antibiotic.

2.   A high fever would develop when an inappropriate antibiotic is being given that is not effective against the invading organism.

3.   Immunosuppression may occur when a client is receiving large dosages of drugs such as steroids, not antibiotics.

Pregnancy Category: D

Client Need: Health Promotion/Maintenance

1-10

(1) **Discharge instructions for clients treated with gentamicin (Garamycin) will include a recommendation to have hearing tests performed at a follow-up visit. Garamycin is ototoxic (destructive to the auditory nerve). Indications of ototoxicity are hearing loss, tinnitus, and vertigo.**

2. Peak and trough blood levels are drawn during the administration of a drug, not after a drug is discontinued. Peak and trough levels are drawn to avoid a drug's toxic effects and maintain therapeutic levels only.

3. A recurrence of symptoms can occur at any time, not just 7 to 10 days after the gentamicin (Garamycin) is discontinued.

4. Infants are too young for yogurt and cottage cheese. The infant should first be observed for symptoms of superinfection, such as mouth lesions, thrush, vaginal irritation, and diaper rash.

Pregnancy Category: D
Client Need: Health Promotion/Maintenance

1-11

(1) **Dapsone and clofazimine (Lamprene) are the regimen of choice for Hansen's disease (leprosy). Dapsone is bactericidal and bacteriostatic against the microorganism causing leprosy (Mycobacterium leprae). Clofazimine (Lamprene) is bactericidal.**

2. Chloramphenicol (Chloromycetin) is a broad-spectrum antibiotic. Because of its association with fatal blood dyscrasias, it is used only in serious infections when other drugs are ineffective.

3. Norfloxacin (Noroxin) is a broad-spectrum antibiotic used in urinary infections and has no impact on leprosy.

4. Pyrazinamide acts against Mycobacterium tuberculosis and can be bactericidal or bacteriostatic. It is not used to treat leprosy.

Pregnancy Category: C
Client Need: Physiological Integrity

1 - 1 2

④ **Clients with roundworms should not prepare meals for others. Pyrantel pamoate (Pin-X) is an anthelmintic (kills parasitic intestinal worms) prescribed for the treatment of pinworms and roundworms. There is a high incidence of familial infestation with this disorder. Preparing meals for the family increases the risk of spreading the condition.**

1. Pyrantel pamoate (Pin-X) may be used for children. The entire family should be treated simultaneously.

2. Neither enemas nor laxatives are recommended after taking pyrantel pamoate (Pin-X). The drug itself may cause nausea, vomiting, diarrhea, and abdominal cramps.

3. Clients taking pyrantel pamoate (Pin-X) for the treatment of roundworms should take the medication as a one-time dosage. The dosage should not exceed 1 gram. If Pin-X is administered to treat pinworms, the dosage should be repeated in 2 weeks.

Pregnancy Category: X
Client Need: Health Promotion/Maintenance

1 - 1 3

③ **Metronidazole (Flagyl) is a trichomonacidal agent and is the treatment of choice for Trichomonas vaginalis. Trichomoniasis is a sexually transmitted disease caused by a protozoan.**

1 and 4. Neither penicillin G or gentamicin are effective in treating Trichomonas vaginalis.

2. Ritonavir is an antiviral used in the treatment of HIV infection. It is not effective in the treatment of trichomoniasis.

Pregnancy Category: C
Client Need: Physiological Integrity

1 - 1 4

① **Fluconazole (Diflucan) is administered to treat fungal infections. Fungal infection is often associated with long-term antibiotic therapy because of the potential for developing superinfection (a new infection caused by an organism different than the one causing the initial infection).**

2. Infections of the upper respiratory tract and urinary tract caused by gram-negative bacilli such as E. coli and Klebsiella enterobacteriaceae are not treated with antifungal medications.

3. Drug sensitivity is often manifested by skin rash and treated by discontinuing the offending drug.

4. Nosocomial infections (infections that develop in a health-care facility as a consequence of poor hygiene, such as inadequate hand-washing or faulty health-care delivery) involve any type of organism, not just fungi.

Pregnancy Category: C
Client Need: Physiological Integrity

1 - 1 5

③ **Nystatin (Mycostatin) is an antifungal. Candidiasis is a yeast-type fungal infection that may be treated effectively by nystatin (Mycostatin). This medication affects the fungal cell's membrane, thus arresting the disease process.**

1. Antivirals are administered to treat specific viral infections; amantadine is used specifically to treat influenza A.

2. Sulfonamides are given to treat bacterial infections.

4. Cephalosporins are a group of antibiotics derived from the fungus Cephalosporium. They are not effective against fungal infections.

Pregnancy Category: NR

Client Need: Health Promotion/Maintenance

1 - 1 6

④ **Ticarcillin (Ticar) contains penicillin and would be contraindicated for clients with penicillin allergy.**

1 and 3. Cefoxitin (Mefoxin) and cefuroxime (Ceftin) are cephalosporin antibiotics and are not necessarily contraindicated for clients with penicillin allergy.

2. Trimethoprim sulfamethoxazole (Septra) is a sulfa antibiotic and would not be contraindicated for clients with penicillin allergy.

Pregnancy Category: B

Client Need: Safe, Effective Care Environment

1 - 1 7

① **A prescription for diphenhydramine (Benadryl) will be anticipated. The client may be having an allergic reaction to penicillin. Diphenhydramine (Benadryl) is an antihistamine used to treat allergic reactions. Because of Benadryl's effective competition for H_1-receptor sites, the histamine response is lessened.**

2, 3, and 4. Ticarcillin (Ticar), cloxacillin (Cloxapen), and oxacillin (Bactocill) are penicillins that may aggravate the situation if given.

Pregnancy Category: B

Client Need: Physiological Integrity

1 - 1 8

① Cefazolin (Ancef) is likely to be administered to a client experiencing a large surface abrasion. Ancef is a cephalosporin anti-infective. It binds to the cell wall of bacteria, causing cell death. It is especially effective in treating serious infections of the skin, bone, and soft tissue, and in general sepsis.

2. Heparin (Liquaemin) is an anticoagulant and has no impact on infection.

3. Verapamil (Calan) is an antiarrhythmic and has no impact on infection.

4. Furosemide (Lasix) is a diuretic and has no impact on infection.

Pregnancy Category: B

Client Need: Physiological Integrity

1 - 1 9

④ You will first check for an allergy to penicillin. There is a possibility of allergy to cephalosporins in persons who are allergic to penicillins. This child will be receiving high dosages of antibiotics because of meningitis; therefore, assessing for drug allergies is essential.

1. Neurological checks should be completed frequently on clients with meningitis, not just in connection with administration of medication.

2. Superinfection occurs during or after a course of antibiotics, not at the onset of administration.

3. The intravenous site should be assessed with each dose of Claforan, not just initially. The intravenous site should be changed every 48 to 72 hours to prevent phlebitis.

Pregnancy Category: B

Client Need: Safe, Effective Care Environment

1 - 2 0

② A client experiencing malaria may be given a prescription for the antimalarial chloroquine (Aralen). It is effective in treating malaria caused by the protozoan parasite Plasmodium.

1. Ampicillin is a penicillin antibiotic and is not effective in treating malaria.

3. Quinidine gluconate is an antiarrhythmic and is not effective in treating malaria.

4. There is no vaccine for malaria.

Pregnancy Category: C

Client Need: Physiological Integrity

1-21

③ **Syphilis may be treated effectively with intramuscular injections of penicillin G. Syphilis is a sexually transmitted infection caused by the spirochete Treponema pallidum. Syphilis may also be spread by contact with infectious lesions and sharing contaminated needles.**

1 and 2. Syphilis is not a viral disease. It is a disease caused by the spirochete bacterium Treponema pallidum. Antiviral medications are therefore inappropriate.

4. Azithromycin by mouth is the treatment of choice for chlamydia disease.

Pregnancy Category: B

Client Need: Psychosocial Integrity

1-22

① **Cefoxitin (Mefoxin) is commonly prescribed for urinary tract infections. It is a broad-spectrum cephalosporin antibiotic. Other uses include treatment of infection in the respiratory tract, on the skin, and in the bones and joints.**

2. Cefoxitin (Mefoxin) is not an antipyretic. It has no effect on body temperature. However, controlling infection may lower body temperature.

3. Systemic fungal infections are treated with the antifungal anti-infectives.

4. Cefoxitin (Mefoxin) is an antibiotic and has no direct effect on pain associated with urination. Dysuria (painful urination) decreases with control of urinary tract infection.

Pregnancy Category: B

Client Need: Physiological Integrity

1-23

③ **It is recommended that tetracycline be taken 1 hour before meals. Tetracycline should be given on an empty stomach because food, milk, and milk products can reduce absorption by 50%.**

1, 2, and 4. Tetracycline should be given on an empty stomach, not in orange juice or with meals. Dairy products are known to bind tetracycline and prevent absorption.

Pregnancy Category: D

Client Need: Health Promotion/Maintenance

1 - 2 4

④ **A major toxic effect of zidovudine (AZT) is bone marrow suppression. This results in severe anemia and reduced white blood count (WBC) and platelet count. Zidovudine (AZT) is an antiviral medication used in the management of human immunodeficiency virus (HIV).**

1. Polycythemia refers to an increase in the total red cell mass of the blood. AZT causes bone marrow suppression and therefore decreases red blood cell production. The client is likely to have anemia.

2 and 3. Watery diarrhea, weight loss, and anorexia are symptoms of HIV and are not necessarily due to the administration of AZT.

Pregnancy Category: C

Client Need: Physiological Integrity

1 - 2 5

③ **You understand that two or more medications from the same drug class (such as rifampin and isoniazid) are administered for their synergistic effect (concomitant treatment). For example, the harmonious action of these two medications produces an effect that neither could produce alone. They produce an effect greater than the total effect of each drug operating alone.**

1. The prophylactic effect of a medication refers to its ability to prevent disease. This client already has tuberculosis. There is no medication that can prevent tuberculosis.

2. Rifampin and isoniazid do not have sedative effects. Adverse reactions include fatigue and drowsiness.

4. Administering rifampin and isoniazid together will not increase their absorption time.

Pregnancy Category: C

Client Need: Health Promotion/Maintenance

1 - 2 6

④ **It is essential for the nurse to maintain a fluid intake between 3000 and 4000 ml daily for clients receiving a sulfonamide such as Gantrisin. Extra fluids promote the excretion of sulfonamides and prevent crystalluria (crystals in the urine) and subsequent stone formation.**

1. Adverse cardiovascular reactions to sulfonamides include tachycardia (pulse rate above 60 beats per minute), palpitations (a rapid throbbing or fluttering of the heart), and syncope (fainting). Bradycardia is not an adverse reaction associated with sulfonamides.

2. Sulfonamides are not associated with blurred vision or mydriasis (pronounced or abnormal dilation of the pupil).

3. Sulfonamides do not adversely affect mental alertness or physical coordination.

Pregnancy Category: C

Client Need: Health Promotion/Maintenance

1-27

③ **The client should use the aerosol device until the chamber is empty. This may take 45 to 60 minutes. A full dosage will not have been given if any of the solution is left in the aerosol chamber.**

1. To administer the aerosol, the nurse will mix the contents of 1 vial of medication with 6 ml of sterile water. Sodium chloride should not be inhaled.
2. Medication should be administered only from a Respigard II nebulizer. The flow rate should be 5 to 7 l/minute from a 40 to 50 psi air or oxygen source.
4. When the medication is given IV, it should be infused slowly with the client lying down. Blood pressure should be closely monitored. When taken as an aerosol, the client should maintain a sitting position (90 degrees).

Pregnancy Category: C
Client Need: Health Promotion/Maintenance

1-28

③ **Before administering levofloxacin (Levaquin), you will obtain a sputum culture. Levofloxacin (Levaquin) is a fluorquinolone antimicrobial medication used in treating respiratory infections. Prior to the administration of any antimicrobial medication, all culture specimens should be obtained. If specimens are obtained after the administration of antimicrobials, the culture results are altered.**

1. Blood pressure is not affected by levofloxacin (Levaquin).
2. Body temperature is not directly affected by levofloxacin (Levaquin). However, once a therapeutic blood level of the medication is established and the infection abates, body temperature should return to normal.
4. There is no justification for maintaining a client on NPO when administering levofloxacin (Levaquin). Fluids should be encouraged to liquefy mucus and avoid dehydration.

Pregnancy Category: C
Client Need: Physiological Integrity

1-29

② **Neomycin sulfate (Neo-Tabs) are administered prior to intestinal surgery to reduce the bacterial count in the client's intestine and minimize the potential for infection.**

1. The surgical site is the colon. The urinary system is not a consideration.
3. Pulmonary complications, such as a pulmonary embolus, would not be affected by the administration of an anti-infective.
4. Anti-infectives cannot reduce metastatic spread.

Pregnancy Category: D
Client Need: Safe, Effective Care Environment

1-30

1. **You will teach the client that all four 500-mg tablets of metronidazole (Flagyl) should be taken at once. The microorganism Trichomonas vaginalis is a resilient flagellum that can be successfully treated with metronidazole. It is important that 2 grams of Flagyl be taken at once for serum levels of the medication to be high enough to kill the microorganisms.**

2. All four 500-mg tablets of metronidazole (Flagyl) should be taken at once, not one a day for 4 days.

3. Alcohol is contraindicated during metronidazole (Flagyl) administration due to the likelihood of nausea and vomiting.

4. Vaginitis caused by the organism Trichomonas vaginalis is a treatable sexually transmitted disease.

Pregnancy Category: B

Client Need: Physiological Integrity

Practice Test 2

Antineoplastic Agents

OVERVIEW

Antineoplastics are administered to destroy or prevent the development, growth, and proliferation of malignant cells. People receiving antineoplastic agents are said to be receiving chemotherapy.

Antineoplastics include:

- **Alkylating agents**
- **Antimetabolites**
- **Antitumor antibiotics**
- **Hormones**
- **Radiation therapy**
- **Miscellaneous antineoplastic agents**

ALKYLATING AGENTS

Alkylating agents interfere with the function of cancer cells by attaching to the protein within them and altering their chemical composition. These agents are extremely toxic and cause very unpleasant and even dangerous side effects.

Conditions treated with alkylating agents include:

- Hodgkin's disease
- Lymphosarcomal leukemias
- Multiple myelomas

ANTIMETABOLITES

Antimetabolites adversely affect cancer cells by interfering in a particular phase of their metabolism. They can cause severe bone marrow depression, which may necessitate their withdrawal.

Conditions treated with antimetabolites include:

- Acute lymphocytic leukemia in children
- Uterine choriocarcinoma
- Lymphosarcoma
- Hodgkin's disease
- Carcinomas of the reproductive tract, pancreas, liver, and gastrointestinal tract
- Tumors of the head, neck, brain, and gallbladder

ANTITUMOR ANTIBIOTICS

Antitumor antibiotics interfere with the RNA synthesis of cancer cells or cause a split in the DNA chains of cancer cells. They should not be confused with anti-infective antibiotics as they do not have anti-infective properties.

Conditions treated by antitumor antibiotics include:

- Wilms' tumor
- Certain lymphomas
- Choriocarcinoma
- Hodgkin's disease
- Solid tumors of the breast, bone, bladder, lung, thyroid gland, and ovaries
- Ewing's sarcoma
- Adenocarcinoma of the stomach, pancreas, colon, and rectum
- Tumors of the head, neck, and cervix

HORMONES

Hormones have a number of uses in the treatment of cancer even though their action is not fully understood. Hormones have produced remissions of certain cancers. Sex hormones have provided palliative treatment for carcinomas of the reproductive tract.

Conditions treated with hormones include:

- Acute lymphocytic leukemia in children
- Carcinoma of the prostate
- Breast cancer in postmenopausal women
- Metastatic breast cancer

RADIATION THERAPY

Radiation is used to treat cancer; in fact, the majority of clients with cancer will receive some form of radiation therapy in addition to chemotherapy. Types of radiation therapy include external and internal therapy.

Conditions treated with external radiation therapy include:

- Salivary gland tumors
- Sarcomas
- Tumors of the lung and prostate

Conditions treated with internal radiation therapy include:

- Tumors of the prostate

MISCELLANEOUS ANTINEOPLASTIC AGENTS

Miscellaneous antineoplastic agents are a heterogeneous group of drugs having various active mechanisms. They include:

Vincristine sulfate (Oncovin)

Conditions treated with vincristine sulfate include:

- Acute leukemia

Vinblastine sulfate (Velban)

Conditions treated with vinblastine sulfate include:

- Choriocarcinoma
- Hodgkin's disease
- Lymphosarcoma

Procarbazine hydrochloride (Matulane)

Conditions treated with procarbazine hydrochloride include:

- Hodgkin's disease (orally)

Mechlorethamine hydrochloride (nitrogen mustard)

Conditions treated with mechlorethamine hydrochloride include:

- Chronic lymphocytic leukemia
- Polycythemia vera

Hydroxyurea (Hydrea)

Conditions treated with hydroxyurea include:

- Chronic granulocytic leukemia
- Malignant melanoma
- Ovarian carcinoma

Azathioprine (Imuran)

Conditions treated with azathioprine include:

- Rejection of kidney transplants

Mitotane (Lysodren)

Conditions treated with mitotane include:

- Adrenocortical carcinoma

Practice Test 2

Questions

2 - 1

A new client arrives at the cancer clinic 10 days post colon resection. A prescription for fluorouracil (5-FU) has been given. Included in your instructions to the client will be the recommendation to:

1. use a soft toothbrush and maintain scrupulous oral hygiene.
2. spend as much time in the sun as possible for the ultraviolet radiation.
3. avoid antiemetics since nausea is a rare side effect of 5-FU.
4. begin taking the medication immediately.

2 - 2

A client with breast cancer is to receive chemotherapy treatments with vinblastine sulfate (VLB). Regarding the administration of this medication, you know that:

1. special precautions are to be taken when mixing and handling.
2. vinblastine is to be given intramuscularly.
3. vinblastine is to be administered intrathecally only.
4. alopecia will not occur.

2 - 3

A client experiencing testicular cancer is to receive plicamycin (mithramycin) intravenously. Prior to the administration of this medication, the nurse will:

1. serve a full meal.
2. force fluids.
3. administer an antiemetic.
4. weigh the client.

2 - 4

A client with cancer is to receive chemotherapy with doxorubicin (Adriamycin). Which statement regarding this medication is true?

1. Doxorubicin (Adriamycin) may only be given subcutaneously.
2. Doxorubicin (Adriamycin) may only be given intramuscularly.
3. Doxorubicin (Adriamycin) has few side effects.
4. Doxorubicin (Adriamycin) may cause severe tissue necrosis.

2 - 5

Clients receiving chemotherapy for cancer should be taught the adverse effects associated with the agents in use. A client receiving bleomycin (Blenoxane) should be taught to report:

1. a decrease in urine output.
2. breathing difficulty and coughing.
3. numbness or tingling in the extremities.
4. weight gain or edema.

2 - 6

Your client is experiencing stomatitis following the administration of methotrexate for the treatment of osteogenic sarcoma. You will assess the oral cavity frequently and recommend:

1. a clear, full-liquid diet.
2. total parenteral nutrition.
3. a high-protein diet.
4. a soft, bland, tepid diet.

2 - 7

A client with cancer is receiving cisplatin (Platinol) intravenous chemotherapy. Which of the following prescriptions should be questioned?

1. a bolus dose of furosemide
2. intravenous fluids at 150 cc per hour
3. metoclopramide (Reglan) 30 to 60 minutes prior to cisplatin
4. a follow-up appointment for a bone marrow test in 2 weeks

2 - 8

A client experiencing leukemia is receiving busulfan (Myleran) and has developed bone marrow suppression. Which nursing diagnosis has the highest priority?

1. activity intolerance
2. altered peripheral tissue perfusion
3. fluid volume deficit: Hemorrhage
4. infection

2 - 9

A client has undergone a mastectomy and has been placed on fluorouracil (5-FU). The side effects of this drug may include the following:

1. constipation
2. ventricular arrhythmias
3. alopecia
4. cystitis

2 - 1 0

A client with advanced cancer of the bladder is receiving cisplatin (Platinol). The latest laboratory results indicate a BUN of 40 mg/dl and a creatinine level of 2.0 mg/dl. You will:

1. document these findings as normal.
2. administer the medication as prescribed.
3. withhold the medication and notify the physician.
4. encourage fluid intake (2 to 3 L daily).

2 - 1 1

Your client is receiving dacarbazine (DTIC-Dome) and is experiencing alopecia. You recognize this adverse reaction to be:

1. the presence of ulcers in the mouth.
2. a loss of appetite.
3. hypersensitivity to sunlight with potential for sunburn.
4. a temporary loss of hair.

2 - 1 2

Your 75-year-old client has squamous-cell carcinoma of the neck and is receiving bleomycin sulfate (Blenoxane) 10 units/m$_2$ IV, twice weekly. You will observe this client closely for the common life-threatening adverse reaction of:

1. pulmonary fibrosis.
2. hyperkeratosis.
3. thrombocytopenia.
4. encephalopathy.

2 - 1 3

Your client is receiving the antineoplastic alkylating drug nitrogen mustard (Mustargen). You know this type of drug is effective against cancer due to its ability to:

1. poison cancer cells.
2. interfere with normal cellular metabolism.
3. alter normal hormonal equilibrium.
4. interfere with DNA or RNA synthesis.

2 - 1 4

A client with Hodgkin's disease is receiving nitrogen mustard (Mustargen) 0.4 mg/kg IV, single dose. You will teach the client to avoid OTC products containing aspirin because:

1. aspirin lowers the platelet count and contributes to bleeding.
2. the anticoagulating effects of aspirin may cause bleeding.
3. aspirin interferes with the Mustargen's ability to destroy cancer cells.
4. aspirin compounds the toxic effects of antineoplastic drugs.

2 - 1 5

Your client is experiencing acute lymphocytic leukemia. Methotrexate (Folex) 3.3 mg/m$_2$/day po has been prescribed. You know to administer this drug:

1. with fruit juices only.
2. with milk.
3. on an empty stomach.
4. immediately before a meal.

2 - 1 6

Providing safe intravenous administration of doxorubicin (Adriamycin) includes your recognition that this drug can cause:

1. severe nausea and vomiting.
2. stomatitis.
3. irreversible alopecia.
4. tissue necrosis.

2 - 1 7

Your client is receiving oral dosages of cyclophosphamide (Cytoxan). To improve toleration of this drug, you will give it with:

1. milk products.
2. cold foods.
3. carbonated drinks.
4. hot drinks.

2-18

Clients receiving potentially myelo-suppressant drugs such as gemcitabine (Gemzar) may become neutropenic. You know the single most important manifestation of infection is:

1. diarrhea.
2. sore throat.
3. anorexia.
4. fever.

2-19

A client has stomatitis after a round of chemotherapy with cyclophosphamide (Cytoxan). To treat this condition, you teach the client to:

1. use a mouthwash containing alcohol after each meal.
2. limit smoking.
3. suck on ice chips periodically.
4. consume soft, bland foods.

2-20

A client's infusion of vincristine sulfate (Oncovin) has infiltrated. To disperse the infiltrated drug, you anticipate administering a local injection of:

1. diphenhydramine.
2. cefazolin sodium.
3. hyaluronidase.
4. famciclovir.

2-21

Which of the following foods should be avoided by clients whose antineoplastic drugs have caused stomatitis?

1. fresh fruits and vegetables
2. milk shakes
3. low-residue foods
4. soft foods

2-22

You know that Hodgkin's disease is treated with nitrogen mustard, Oncovin, procarbazine, and prednisone (MOPP) given every 28 days for a minimum of:

1. 2 cycles.
2. 4 cycles.
3. 6 cycles.
4. 8 cycles.

Practice Test 2

Answers, Rationales, and Explanations

2 - 1

(1) **Clients receiving fluorouracil (5-FU) should be taught to use a soft toothbrush. 5-FU is an antineoplastic drug and has a high incidence of stomatitis (inflammation of the mouth). A soft toothbrush will prevent additional irritation and discomfort.**

2. Photosensitivity is among the side effects of fluorouracil (5-FU). Persons taking 5-FU should avoid direct sunlight and ultraviolet lamp treatments. Photosensitivity subsides 2 to 3 months after the last dosage.

3. 5-FU very frequently causes nausea. Antiemetics may be prescribed before and after 5-FU administration.

4. 5-FU therapy is generally contraindicated within 1 month of major surgery due to leukopenia (WBC below $3500/mm_3$) and the likelihood of infection.

Pregnancy Category: D

Client Need: Safe, Effective Care Environment

2 - 2

(1) **Special precautions are taken when mixing and handling vinblastine sulfate (VLB) to prevent any possible entry into the caregiver. Vinblastine sulfate (VLB) is an anti-neoplastic drug that has a carcinogenic risk for handlers.**

2. Vinblastine sulfate (VLB) attacks cell division and is only to be given intravenously into a large vein.

3. Vinblastine is fatal if given intrathecally. It is only for IV use.

4. Alopecia (hair loss) is common with this type of chemotherapy, but is usually temporary.

Pregnancy Category: D

Client Need: Safe, Effective Care Environment

2 - 3

(3) **Administration of an antiemetic is appropriate prior to receiving plicamycin (mithramycin). Mithramycin is an antineoplastic agent that commonly causes nausea and vomiting. Many protocols recommend that an antiemetic be administered prior to the infusion of mithramycin to help prevent nausea and vomiting.**

1 and 2. Most clients prefer to have an empty stomach prior to receiving mithramycin therapy because of the nausea and vomiting that commonly occurs.

4. There is no indication that clients receiving mithramycin should be weighed prior to the administration of this medication.

Pregnancy Category: X

Client Need: Health Promotion/Maintenance

2 - 4

④ **Doxorubicin (Adriamycin) may cause severe tissue necrosis. It is an antineoplastic agent that is a vesicant (very irritating to tissue). If the drug infiltrates, it may cause necrosis and sloughing of tissue. The intravenous site must be precisely monitored.**

1, 2, and 3. This medication may only be given intravenously. It has many side effects, including nausea, vomiting, cardiac arrhythmias, and alopecia (hair loss).

Pregnancy Category: D

Client Need: Safe, Effective Care Environment

2 - 5

② **Clients receiving the antineoplastic medication bleomycin (Blenoxane) should be taught to report breathing difficulty and/or coughing. An adverse effect unique to bleomycin is pulmonary fibrosis. This is usually a late effect and is more frequent in the elderly.**

1. Renal toxicity is most likely to occur with the antineoplastic drugs cisplatin, cyclophosphamide, and methotrexate, not Blenoxane.
3. Neurotoxicity, especially of the peripheral nerves, is most likely to occur with the antineoplastic drug vincristine, not Blenoxane.
4. Cardiotoxicity resulting in fluid retention is most likely to occur with the antineoplastic drugs doxorubicin and daunorubicin, not Blenoxane.

Pregnancy Category: D

Client Need: Physiological Integrity

2 - 6

④ **Special nursing care for stomatitis includes a soft, bland, tepid diet and frequent assessment of the oral cavity. Methotrexate is an antimetabolite chemotherapy agent that destroys cancer cells by blocking synthesis of DNA and RNA. Major side effects include: Stomatitis, kidney impairment, skin rashes, nausea, vomiting, diarrhea, allergic reactions, conjunctivitis, and encephalopathy.**

1. It is not necessary to limit clients with stomatitis to clear, full-liquid diets.
2. Total parenteral nutrition is not recommended as long as clients are able to consume a soft, bland, tepid diet.
3. A high-protein diet would be irritating to painful ulcerations in the mouth and is not recommended.

Pregnancy Category: X

Client Need: Health Promotion/Maintenance

2 - 7

① **A prescription for furosemide should be questioned. Both cisplatin and furosemide are ototoxic (damaging to auditory nerves) and concurrent use should be avoided. Renal toxicity may also occur with cisplatin, but may be prevented by "pushing fluids" (parenteral and oral) and by administering a bolus of mannitol to help ensure diuresis.**

2. The administration of extra fluids helps decrease renal toxicity. Desired output is 100 to150 cc per hour.

3. Severe nausea and vomiting can occur with cisplatin. Administration of an antiemetic such as Reglan can be very beneficial.

4. Bone marrow suppression can occur with cisplatin. Follow-up testing should be completed.

Pregnancy Category: C

Client Need: Safe, Effective Care Environment

2 - 8

④ **Infection, especially a viral infection, can be life threatening and therefore has the highest priority. Bone marrow is responsible for producing red and white blood cells. When bone marrow is suppressed, the client becomes open to infection and may experience anemia.**

1. Activity intolerance is not life threatening and can be treated with red blood cells.

2. Volume expanders can be administered when tissue perfusion is a problem.

3. In the event of fluid volume deficit, platelets can be administered.

Pregnancy Category: D

Client Need: Health Promotion/Maintenance

2 - 9

③ **The side effects of fluorouracil (5-FU) therapy include reversible alopecia (loss of hair). Fluorouracil is an antineoplastic agent whose impact on chromosomal structure contributes to numerous side effects including: Nausea, vomiting, diarrhea, leukopenia (low white blood cell count), and alopecia.**

1. Fluorouracil (5-FU) may cause diarrhea, not constipation. Other side effects include nausea, vomiting, and stomatitis.

2. Fluorouracil (5-FU) does not cause ventricular arrhythmias. It may cause hypotension and bradycardia.

4. Fluorouracil (5-FU) does not cause cystitis (inflammation of the urinary bladder), but it may cause urinary retention.

Pregnancy Category: D (injection); X (topical form)

Client Need: Physiological Integrity

2-10

③ **The cisplatin (Platinol) should be withheld and the physician notified. The normal BUN for an adult is 7 to 18 mg/dl, and the normal creatinine is 0.6 to 1.2 mg/dl. This client's laboratory values indicate renal failure (BUN 40 mg/dl and creatinine 2.0 mg/dl). Additional dosages of cisplatin (Platinol) should not be given until renal function has returned to normal.**

1. The normal adult BUN is 7 to 18 mg/dl. The normal creatinine is 0.6 to 1.2 mg/dl.
2. The medication should be withheld until kidney function has returned to normal.
4. Simply increasing the fluid intake will not be adequate inasmuch as the medication is the problem. It should be withheld and the physician notified.

Pregnancy Category: D

Client Need: Health Promotion/Maintenance

2-11

④ **Alopecia (hair loss) is one of the many adverse reactions associated with dacarbazine (DTIC-Dome) administration. The client should be taught that hair loss is probable but temporary.**

1. Stomatitis (ulcers in the mouth) is an adverse reaction to dacarbazine (DTIC-Dome).
2. Anorexia (loss of appetite) with severe nausea and vomiting are adverse reactions associated with dacarbazine (DTIC-Dome).
3. Phototoxicity (hypersensitivity to sunlight) is an adverse effect of dacarbazine (DTIC-Dome). Clients should be taught to wear protective clothing when exposed to sunlight.

Pregnancy Category: C

Client Need: Psychosocial Integrity

2-12

① **You will observe the client for the common life-threatening adverse reaction of pulmonary fibrosis (abnormal formation of fibrous tissue in the lung). Clients over 70 are more likely to experience this reaction.**

2. Hyperkeratosis (a skin condition characterized by excessive horny growth) is an uncommon adverse reaction to bleomycin sulfate (Blenoxane).
3. Thrombocytopenia (an abnormal decrease in blood platelets) is not associated with bleomycin sulfate (Blenoxane). It is a common life-threatening reaction associated with methotrexate (Folex).
4. Encephalopathy (dysfunction of the brain) is not associated with bleomycin sulfate (Blenoxane). It is associated with methotrexate (Folex).

Pregnancy Category: D

Client Need: Health Promotion/Maintenance

2 - 1 3

① Antineoplastic alkylating drugs such as nitrogen mustard (Mustargen) are effective against cancer due to their ability to attach to the proteins within the cancerous cells and poison them.

2. Antineoplastic antimetabolites are effective against cancer due to their ability to interrupt normal cellular metabolism within cancer cells.

3. Antineoplastic hormones are effective against cancer due to their ability to alter normal hormonal equilibrium.

4. Antineoplastic antibiotics are effective against cancer due to their ability to alter DNA or RNA synthesis.

Pregnancy Category: D
Client Need: Physiological Integrity

2 - 1 4

② Clients receiving nitrogen mustard (Mustargen) should be taught to avoid OTC drugs containing aspirin. Aspirin has anticoagulating effects and may contribute to hemorrhage if the client's platelet count falls below 100,000/mm$_3$.

1. Aspirin does not lower the platelet count. Nitrogen mustard (Mustargen) lowers the platelet count.

3. Aspirin does not interfere with the ability of nitrogen mustard (Mustargen) to destroy cancer cells.

4. Aspirin does not compound the toxic effects of antineoplastic drugs.

Pregnancy Category: D
Client Need: Health Promotion/Maintenance

2 - 1 5

③ Clients should receive methotrexate (Folex) on an empty stomach. All foods are likely to delay the absorption of this medication and reduce its peak concentration.

1, 2, and 4. All foods will affect the absorption and concentration of methotrexate (Folex) and should not be taken concurrently.

Pregnancy Category: X
Client Need: Physiological Integrity

2-16

④　**Doxorubicin (Adriamycin) is a severe vesicant. Should extravasation occur, tissue necrosis may develop.**

1 and 2. Common side effects of doxorubicin (Adriamycin) include severe nausea, vomiting, and stomatitis. However, this occurs regardless of which method of administration is used, not just intravenous administration.

3.　Alopecia (hair loss) is a common side effect of doxorubicin (Adriamycin) and is usually reversible.

Pregnancy Category: D

Client Need: Health Promotion/Maintenance

2-17

②　**Cold foods improve a client's tolerance of the oral preparations of cyclophosphamide (Cytoxan). Cold foods do not stimulate the secretion of gastric juices and are not as likely to contribute to nausea and vomiting.**

1, 3, and 4. Milk products, carbonated drinks, and hot drinks are not recommended in facilitating the administration of Cytoxan.

Pregnancy Category: D

Client Need: Health Promotion/Maintenance

2-18

④　**Fever is the single most important manifestation of infection associated with neutropenia (an abnormally small number of neutrophils, or white blood cells).**

1 and 3. Diarrhea and anorexia are common side effects associated with the administration of antineoplastic drugs. However, neither confirm infection.

2.　A sore throat should be monitored closely. However, until fever is assessed, one cannot conclude that an infection is present.

Pregnancy Category: D

Client Need: Health Promotion/Maintenance

2-19

④　**Soft, bland foods that do not irritate the mucosa should be encouraged when caring for clients with stomatitis.**

1.　Mouthwashes containing alcohol should be avoided since they irritate the mucosa.

2.　All smoking should be discouraged (not just limited) since smoke and tobacco irritate the mucosa.

3.　Extreme temperatures (cold/hot) should be avoided since they further traumatize the mucosa.

Pregnancy Category: D

Client Need: Health Promotion/Maintenance

2-20

③ **The enzyme hyaluronidase may be injected locally to help disperse th cristine sulfate. The action of hyaluronidase increases absorption and other injected or infiltrated drugs.**

1. Diphenhydramine (Benadryl) is an antihistamine/antitussive and would no to disperse infiltrated drugs such as Oncovin.

2. Cefazolin sodium (Ancef) is an anti-infective. There is no indication that th efit from an anti-infective at this time.

4. Famciclovir (Famvir) is an antiviral. There is no indication that the client wo an antiviral at this time (also, Famvir comes only as a tablet).

Pregnancy Category: D
Client Need: Health Promotion/Maintenance

2-21

① **Fresh fruits and vegetables should be avoided because many are acid chew. Fresh fruits and vegetables are also difficult to clean and are no infection.**

2. Milk shakes are appropriate due to their soft texture and cool temperature.

3. Low-residue diets are appropriate inasmuch as they are not irritating to the

4. Soft foods are less irritating and should be included in the diet.

Pregnancy Category: Varies with specific drug
Client Need: Health Promotion/Maintenance

2-22

③ **The MOPP Regimen for Hodgkin's disease is administered every 28 (mum of 6 cycles.**

1. 2 cycles is under the minimum of 6 cycles.

2. 4 cycles is under the minimum of 6 cycles.

4. 8 cycles is greater than the minimum of 6 cycles.

Pregnancy Category: prednisone, C; nitrogen mustard, Oncovin, and procarb
Client Need: Physiological Integrity

Practice Test 3

Cardiovascular Agents

OVERVIEW

Cardiovascular agents treat and/or prevent various conditions affecting the heart's ability to pump oxygenated blood to the tissues and provide the tissues with other nutrients. Cardiovascular agents also treat and/or prevent conditions affecting the removal of carbon dioxide and other waste products from the body.

Cardiovascular agents include:

- Antianginals
- Antiarrhythmics
- Antihypertensives
- Antilipemics
- Inotropics

ANTIANGINALS

Antianginals are vasodilating substances, such as nitrates and calcium channel blockers, that relax the smooth muscle layer of arterial blood vessels.

Conditions treated with antianginals include:

- Angina pectoris (acute)
- Angina pectoris (as a prophylaxis)

ANTIARRHYTHMICS

Antiarrhythmic substances are generally administered to treat clients with heart disease or a disease that affects cardiovascular function. Arrhythmias include any heart rate or rhythm other than the normal sinus rhythm.

Conditions treated with antiarrhythmics include:

- Atrial fibrillation
- Paroxysmal atrial tachycardia
- Premature ventricular contractions (PVC)
- Ventricular tachycardia

ANTIHYPERTENSIVES

Antihypertensives are administered to lower blood pressure. Many antihypertensives lower blood pressure by dilating arterial blood vessels. Dilating the arterial blood vessels will increase the amount of space available for the circulating blood. An increase in available space for circulating blood will lower blood pressure.

Conditions treated with antihypertensives include:

- Essential hypertension
- Hypertension (mild, moderate, severe)

ANTILIPEMICS

Antilipemics are used in conjunction with diet and exercise to reduce blood lipids (fats or fatlike substances in the blood).

Conditions treated with antilipemics include:

- Primary hypercholesterolemia
- Pruritus caused by partial bile obstruction

INOTROPICS (CARDIOTONIC SUBSTANCES)

Inotropics (cardiotonic substances) increase the force of contraction of the heart muscle (myocardium). As a result of the increased contractility of the myocardium, cardiac output is increased, blood flow to the kidneys and periphery is improved, venous pressure is improved, and excess fluid (edema) is excreted.

Conditions treated with inotropics (cardiotonic substances) include:

- Atrial fibrillation
- Atrial flutter
- Congestive heart failure
- Paroxysmal atrial tachycardia

Practice Test 3

Questions

3 - 1

A client was admitted for tachycardia and is being discharged with a prescription for digoxin 0.25 mg, by mouth, at 9 a.m. Your discharge teaching will include:

1. "Take antacids daily, since nausea is an expected side effect of digoxin."
2. "Take medication only on the days when "palpitations" are felt."
3. "Check the radial pulse rate prior to taking the medication."
4. "Double the dosage if one day is missed."

3 - 2

A client is admitted with chest pain. Nitroglycerin translingual spray is prescribed. The administration of nitroglycerin spray includes:

1. spraying 5 times rapidly to the oral mucosa.
2. shaking the container vigorously prior to spraying.
3. instructing the client to inhale the spray.
4. spraying once onto or under the tongue.

3 - 3

A client is experiencing a hypertensive crisis. Blood pressure is 227/133 mmHg. Prescription reads: Diazoxide (Hyperstat) 100 mg intravenously. You know the action of this drug will:

1. decrease the heart rate by vagal stimulation.
2. directly relax vascular smooth muscle in peripheral arterioles.
3. promote diuresis.
4. block calcium channels.

3 - 4

The safe dosage range for digoxin is 0.08 to 0.10 mg/kg. Which of the following would be the maximum safe dosage for a child weighing 20 pounds?

1. 0.2 mg
2. 0.9 mg
3. 2.0 mg
4. 9.0 mg

3 - 5

Your client is receiving nitroglycerin sublingually. Which of the following statements is correct and should be included in your teaching plan?

1. "Nitroglycerin should relieve pain within 1 minute. Four consecutive dosages of nitroglycerin may be taken at 3-minute intervals."
2. "Nitroglycerin should relieve pain within 3 minutes. After the initial dose, two additional dosages can be taken at 5-minute intervals."
3. "Nitroglycerin should be taken daily upon arising. If pain occurs during the day, additional dosages may be taken."
4. "Rapid tolerance to nitroglycerin develops and the dosage may need to be increased."

3 - 6

A client is to be digitalized. Prior to administering a digitalis derivative, which of the following pulses will the nurse count?

1. temporal
2. carotid
3. apical
4. radial

3 - 7

What assessment finding would indicate that the medication Tridil is effective?

1. Chest pain is relieved.
2. Heart rate decreases to 80 beats per minute.
3. Blood pressure increases to 110/70.
4. Breath sounds are clear at auscultation.

3 - 8

A client should be taught to take an oral liquid digitalis preparation:

1. after breakfast if on a once-a-day regimen.
2. with a calcium-containing beverage.
3. accompanied by a high-fiber food.
4. well diluted in a full glass of fluid.

3 - 9

A client taking a digitalis preparation is suspected of suffering toxic effects from the medication. You should withhold the medication and:

1. prepare a dose of digoxin immune Fab (ovine) (Digibind).
2. offer the client a glass of orange or tomato juice.
3. start intravenous 5% dextrose in water (D5W).
4. administer an adrenocorticosteroid preparation.

3 - 1 0

A client receiving nitroglycerin should be instructed to:

1. report symptoms of shakiness, sweating, and hunger.
2. notify the nurse if a rash occurs.
3. consume a high-fiber diet to help avoid the common side effect of constipation.
4. change positions slowly, especially if dizziness occurs.

3 - 1 1

A client taking sublingual nitroglycerin reports all of the following. Which action by the client indicates a need for further teaching?

1. The client carries a bottle of tablets whenever away from home.
2. The client keeps the medicine in a locked suitcase in another room when grandchildren visit.
3. When the grandchildren are not visiting, the client stores the "pills" in the refrigerator, away from heat and light.
4. The client gets new tablets every 6 months.

3 - 1 2

You understand that the action of pentoxifylline (Trental) will:

1. dilate the bronchus.
2. dissolve blood clots.
3. treat cardiac dysrhythmia.
4. increase peripheral circulation.

3 - 1 3

A client is exhibiting left-sided weakness. The blood pressure reading is 224/138 mmHg. Which of the following medications may be administered?

1. atropine sulfate
2. dopamine
3. norepinephrine
4. labetalol (Normodyne)

3 - 1 4

Your client has been taking the calcium channel blocker verapamil (Calan) to control moderate hypertension. The client is now experiencing postural hypotension. Nursing management will include:

1. encouraging the client to lie on the left side.
2. doubling the dosage of the channel blocker.
3. checking the blood pressure while the client is supine.
4. assisting the client in changing positions slowly.

3 - 1 5

A client is to receive antilipemic cholestyramine (Questran) for elevated serum cholesterol levels. The nurse will teach the client that the stabilizing effects of this medication may not be achieved for:

1. 48 hours.
2. 1 week.
3. 1 month.
4. 12 months.

3 - 1 6

Your client is taking the beta-adrenergic blocker propranolol (Inderal) for hypertension. Which nursing intervention is most appropriate for clients receiving this medication?

1. Weigh daily.
2. Supplement the diet with potassium-rich foods.
3. Instruct the client not to stop the medication suddenly.
4. Suggest chewing gum to relieve dry mouth.

3 - 1 7

A client is admitted to the hospital with mild congestive heart failure. Digoxin (Lanoxin 0.25 mg) is prescribed. Available are scored tablets of Lanoxin labeled 0.125 mg. How many tablets will the nurse give?

1. 1/4 tablet
2. 1/2 tablet
3. 1 1/2 tablets
4. 2 tablets

3 - 1 8

Your client is complaining of chest pain. Which action would be most appropriate prior to the administration of sublingual nitroglycerin (Nitrostat)?

1. Monitor the client's blood pressure.
2. Encourage a full glass of water with the medication.
3. Administer acetaminophen first, then give the nitroglycerin if there is no relief.
4. Assist the client to a standing position.

3 - 1 9

A client continues to have chest pain after returning from the special procedures laboratory. A Tridil drip is prescribed. What is the common side effect of this medication?

1. nausea
2. headache
3. drowsiness
4. hypertension

3 - 2 0

Which of the following groups of medications would be administered to prevent thrombus formation in a postoperative client?

1. antithrombolytics
2. anticoagulants
3. antiarrhythmics
4. analgesics

3 - 2 1

What abnormal signs and symptoms are indicative of digoxin toxicity?

1. convulsions
2. colored vision
3. muscle cramping
4. orthostatic hypotension

3 - 2 2

A client comes to the emergency department experiencing "crushing" chest pain. Which of the following may be prescribed?

1. nizatidine (Axid)
2. nifedipine (Procardia)
3. nortriptyline hydrochloride (Aventyl)
4. nystatin (Mycostatin)

3 - 2 3

Several of the clients to whom you will administer medications are to receive verapamil (Cardizem) po as part of their morning medications. For whom would you withhold the verapamil and notify the physician?

1. a 45-year-old female who is also taking furosemide
2. a 70-year-old male who has a cough and a fever of 101.1° F
3. a 61-year-old female who has been recently diagnosed with Type 2 diabetes
4. a 62-year-old male with an apical pulse rate of 54 beats per minute

3 - 2 4

You will administer ramipril (Altace) to a client experiencing hypertension. You know the action of this medication will lower the client's blood pressure by:

1. dilating the arteriolar lumen.
2. constricting the arteriolar lumen.
3. decreasing the total circulating volume.
4. inhibiting the formation of angiotensin II.

3 - 2 5

Your client is receiving a loading dose of digoxin 0.5 mg po in divided dosages over a 24-hour period. You will recognize the most common and earliest adverse reaction to digoxin as:

1. paresthesia.
2. nausea and anorexia.
3. blurred vision.
4. dizziness and vertigo.

3 - 2 6

An electrocardiogram shows a supra-ventricular tachycardia at 198 beats per minute. Which medication will you anticipate administering?

1. adenosine 6 mg intravenously
2. adenosine 6 mg by mouth
3. atropine 1 mg by mouth
4. atropine 1 mg intravenously

3 - 2 7

Which of the following medications prolong partial thromboplastin time (PTT)?

1. digoxin
2. aminophylline
3. acetaminophen
4. heparin

3 - 2 8

A client experiences chest pain. Laboratory results reveal a hemoglobin of 7.5 gm/dl. Which of the following treatments would be given?

1. norepinephrine (Levophed)
2. oxygen (O_2)
3. potassium chloride (K-Dur)
4. alprazolam (Xanax)

3 - 2 9

Your client has a history of atrial fibrillation and subsequent pulmonary embolus. Because of this, your client is taking a maintenance dosage of warfarin (Coumadin). You know that the purpose of this medication is to:

1. convert atrial fibrillation to sinus rhythm.
2. prevent arrhythmia-related congestive heart failure by diuresis.
3. decrease heart rate.
4. prevent blood clot formation.

3 - 3 0

Your client has peripheral arterial disease (PAD). The physician has prescribed the antiplatelet medication:

1. dipyridamole (Persantine).
2. dobutamine (Dobutrex).
3. atorvastatin calcium (Lipitor).
4. penbutolol sulfate (Levatol).

Practice Test 3

Answers, Rationales, and Explanations

3 - 1

③ **Clients should check their radial pulse rate prior to taking digoxin. They should be taught how to count the pulse rate and should be instructed to withhold the digoxin if the pulse rate is < 60 or > 100 beats per minute (BPM).**

1. Nausea might be a toxic side effect of digoxin and should be reported.
2. To be effective, digoxin levels must be maintained with regular dosages. The medication should not be taken only when palpitations are felt.
4. Missed dosages should be taken within 12 hours or not at all. Doubling the dosage could decrease the heart rate dramatically.

Pregnancy Category: C

Client Need: Health Promotion/Maintenance

3 - 2

④ **Nitroglycerin translingual spray is administered initially by spraying once onto or under the tongue. Translingual nitroglycerin is a metered spray (0.4 mg/spray). Spraying once onto the oral mucosa for an initial dose is an appropriate dosage. Clients should be taught not to swallow immediately after the spray is administered. No more than 3 metered doses should be taken within 15 minutes.**

1. Spraying 5 times rapidly to the oral mucosa is an excessive initial dose.
2. A container of nitroglycerin spray should not be shaken.
3. Nitroglycerin spray is not an inhalant.

Pregnancy Category: C

Client Need: Physiological Integrity

3 - 3

② **Diazoxide (Hyperstat) lowers blood pressure by directly relaxing vascular smooth muscle in peripheral arterioles.**

1. Diazoxide (Hyperstat) does not affect the vagus nerve.
3. Diazoxide (Hyperstat) is not a diuretic (an agent that increases the secretion of urine).
4. Diazoxide (Hyperstat) is not a calcium channel blocker (a drug that lowers blood pressure by decreasing arterial resistance).

Pregnancy Category: C

Client Need: Physiological Integrity

3 - 4

② **The maximum safe dosage of digoxin for a child weighing 20 pounds is 0.9 mg.**

Formula: 2.2 kg : 1 pound :: X kg : 20 pounds

X = 9.09 kg

0.10 mg : each kg :: X mg : 9.09 kg

X = .909 kg (0.1 x 9 = 0.9)

1, 3, and 4 are incorrect calculations.

Pregnancy Category: NA

Client Need: Safe, Effective Care Environment

3 - 5

② **Nitroglycerin should relieve pain within 3 minutes after the initial dose. If the pain is not relieved after the first dose, two additional dosages can be taken at 5-minute intervals. Nitroglycerin is a vasodilator and is prescribed to treat acute angina pectoris.**

1. No more than 3 consecutive dosages of nitroglycerin should be taken at 5-minute intervals. If pain is not relieved, the client should seek medical attention.

3. Nitroglycerin should be placed under the tongue at the first indication of an attack or prior to situations that precipitate angina; e.g., exercising, eating a large meal, or sexual intercourse.

4. Tolerance to nitroglycerin does not occur when taken as directed. Therefore, the dosage will not need to be increased.

Pregnancy Category: C

Client Need: Health Promotion/Maintenance

3 - 6

③ **The apical pulse will be counted prior to administering a digitalis derivative. The apical pulse is taken at the point of maximum impulse, at the fourth, fifth, or sixth intercostal space to the left of the sternum (at the apex of the heart). Counting the apical pulse is the only way the nurse can ensure against a pulse deficit interfering with the assessment for beats per minute. A pulse deficit is a condition in which the number of pulse beats counted at the wrist is lower than those counted in the same minute of time at the heart. Many clients receiving digitalis will have a pulse deficit. Digitalis should be withheld and the physician notified if the client's apical pulse is < 60 or > 100 beats per minute.**

1, 2, and 4. The temporal, carotid, and radial pulses are located at various distances from the heart and therefore will not give an accurate measurement of the heart's beats per minute (BPM) if there is a pulse deficit.

Pregnancy Category: C

Client Need: Physiological Integrity

3 - 7

① Tridil is given to relieve chest pain. Tridil is a vasodilator and the intravenous form of nitroglycerin. Side effects include a decrease in blood pressure and headaches.

2 and 3. Adverse cardiovascular side effects of Tridil include tachycardia, palpitations, and postural hypotension.

4. Administration of Tridil does not directly affect the respiratory system.

Pregnancy Category: C

Client Need: Physiological Integrity

3 - 8

① The oral liquid digitalis preparation should be taken routinely at the same time each day. Taking it every morning after breakfast is recommended. Digitalis can irritate the gastric mucosa and should not be taken on an empty stomach. It should be taken at the same time daily and at a convenient time to decrease the chance of forgetting a dose. Generally, missed dosages should not be made up. Since anorexia is an indication of toxicity, scheduling dosages after a meal would allow for evaluation of appetite prior to administration.

2. Taking a beverage containing calcium has no effect on digitalis administration.

3. It is not recommended that digitalis be accompanied by high-fiber foods since this will decrease its absorption.

4. It is not necessary to dilute oral digitalis in a full glass of liquid.

Pregnancy Category: C

Client Need: Health Promotion/Maintenance

3 - 9

② Offer the client a glass of orange or tomato juice. A common cause of digitalis toxicity is low serum potassium. Either of these juices would furnish potassium and would help decrease toxicity along with withholding the dose of digitalis. Even a therapeutic level of digitalis can be toxic if serum potassium is low.

1. Digibind is used only for clients with normal or elevated potassium levels. A common cause of digitalis toxicity is low serum potassium.

3. There is no indication that extra fluids or immediate intravenous access are needed in this situation.

4. Adrenocorticosteroid preparations are not used to treat digitalis toxicity and could contribute to toxicity.

Pregnancy Category: C

Client Need: Safe, Effective Care Environment

3 - 1 0

④ **When taking nitroglycerin, clients should be taught to change positions slowly. Nitroglycerin is a vasodilator. Vasodilation can cause postural hypotension, which can cause potential injury.**

1. Shakiness, sweating, and hunger are signs often associated with low blood sugar, not vasodilation.

2. A rash does not usually occur except from local irritation with transdermal applications of nitroglycerin. There is no indication that this client is taking the transdermal form of nitroglycerin.

3. Constipation is not a common side effect of nitroglycerin.

Pregnancy Category: C

Client Need: Safe, Effective Care Environment

3 - 1 1

③ **Nitroglycerin tablets should not be stored in the refrigerator because the humidity in the refrigerator causes the nitroglycerin to lose its potency. A tightly sealed brown glass bottle at room temperature is good storage practice since nitroglycerin tablets lose potency in plastic or cardboard containers or when exposed to sunlight.**

1. It is good practice for clients to take their nitroglycerin with them. They should carry the medication away from body heat because heat causes nitroglycerin tablets to lose their potency.

2. Keeping all medicines away from children is a good practice and helps prevent accidental ingestion.

4. Purchasing new nitroglycerin tablets every 6 months would help assure adequate potency of the medication.

Pregnancy Category: C

Client Need: Health Promotion/Maintenance

3 - 1 2

④ **Pentoxifylline (Trental) increases peripheral circulation. Trental is administered to treat intermittent claudication. The action is not well-defined, but it seems to enhance flexibility of red blood cells, thus increasing circulation in the smaller blood vessels. Blood viscosity seems to be decreased as well.**

1. Pentoxifylline (Trental) is a hemorrheologic agent, not a bronchodilator.

2. Pentoxifylline (Trental) does not dissolve (lyse) blood clots.

3. Pentoxifylline (Trental) is not used to treat cardiac dysrhythmia.

Pregnancy Category: C

Client Need: Physiological Integrity

3 - 1 3

④ **Labetalol (Normodyne) may be administered. It is an antihypertensive medication whose impact on the sympathetic nervous system reduces peripheral vascular resistance. For treatment of severe hypertension, the drug is administered intravenously.**

1, 2, and 3. Atropine, dopamine, and norepinephrine stimulate the cardiovascular system in different ways and would tend to increase blood pressure.

Pregnancy Category: C
Client Need: Physiological Integrity

3 - 1 4

④ **Clients taking calcium channel blockers such as verapamil (Calan) should change positions slowly to avoid fainting and to prevent injuries from falls. Verapamil (Calan) decreases total peripheral vascular resistance and reduces arterial blood pressure by dilating peripheral arterioles. Calcium channel blockers such as verapamil may cause postural hypotension (a drop in blood pressure when the client changes positions quickly from supine to standing).**

1. There is no reason why clients taking antihypertensives may not lie on their left sides.
2. Because hypotension has occurred, the dosage may need to be decreased, not increased.
3. Blood pressure should be checked while the client is lying, sitting, and standing, to identify any drop in blood pressure when changing positions.

Pregnancy Category: C
Client Need: Physiological Integrity

3 - 1 5

④ **It may take up to 12 months for the antilipemic cholestyramine (Questran) to stabilize. Antilipemics should begin to decrease cholesterol levels in 48 hours. Antilipemics bind with bile acids in the gastrointestinal tract and are then excreted; thus, the liver must utilize circulating cholesterol to form new acids. A gradual reduction of serum cholesterol is the result of this process.**

1, 2, and 3. The stabilizing effects of cholestyramine may take up to 1 year.

Pregnancy Category: NR
Client Need: Physiological Integrity

3 - 1 6

③ **You will instruct clients not to stop the medication propranolol (Inderal) suddenly. Sudden withdrawal of Inderal can result in overstimulation of the sympathetic nervous system and precipitate life-threatening hypertension, arrhythmias, and myocardial ischemia. Inderal should be gradually decreased and discontinued under a physician's supervision. Inderal is contraindicated for anyone with a history of congestive heart failure, chronic obstructive pulmonary disease, heart block, asthma, or diabetes mellitus.**

1. A client on diuretics needs to be weighed daily to monitor fluid retention and weight reduction. Clients on Inderal need to be weighed only 2 to 3 times a week.

2. Clients on thiazide diuretics, not beta-adrenergic blockers, need to supplement their diet with potassium-rich foods, since potassium is depleted in the diuretic process.

4. Inderal does not cause dry mouth. Centrally acting alpha-blockers like Catapres cause dry mouth. Chewing gum may help to relieve dry mouth.

Pregnancy Category: C
Client Need: Safe, Effective Care Environment

3 - 1 7

④ **Two tablets of digoxin (Lanoxin) should be administered.**

Formula: 0.25 mg : 1 tab :: 0.125 mg : X

X = 2 tablets

1, 2, and 3 are incorrect calculations.

Pregnancy Category: C
Client Need: Physiological Integrity

3 - 1 8

① **You will monitor the client's blood pressure. Nitroglycerin (Nitrostat) is an anti-anginal vasodilator used in the relief of ischemic chest pain. Because of the vasodilatory action of the medication, blood pressure may be lowered. Although protocols regarding this medication may vary, it is generally considered prudent to withhold the medication if the blood pressure is less than 90 to 100 mmHg systolic. Blood pressure should be measured prior to this medication's administration.**

2. Sublingual (under the tongue) nitroglycerin is not taken with water.

3. Anginal pain will not be relieved with analgesics such as acetaminophen.

4. Clients should be in an upright position when receiving this medication because of the risk of postural hypotension.

Pregnancy Category: C
Client Need: Physiological Integrity

3 - 1 9

② Headache is a common side effect of Tridil administration. Tridil is the intravenous form of nitroglycerin and promotes vasodilation. It is the vasodilating action of Tridil that causes the frequent side effect of headache.

1. Nausea may occur; however, it is not a common side effect of Tridil.

3. Drowsiness is not a common side effect of Tridil.

4. Hypotension, not hypertension, is among the most common side effects of Tridil administration.

Pregnancy Category: C
Client Need: Physiological Integrity

3 - 2 0

② Anticoagulants are administered to prevent thrombus formation postoperatively. Anticoagulants, which include heparin and warfarin (Coumadin), delay the time required for blood to clot by their impact on thrombin formation or platelet aggregation.

1. Antithrombolytics such as streptokinase are used to dissolve clots already formed and are usually contraindicated in the postoperative client.

3. Antiarrhythmics are used to treat cardiac arrhythmias and have no direct impact on thrombus formation.

4. Analgesics are used to treat pain and have no impact on thrombus formation.

Pregnancy Category: heparin, C; Coumadin, D
Client Need: Health Promotion/Maintenance

3 - 2 1

② Signs and symptoms of digoxin toxicity include headaches, colored, blurred, or double vision, drowsiness, restlessness, muscle weakness, anorexia, nausea, vomiting, diarrhea, and various cardiac arrhythmias.

1. Convulsions are not associated with digoxin administration. CNS adverse effects include: Fatigue, muscle weakness, headaches, dizziness, and paresthesia (sensation of numbness or tingling).

3. Muscle cramps are not associated with digoxin administration.

4. Orthostatic hypotension is not associated with digoxin administration.

Pregnancy Category: C
Client Need: Health Promotion/Maintenance

3 - 2 2

② **The nurse will anticipate a prescription for nifedipine (Procardia). Procardia is a calcium channel blocker that has coronary vasodilatory action. Vasodilation allows more oxygen to travel to the myocardial cells, thus relieving pain associated with ischemia (lack of oxygen). Procardia is administered for the treatment of angina pectoris (chest pain) caused by coronary insufficiency or vasospasm.**

1. Nizatidine (Axid) is an antiulcer agent and has no impact on chest pain.
2. Nortriptyline hydrochloride (Aventyl) is a tricyclic antidepressant and has no impact on chest pain.
3. Nystatin (Mycostatin) is an antifungal agent and has no impact on chest pain.

Pregnancy Category: C
Client Need: Physiological Integrity

3 - 2 3

④ **Verapamil (Cardizem) should be withheld and the physician notified if a client's pulse rate is < 60 beats per minute (BPM). Verapamil (Cardizem) belongs to a group of medications called calcium channel blockers. Calcium channel blockers slow the heart's rate and decrease blood pressure by affecting calcium ion flow in the tissue. A client whose heart rate is < 60 beats per minute (BPM) should not receive calcium channel blockers.**

1. There is no reason to withhold verapamil from a 45-year-old female who is also taking furosemide (Lasix).
2. Having a fever of 101 F° and a cough would not inhibit the administration of verapamil (Cardizem).
3. There is no reason why clients with Type 2 diabetes cannot take verapamil (Cardizem).

Pregnancy Category: C
Client Need: Safe, Effective Care Environment

3 - 2 4

④ **Ramipril (Altace) lowers blood pressure by inhibiting the formation of angiotensin II. Altace is an angiotensin converting enzyme (ACE) inhibitor. ACE inhibitors inhibit the conversion of angiotensin I to angiotensin II, which is a potent vasoconstrictor.**

1. Medications such as diazoxide (Hyperstat IV) lower blood pressure directly by relaxing the arteriolar lumen.
2. Blood pressure would rise if a medication were administered that constricted the arteriolar lumen. Constricted blood vessels would increase vascular resistance.
3. Ramipril (Altace) does not decrease total circulatory volume. Diuretics such as furosemide (Lasix) can lower blood pressure by decreasing circulatory volume.

Pregnancy Category: C; D (in second trimester)
Client Need: Physiological Integrity

3 - 2 5

② **Nausea and anorexia are common early adverse reactions to digoxin (Lanoxin) administration.**

1. Paresthesia (a sensation of numbness or tingling) is an uncommon adverse reaction to digoxin (Lanoxin) administration.

3. Blurred vision is an uncommon adverse reaction to digoxin (Lanoxin) administration. However, it may occur, along with yellow-green halos around images, flashes of light, diplopia (double vision), and photophobia (unusual intolerance to light).

4. Dizziness and vertigo are uncommon adverse reactions to digoxin (Lanoxin) administration.

Pregnancy Category: C

Client Need: Health Promotion/Maintenance

3 - 2 6

① **You will anticipate administering adenosine (Adenocard) 6 mg intravenously. Adenosine is an antiarrhythmic medication whose tendency to slow conduction makes it a treatment of choice in supraventricular tachyarrhythmias. Because of its extremely short half-life, it must be given in rapid intravenous boluses in dosages of 6 mg or 12 mg per bolus.**

2. Adenosine is not given orally.

3 and 4. Atropine is used to treat bradyarrhythmias, not tachycardia.

Pregnancy Category: C

Client Need: Physiological Integrity

3 - 2 7

④ **Heparin prolongs partial thromboplastin time (PTT). Heparin is an anticoagulant whose actions prevent fibrin formation during the blood-clotting process.**

1. Digoxin is a cardiac glycoside and has no impact on blood clotting.

2. Aminophylline is a bronchodilator and has no impact on blood clotting.

3. Acetaminophen is an analgesic and has no impact on blood clotting.

Pregnancy Category: C

Client Need: Physiological Integrity

3 - 2 8

② **The client will be treated with supplemental oxygen. Hemoglobin is the iron-containing pigment of the red blood cells. It carries oxygen from the lungs to the tissues. Low hemoglobin levels compromise the body's oxygen transport capacity. A normal hemoglobin is 12 to 16 gm/dl. A hemoglobin of 7.5 gm/dl is too low.**

1. Norepinephrine (Levophed) is a pressor agent (it restores blood pressure in acute hypotensive conditions). It has no impact on chest pain.
3. Potassium chloride (K-Dur) is an electrolyte and has no impact on chest pain.
4. Alprazolam (Xanax) is an antianxiety medication and has no impact on chest pain that is associated with low hemoglobin levels.

Pregnancy Category: Not Known
Client Need: Physiological Integrity

3 - 2 9

④ **The purpose of warfarin (Coumadin) is to prevent blood clot formation. Warfarin is an anticoagulant that affects the formation of clotting factors. It is used to increase prothrombin time, which prevents the formation of blood clots. This client may be prone to blood clots that could form in the atria, as the atria do not empty completely while fibrillating.**

1, 2, and 3. Warfarin (Coumadin) is not an antiarrhythmic agent or a diuretic.

Pregnancy Category: NR
Client Need: Health Promotion/Maintenance

3 - 3 0

① **Dipyridamole (Persantine) is an antiplatelet agent that is often prescribed, along with acetylsalicylic acid, to minimize the potential for thrombus formation.**

2. Dobutamine hydrochloride (Dobutrex) is a beta-adrenergic used to improve cardiac contractility and increase cardiac output. It is not an antiplatelet.
3. Atorvastatin calcium (Lipitor) is an antilipemic used as an adjunct to diet to lower low-density lipoprotein (LDL). It is not an antiplatelet.
4. Penbutolol sulfate (Levatol) is an antihypertensive administered to treat mild to moderate hypertension. It is not an antiplatelet.

Pregnancy Category: B
Client Need: Health Promotion/Maintenance

Practice Test 4

Fluid and Electrolytic Agents

OVERVIEW

Fluid and electrolytic agents magnify the ability of the renal system to selectively excrete electrolytes and water. They replace lost electrolytes and maintain the body's acid/base balance.

Fluid and electrolytic agents include:

- Acidifiers and alkalinizers
- Antidiuretics
- Diuretics
- Electrolytes and electrolyte modifiers

ACIDIFIERS AND ALKALINIZERS

ACIDIFIERS increase the acidity of substances to which they are added or exposed.

Acidifiers include:

- Ammonium chloride

Conditions treated with acidifiers include:

- Metabolic alkalosis

ALKALINIZERS increase the alkalinity of substances to which they are either added or exposed.

Alkalinizers include:

- Sodium bicarbonate
- Sodium lactate
- Tromethamine

Conditions treated with alkalinizers include:

- Metabolic acidosis
- Metabolic acidosis associated with cardiac bypass surgery

ANTIDIURETICS

Antidiuretics decrease urinary output by suppressing the rate of urine formation or by promoting the reabsorption of water. Hormones such as vasopressin regulate the reabsorption of water by the kidneys. Vasopressin is secreted by the posterior pituitary gland when body fluids must be conserved.

Conditions treated with vasopressin and its derivatives include:

- Diabetes insipidus
- Postoperative distention

DIURETICS

Diuretics facilitate the excretion of water and electrolytes from the body and thereby reduce the amount of excess fluid in the tissues. Diuretics include thiazides, loop diuretics, osmotic diuretics, and potassium-sparing diuretics.

Conditions treated with diuretics include:

- Endocrine disorders
- Heart failure
- Kidney and liver disease

ELECTROLYTES AND ELECTROLYTE MODIFIERS

Electrolytes disunite, or separate, into ions (particles carrying an electric charge) when fused or in solution. By doing so, they become capable of conducting electricity.

Electrolytes and electrolyte modifiers include:

- Bicarbonate (HCO_3)
- Calcium ($Ca2^+$)
- Magnesium ($Mg2^+$)
- Potassium (K^+)
- Sodium (Na^+)

Conditions treated with electrolytes and electrolyte modifiers include:

- Hypocalcemia
- Hypokalemia
- Hyponatremia
- Metabolic acidosis
- Prevention and control of seizures

Practice Test 4

Questions

4 - 1

Your client is scheduled for a thyroidectomy. What pharmacologic agent should be available at the bedside when the client returns from surgery?

1. parenteral calcium gluconate preparation
2. parenteral potassium preparation
3. calcitonin (Calcimar)
4. parenteral liothyronine (Cytomel)

4 - 2

A client with iron deficiency anemia is taking a prescription for ferrous sulfate (Slow-Fe) 390 mg daily. When teaching the client, the nurse should include which information regarding this iron replacement?

1. "If a dosage is missed, the next dose should be doubled."
2. "To increase absorption, take the medication with orange juice."
3. "The tablet can be crushed if the client has difficulty in swallowing."
4. "Take the medication with milk or an antacid to avoid gastric discomfort."

4 - 3

A client has developed chronic renal failure and is taking calcium carbonate (Os-Cal). The nurse explains to the client that calcium is needed to:

1. lower the serum phosphate level.
2. reduce gastric irritation.
3. control blood pressure.
4. regulate bowel function.

4 - 4

An adult client's prescriptions include iron dextran (DexFerrum) 100 mg intramuscularly as a one-time dose. The ampule of DexFerrum supplied contains 50 mg/ml. The best method of administering this medication is to give:

1. 2 ml deep intramuscularly in the posterior gluteal site with a 23-gauge, 1-inch needle.
2. 1 ml in each deltoid site using a 21-gauge, 1 1/2-inch needle.
3. 1 ml in each anterior thigh site using the Z-track technique and a 20-gauge, 1 1/2-inch needle.
4. 1 ml in each posterior gluteal site using the Z-track technique and a 19-gauge, 2-inch needle.

4 - 5

Your client has begun vomiting copious amounts of bright red blood and is exhibiting signs of shock. Hetastarch (Hespan) has been prescribed. You know this medication is given:

1. to replace the sodium lost due to vomiting.
2. to help stop the bleeding by affecting clotting time.
3. as a preoperative antibiotic.
4. as a fluid volume expander, which is helpful in treating shock.

4 - 6

A client is receiving hydrochlorothiazide (Ezide) to treat hypertension. You will instruct the client that dietary intake should be high in which of the following?

1. magnesium
2. iron
3. potassium
4. calcium

4 - 7

A client is receiving medication to reduce intraocular pressure. Which drug will have the side effects of numbness and tingling?

1. pilocarpine
2. neostigmine
3. Dramamine
4. Diamox

4 - 8

You plan to irrigate a Stage III pressure ulcer. Which of the following solutions would you select?

1. Dakin's solution
2. Betadine solution
3. hydrogen peroxide solution
4. normal saline solution

4 - 9

Which fluid can be administered with packed red blood cells?

1. lactated Ringer's
2. sodium chloride
3. dextrose 5%
4. dextrose 5% in 1/2 normal saline

4 - 1 0

A client experiencing lymphedema is to receive a hypertonic intravenous solution. Which of the following would be appropriate?

1. 0.9% sodium chloride
2. 0.45% sodium chloride
3. 5% dextrose in water
4. 5% dextrose in normal saline

4 - 1 1

A client has experienced extensive burns and is hyponatremic. The intravenous fluid of choice to correct this imbalance would be:

1. 5% dextrose in water.
2. 0.45% saline.
3. 0.9% saline.
4. 3% saline.

4 - 1 2

A client has cardiac insufficiency and is experiencing marked peripheral edema. For which of the following medications do you anticipate a prescription?

1. furosemide (Lasix)
2. allopurinol (Zyloprim)
3. ranitidine (Zantac)
4. cefotaxime (Claforan)

4 - 1 3

A client is experiencing a fluid volume deficit and is to receive 1000 ml of normal saline solution to begin at 10 a.m. and infuse for 8 hours. How many drops per minute will the client receive if the drop factor is 10 gtts/ml?

1. 17
2. 21
3. 42
4. 53

4 - 1 4

A client has developed intracranial pressure and the heart rate is dropping. Mannitol 1.5 gm/kg of body weight is administered intravenously over 60 minutes as prescribed. This medication will:

1. increase the heart rate.
2. lower the blood pressure.
3. help reduce intracranial pressure.
4. act as an antimicrobial.

4 - 1 5

An elderly client is admitted to your unit in dehydration. History reveals: Vomiting and diarrhea for 4 days. Laboratory values indicate a potassium level of 2.8 mEq/l. You know that:

1. potassium chloride may be given intramuscularly if there is no intravenous site available.
2. potassium chloride may be given undiluted in a rapid intravenous bolus.
3. potassium chloride may not be given intravenously.
4. potassium chloride is usually limited to 40 mEq/l of intravenous fluid.

4 - 1 6

The parathyroid glands were inadvertently removed during a thyroidectomy. Which of the following medications would be prescribed?

1. potassium chloride
2. glucose
3. sodium chloride
4. calcium gluconate

4 - 1 7

Your client is experiencing renal failure. Laboratory values reveal: Sodium 155 mEq/l, potassium 5.6 mEq/l, blood urea nitrogen (BUN) 23, and creatinine 2.4. You will anticipate a prescription for:

1. 0.9% sodium chloride solution.
2. Kayexalate.
3. diuretics.
4. potassium chloride.

4 - 1 8

A 2-year-old is to receive 320 cc of normal saline intravenously over an 8-hour period due to dehydration. The intravenous equipment used delivers 60 microdrops per cc. How many microdrops per minute will the client receive?

1. 20
2. 40
3. 60
4. 80

4-19

A client has taken hydrochlorothiazide (Ezide) for several years and is complaining of anorexia, muscle cramps, and confusion. These symptoms indicate:

1. hypokalemia.
2. hyponatremia.
3. hypovolemia.
4. drug toxicity.

4-20

A client taking a digitalis preparation should be assessed for toxicity when:

1. taking phenytoin (Dilantin).
2. taking furosemide (Lasix).
3. taking nonsteroidal anti-inflammatory drugs (NSAIDs).
4. symptoms of hyperlipidemia are present.

4-21

Your client is experiencing acute congestive heart failure. You will anticipate a prescription for:

1. atenolol (Tenormin).
2. furosemide (Lasix).
3. cimetidine (Tagamet).
4. cefprozil (Cefzil).

4-22

A client enters the hospital in acute renal failure. The client complains of drowsiness and nausea and has Kussmaul's respiration. Laboratory tests show a serum potassium of 6.8, serum sodium of 120, and blood pH 7.2. Which of the following physician's prescriptions should the nurse question?

1. Polystyrene sodium sulfonate (Kayexalate) 50 gm per rectum as enema.
2. 2000-calorie, high-carbohydrate, high-protein diet when nausea subsides.
3. Hypertonic glucose (25%) 300 cc with units of Regular insulin per intravenous infusion over 1 hour.
4. Limit po fluids per 8 hours to no more than 100 cc more than urinary output for the previous 8 hours.

4 - 2 3

A client is experiencing vomiting and gastrointestinal bleeding. You and the registered nurse will prepare an intravenous infusion containing potassium chloride. The purpose of administering potassium chloride is to:

1. replace potassium that is lost in urine.
2. restore lost potassium reserves.
3. provide potassium to promote excretion of sodium.
4. replace the potassium that is being lost through vomiting.

4 - 2 4

A client is in hypovolemic shock. The prescription reads: Intravenous 2000 ml normal saline to begin at 3 p.m. and infuse for 24 hours. How many drops per minute should the client receive if the drop factor is 20 gtts/ml?

1. 28
2. 31
3. 44
4. 52

Practice Test 4

Answers, Rationales, and Explanations

4 - 1

① Parenteral calcium gluconate preparation should be available at the bedside to treat the potential for tetany following a thyroidectomy. During a thyroidectomy, the parathyroid glands may be damaged or removed, causing an upset in calcium metabolism (hypocalcemia).

2. Potassium is not affected by a thyroidectomy.

3. Calcitonin is a hypocalcemic used in the management of hypercalcemia.

4. Cytomel is a hormone replacement used with diminishing or absent thyroid functioning. Cytomel is usually given as an oral preparation.

Pregnancy Category: C

Client Need: Safe, Effective Care Environment

4 - 2

② To increase absorption of iron, it should be taken with a beverage containing vitamin C, such as orange juice. Vitamin C increases absorption of iron in the intestine. Ferrous sulfate is an antianemic iron supplement.

1. The dosage should not be doubled. Doubling the dosage may contribute to overdose.

3. Slow-Fe is an extended release iron tablet and should not be crushed or chewed to avoid alterations in dosages.

4. Milk and antacids decrease iron absorption.

Pregnancy Category: A

Client Need: Physiological Integrity

4 - 3

① Calcium carbonate (Os-Cal) lowers serum phosphate levels. Calcium binds with phosphates to decrease its absorption, thus lowering serum phosphate levels.

2. Reducing gastric irritation is not a primary concern in chronic renal failure.

3. Calcium carbonate has no direct effect on blood pressure.

4. Calcium salt is used as a laxative, but the primary action of calcium carbonate, when given to treat chronic renal failure, is to regulate phosphate levels.

Pregnancy Category: C

Client Need: Health Promotion/Maintenance

4 - 4

④ **The best method of administering a thick intramuscular preparation like iron dextran (DexFerrum) is to give 1 ml in each posterior gluteal site using the Z-track technique and a 19-gauge, 2-inch needle. DexFerrum will be given using the Z-track technique to prevent iron compounds from leaking back into the subcutaneous tissue and causing irritation and staining of the skin.**

1. DexFerrum should be given deep intramuscularly to prevent irritation of subcutaneous tissue. A 19-gauge, 2-inch needle should be used.

2 and 3. The posterior gluteal area of the buttock is the site of choice for an adult because it is a large muscle and not as likely to abscess when injected with a thick preparation such as DexFerrum.

Pregnancy Category: B

Client Need: Safe, Effective Care Environment

4 - 5

④ **Hetastarch (Hespan) is given to expand fluid volume. It is a plasma volume expander and is sometimes used to treat shock until blood products are available.**

1. Hespan does not replace serum sodium.
2. Hespan does not decrease clotting time.
3. Hespan is not an anti-infective agent.

Pregnancy Category: C

Client Need: Health Promotion/Maintenance

4 - 6

③ **A client receiving hydrochlorothiazide (Ezide) should be instructed to consume high amounts of potassium in the diet. Thiazide drugs such as Ezide are potassium depleting. Potassium is necessary for transmission of electrical impulses and contractions of smooth, cardiac, and skeletal muscles.**

1. Thiazide drugs such as Ezide deplete potassium, not magnesium. The chief functions of magnesium are bone mineralization, enzyme action, building of protein, normal muscle contractions, transmission of nerve impulses, and maintenance of teeth. Adverse reactions are seldom seen, unless related to overdose.

2. Thiazide drugs such as Ezide deplete potassium, not iron. Iron is in cells and carries oxygen to the cells of the body. Ferrous sulfate and ferrous gluconate are used in the treatment of iron-deficiency anemia.

4. Thiazide drugs such as Ezide deplete potassium, not calcium. Calcium is involved in the functioning of nerves and muscles, clotting of blood, and building of bones and teeth. Calcium is given for the treatment of hypocalcemia seen in parathyroid disorders. Calcium may also be given during pregnancy due to an increased need.

Pregnancy Category: B

Client Need: Health Promotion/Maintenance

4 - 7

④ **Acetazolamide (Diamox) has side effects that include numbness and tingling. Its diuretic action decreases secretions of aqueous humor and thereby reduces pressure in angle-closure glaucoma. Adverse side effects include parethesias (abnormal sensations such as burning or prickling), especially of the tongue, lips, anus, and extremities.**

1. Pilocarpine is effective in treating glaucoma by facilitating the outflow of aqueous humor. Side effects include blurring of vision, headache, nausea, and diarrhea. It is not associated with numbness and tingling.

2. Neostigmine is a cholinergic used to increase muscle strength in the symptomatic treatment of myasthenia gravis. Adverse side effects include: Nausea, vomiting, abdominal cramps, increased salivation, and lacrimation. It is not prescribed to treat intraocular pressure and it is not associated with numbness and tingling.

3. Dramamine is an antiemetic used in the treatment of ear conditions involving vertigo. It is not prescribed to treat intraocular pressure. Dramamine is also effective in treating motion sickness. Adverse side effects include: Headache, blurred vision, and dry mouth.

Pregnancy Category: C
Client Need: Safe, Effective Care Environment

4 - 8

④ **Normal saline should be used to irrigate Stage III pressure ulcers. The composition of normal saline approximates our own body fluids. Because normal saline is not a chemical, it does not disrupt the normal healing process. Allowing enzymes to promote healing is referred to as autolytic healing. Deep wounds (Stage III pressure ulcers) exude fluid that contains enzymes. These enzymes destroy microorganisms and thereby promote healing. When chemical solutions are poured into these wounds (Dakin's, Betadine, hydrogen peroxide), they negate the effect of these enzymes and disrupt healing.**

1, 2, and 3. Dakin's, Betadine, and hydrogen peroxide may be administered when Stage III pressure ulcers are grossly infected.

Pregnancy Category: NR
Client Need: Physiological Integrity

4 - 9

② **The only fluid that can be administered with blood components is sodium chloride (normal saline). Anything other than normal saline can cause rupture of erythrocytes. Normal saline is isotonic (same osmotic pressure as blood serum). Sodium chloride is most like the body's fluids.**

1. Solutions containing calcium, such as lactated Ringer's, can cause clotting.

3 and 4. Solutions containing dextrose can cause hemolysis (red blood cells fill with fluid, the membranes rupture, and the cells are destroyed).

Pregnancy Category: NR
Client Need: Safe, Effective Care Environment

4 - 1 0

④ **Dextrose 5% in normal saline is an appropriate hypertonic intravenous solution to administer to a client experiencing lymphedema (swelling of tissues due to the increase in lymph). Hypertonic fluids, like dextrose 5% in normal saline, reduce lymphedema by increasing osmotic pressure, which moves lymph into the bloodstream.**

1. NaCl 0.9% is an isotonic solution and therefore does not increase osmotic pressure and move lymph into the bloodstream.
2. NaCl 0.45% is a hypotonic solution and therefore does not increase osmotic pressure and move lymph into the bloodstream.
3. Dextrose 5% in water is an isotonic solution and therefore does not increase osmotic pressure and move lymph into the bloodstream.

Pregnancy Category: NR
Client Need: Physiological Integrity

4 - 1 1

④ **The intravenous fluid of choice for correcting hyponatremia due to extensive burns is 3% saline. Burn victims lose large amounts of sodium in edema and exudate. Because of this, hyponatremia (low serum sodium) develops. Sodium is replaced by intravenous fluid in concentrations above isotonic, which is 0.9%.**

1. Dextrose 5% in water contains no saline and would not significantly elevate sodium levels.
2. Saline 0.45% is hypotonic and would not elevate serum sodium levels.
3. Saline 0.9% is isotonic and would not significantly elevate sodium levels.

Pregnancy Category: NR
Client Need: Physiological Integrity

4 - 1 2

① **You will anticipate a prescription for the diuretic furosemide (Lasix). The action of Lasix occurs mainly in the loop of Henle (hence, "loop diuretic"). Lasix increases urine output by affecting osmotic pressure in the loop portion of the kidney. Diuresis aids in reducing fluid volume collected in the pulmonary vasculature and the periphery, thus reducing peripheral edema.**

2. Allopurinol (Zyloprim) is prescribed for the treatment of gout and has no impact on peripheral edema.
3. Ranitidine (Zantac) is an antiulcer medication and has no impact on peripheral edema.
4. Cefotaxime (Claforan) is a cephalosporin antibiotic and has no impact on peripheral edema.

Pregnancy Category: C
Client Need: Physiological Integrity

4 - 1 3

② The client will receive 21 drops per minute.

Formula: $\dfrac{\text{amount} \times \text{drop factor}}{\text{time (in minutes)}}$

$\dfrac{\text{normal saline 1000 ml} \times \text{10 gtts}}{\text{8 hours (in minutes)}}$
= 10,000 ml / 480 minutes
= 20.8 = 21 drops (rounding up)

1, 3, and 4 are incorrect calculations.

Pregnancy Category: NR
Client Need: Health Promotion/Maintenance

4 - 1 4

③ **The nurse knows that mannitol will reduce intracranial pressure. Mannitol is an osmotic diuretic that reduces intracranial pressure by reducing circulating volume.**

1. Mannitol is an osmotic diuretic and has no impact on heart rate.

2. Mannitol is an osmotic diuretic and is not given to decrease blood pressure, although this may occur as fluid volume decreases.

4. Mannitol is not an antimicrobial medication.

Pregnancy Category: B
Client Need: Health Promotion/Maintenance

4 - 1 5

④ **You know that potassium chloride is usually limited to 40 mEq/l of intravenous fluid. A potassium chloride mixture of 40 mEq/l should be given at a controlled and moderate rate in order to observe for side effects. (The normal value of potassium is 3.5 mEq/l or 3.5 to 5.0 mmol/l).**

1 and 3. Potassium chloride can only be given by mouth and intravenously.

2. Rapid administration of intravenous potassium chloride will cause lethal arrhythmias and should never be done.

Pregnancy Category: C
Client Need: Physiological Integrity

4 - 1 6

④ Calcium gluconate would be prescribed for clients whose parathyroid glands have been removed. The hormone secreted by the parathyroid gland (parathormone) causes calcium to be absorbed from the gastrointestinal tract and from bone. Because serum levels of calcium are dependent on parathormone's presence, the calcium will need to be replaced.

1, 2, and 3. Potassium chloride, glucose, and sodium chloride are not directly affected by the parathyroid's hormone.

Pregnancy Category: C

Client Need: Physiological Integrity

4 - 1 7

② You will anticipate a prescription for Kayexalate. Kayexalate lowers serum potassium. The normal potassium value is 3.5 to 5.5 mEq/L. A value of 5.6 mEq/L suggests hyperkalemia. Kayexalate is an electrolyte modifier (cation exchange resin) administered to lower serum potassium levels. Each gram of Kayexalate is exchanged for 0.5 to 1 mEq of potassium.

1. Infusing an isotonic solution (0.9%) of sodium chloride would increase sodium retention, which is contraindicated in renal failure.

3. Loop diuretics are the treatment of choice to increase sodium and fluid excretion, but they do not treat hyperkalemia.

4. The client has hyperkalemia. Therefore, potassium is contraindicated.

Pregnancy Category: C

Client Need: Physiological Integrity

4 - 1 8

② The child will receive 40 microdrops per minute.

Formula: $\dfrac{\text{amount} \times \text{gtt factor}}{\text{time (in minutes)}}$

$$\frac{320 \text{ cc} \times 60 = 19,200}{8 \times (60) = 480}$$

$= 40$ **microdrops per minute**

1, 3, and 4 are all incorrect calculations.

Pregnancy Category: NR

Client Need: Health Promotion/Maintenance

4 - 1 9

(1) The client's symptoms are characteristic of hypokalemia (potassium depletion). Hydrochlorothiazide (Ezide) is a diuretic (thiazide) that increases excretion of water and sodium by preventing sodium reabsorption in the distal tubules. In addition, excretion of chloride, bicarbonate, magnesium, and potassium takes place. The loss of too much potassium results in hypokalemia and should be treated. Symptoms of hypokalemia include anorexia, muscle cramps, numbness and tingling of the lower extremities, confusion, and coma.

2. Major symptoms of hyponatremia (sodium depletion) include anxiety, drowsiness and stupor, muscle weakness, convulsions, oliguria, and anuria.

3. Major symptoms of hypovolemia (abnormally decreased volume of circulating fluid) include oliguria, hypotension, and dry skin.

4. Symptoms of Ezide toxicity include hypotension and tachycardia.

Pregnancy Category: B

Client Need: Health Promotion/Maintenance

4 - 2 0

(2) Clients taking a digitalis preparation and the diuretic furosemide (Lasix) concurrently should be assessed for digitalis toxicity. Furosemide (Lasix) is a potassium-depleting diuretic. Low serum levels of potassium (hypokalemia) increase the action of digitalis, and digitalis toxicity can occur.

1. There is no interaction between digitalis and phenytoin (Dilantin) administration.

3. There is no interaction with nonsteroidal anti-inflammatory drugs (NSAIDs) and digitalis toxicity. Toxicity is more likely to occur with corticosteroids.

4. There is no association between digitalis toxicity and hyperlipemia (increased lipids in the plasma).

Pregnancy Category: C

Client Need: Health Promotion/Maintenance

4 - 2 1

(2) You will anticipate a prescription for furosemide (Lasix) for a client experiencing acute congestive heart failure. Furosemide (Lasix) is a loop diuretic whose impact on the reabsorption of some electrolytes within the nephron causes an increase in urinary excretion of water, as well as some electrolytes. Heart failure is relieved as circulatory volume is diminished.

1. Atenolol (Tenormin) is a beta-blocker administered to treat tachycardia.

3. Cimetidine (Tagamet) is an antiulcer drug. It has no impact on congestive heart failure.

4. Cefprozil (Cefzil) is an anti-infective and has no impact on congestive heart failure.

Pregnancy Category: C

Client Need: Physiological Integrity

4-22

② **A high-protein diet should be questioned for clients experiencing renal failure. Dietary protein is usually limited in acute renal failure to decrease nitrogenous metabolic waste products.**

1. Kayexalate reduces serum potassium by exchanging sodium for potassium ions in the gastrointestinal tract. As the client is hyperkalemic and hyponatremic, this is a reasonable prescription.

3. Hypertonic glucose and insulin promote movement of potassium into the cells, reducing hyperkalemia.

4. Fluid balance must be carefully monitored. Intake should be slightly more than output per 24 hours as rapid changes may occur. Intake is frequently based on prior 8-hour output.

Pregnancy Category: NR
Client Need: Health Promotion/Maintenance

4-23

④ **Potassium is one of the electrolytes contained in gastric secretions. When excessive vomiting or suctioning of gastric contents occurs, clients lose potassium (K^+), and if it is not replaced, this can lead to hypokalemia and dysrhythmia.**

1. Potassium is usually lost in urine during diuretic therapy.

2. Potassium cannot be stored in the body. An amount of 40 mEq of potassium must be consumed daily. Normal potassium is 3.5 mEq/l to 5.5 mEq/l.

3. Potassium does not promote excretion of sodium. When potassium is lost from cells, sodium shifts into the cells to replace lost K^+.

Pregnancy Category: C
Client Need: Health Promotion/Maintenance

4-24

① **The client will receive 28 drops per minute.**

Formula: $\dfrac{\text{amount} \times \text{gtt factor}}{\text{time (in minutes)}}$

$\dfrac{\text{normal saline } 2000 \times 20 \text{ gtts}}{60 \text{ min} \times 24} = \dfrac{40{,}000 \text{ gtts}}{1440 \text{ min.}}$

$40{,}000 / 1440 = 27.7$ gtts = **28 drops per minute (rounding up)**

2, 3, and 4 are incorrect calculations.

Pregnancy Category: C
Client Need: Physiological Integrity

Practice Test 5

Gastrointestinal Tract Agents

OVERVIEW

Gastrointestinal tract agents treat, inhibit, and prevent conditions that interfere with the process of digestion: the breakdown, absorption, and elimination of food.

Gastrointestinal tract agents include:

- Adsorbents
- Antacids
- Antidiarrheals
- Antiemetics
- Antiflatulents
- Antiulcer substances
- Digestive enzymes
- Gallstone solubilizers
- Laxatives

ADSORBENTS

Adsorbents easily adhere to other substances. For example, activated charcoal may be administered for its ability to adhere to drugs and poisons and prevent them from being absorbed into the gastrointestinal tract. Adsorbents are generally administered as antagonists (substances that counteract the actions of something else) or antidotes (substances that neutralize poisons or their effects).

Conditions treated with adsorbents include:

- Drug overdoses
- Poisoning

ANTACIDS

Antacids neutralize or reduce acidity in the digestive tract. Antacids elevate gastrointestinal pH, which reduces pepsin effects, which in turn increases esophageal sphincter tone and maintains a strong gastric mucosal barrier.

Conditions treated with antacids include:

- Peptic, duodenal, and gastric ulcers (as adjunctive therapy)
- Esophageal reflux
- Hyperacidity
- Indigestion
- Hyperphosphatemia (for clients in chronic renal failure)

ANTIDIARRHEALS

Antidiarrheals are administered to prevent or treat diarrhea (frequent passage of unformed, watery bowel movements).

Conditions treated with antidiarrheals include:

- Acute nonspecific diarrhea
- Diarrhea associated with carcinoid tumors (tumors located in the intestinal tract, bile ducts, pancreas, bronchus, or ovaries)
- Mild nonspecific diarrhea

ANTIEMETICS

Antiemetics are used to treat or prevent nausea and vomiting. Nausea and vomiting are generally associated with the side effects of drug and radiation therapy as well as some metabolic conditions. Antiemetics inhibit stimulation of the vomiting center in the brain and depress the sensitivity of the vestibular apparatus in the inner ear.

Conditions treated with antiemetics include:

- Motion sickness (prevention and treatment)

- Nausea associated with chemotherapy for cancer (as a preventive)
- Vertigo
- Antiemetics are also used as a preoperative preparation, to prevent nausea or vomiting.

ANTIFLATULENTS

Antiflatulents relieve the painful effects of excess gas in the gastrointestinal tract.

Conditions treated with antiflatulents include:

- Dyspepsia
- Flatulence
- Gastric bloating

ANTIULCER SUBSTANCES

Antiulcer substances are administered to clients who have gastrointestinal ulcers, such as peptic and duodenal ulcers. Antiulcer substances:

- Destroy H. pylori in the gastrointestinal tract
- Inhibit acid secretions
- Neutralize or buffer hydrochloric acid
- Strengthen the mucosal barrier

Conditions treated with antiulcer substances include:

- Duodenal ulcer
- Gastroesophageal reflux
- Heartburn
- Pathologic hypersecretory conditions

DIGESTIVE ENZYMES

Digestive enzymes are normally secreted by the mouth, stomach, and intestines. They are responsible for the decomposition and digestion of food. Enzymes present in digestive juices act upon food to break it down into simpler compounds.

Conditions treated with digestive enzymes include:

- Pancreatic secretion insufficiency
- Steatorrhea (fatty stools as seen in pancreatic diseases)

GALLSTONE SOLUBILIZERS

Gallstone solubilizers dissolve gallstones that are retained in the biliary tract following a cholecystectomy. The most common gallstones are cholesterol-containing stones. Gallstones form when the bile contains more cholesterol than can be maintained in a solution.

Conditions treated with gallstone solubilizers include:

- Gallstones

LAXATIVES

Laxatives are foods or chemicals administered to treat or prevent constipation. The actions of various laxatives are different, but all are administered to relieve constipation.

Laxatives include:

- Bulk-forming substances
- Fecal softeners
- Hyperosmolar substances
- Saline substances
- Stimulants

Conditions treated with laxatives include:

- Chronic constipation
- Laxatives are also used to prepare clients for bowel examination, delivery, and surgery.

Practice Test 5

Questions

5 - 1

Which of the following helps reduce "heartburn" by decreasing gastric acid secretion?

1. calcium carbonate (Tums)
2. ranitidine (Zantac)
3. psyllium (Fiberall)
4. aluminum hydroxide (Nephrox)

5 - 2

A client has been admitted with a foreign body obstruction in the colon and is awaiting surgery. Which medications would be contraindicated?

1. narcotic analgesics
2. antibiotics
3. antianxiety drugs
4. laxatives

5 - 3

Your 92-year-old client has gallstones but is not a candidate for surgery. You anticipate a prescription for:

1. simethicone.
2. magaldrate.
3. ursodiol.
4. Pancreatin.

5 - 4

A client with diverticulosis will begin a bulk-forming laxative regimen, which will include a drug such as:

1. psyllium (Metamucil)
2. docusate sodium (Colace)
3. loperamide (Imodium)
4. cimetidine (Tagamet)

5 - 5

A client receiving long-term hemodialysis asks you why aluminum hydroxide (Amphojel) has been prescribed 3 times a day. Your answer demonstrates your understanding that:

1. the dosage is preventive since the anxiety of undergoing dialysis may lead to stress ulcers.
2. aluminum salt combines with phosphates for excretion since clients on dialysis develop hyperphosphatemia.
3. the client is likely to develop indigestion because of dialysis.
4. the drug is a strong acid neutralizer needed by clients receiving dialysis.

5 - 6

A client has frequent watery stools. Which medication would be administered to treat this condition?

1. dimenhydrinate (Dramamine)
2. metoclopramide (Reglan)
3. loperamide (Imodium)
4. lactulose (Cephulac)

5 - 7

A client is taking aluminum hydroxide to control the development of renal osteodystrophy. The nurse should teach the client that a frequent side effect of this medication is:

1. diarrhea.
2. constipation.
3. flatulence.
4. vomiting.

5 - 8

As you prepare to administer sucralfate (Carafate), your client asks if this medication is another type of antacid. You explain that this medication:

1. is classified as an antacid.
2. helps to hasten the absorption of medications.
3. blocks histamine receptor sites in the stomach.
4. forms a paste that protects ulcers.

5 - 9

A client receiving treatment for gastric ulcers has become confused. Which medication is likely to have caused this side effect?

1. ranitidine (Zantac)
2. acetaminophen (Tylenol)
3. sucralfate (Carafate)
4. dihydroxyaluminum sodium carbonate (Rolaids)

5 - 1 0

A client tells you about taking paregoric (camphorated tincture of opium) for diarrhea. You will teach the client that this medication:

1. is not indicated for diarrhea.
2. may be taken daily, indefinitely.
3. may cause respiratory depression.
4. may be taken by persons allergic to morphine.

5 - 1 1

A client received metoclopramide (Reglan) in the recovery room. You know this drug helps to:

1. reduce postoperative pain.
2. stimulate respiration.
3. decrease risk of thrombus formation.
4. prevent postoperative nausea.

5 - 1 2

Your postoperative client is to receive a stool softener. You know to administer:

1. magnesium hydroxide (milk of magnesia).
2. docusate sodium (Colace).
3. loperamide (Imodium).
4. bismuth subsalicylate (Pepto-Bismol).

5 - 1 3

Which class of medications is used to treat gastroesophageal reflux disease (GERD)?

1. H$_2$ blockers
2. calcium channel blockers
3. beta blockers
4. potassium blockers

5 - 1 4

Which of the following medications would be administered to treat Curling's ulcers?

1. digoxin (Lanoxin)
2. erythromycin (Erythrocin)
3. ranitidine (Zantac)
4. ganciclovir (Cytovene)

5 - 1 5

A client is taking diphenoxylate and atropine (Lomotil) for diarrhea. Because of the atropine in this medication, you know to assess the client for:

1. bradycardia.
2. excess salivation.
3. tachycardia.
4. urinary incontinence.

Practice Test 5

Answers, Rationales, and Explanations

5 - 1

② Ranitidine (Zantac) reduces "heartburn" by decreasing gastric acid secretion. Raniti-dine's competitive inhibition of the chemical receptors responsible for gastric acid secretion has a direct impact on the amount of gastric acid secreted. Unlike neutralizing agents, medications like ranitidine (Zantac) actually reduce the quantity of gastric acid secreted.

1 and 4. Calcium carbonate (Tums) and aluminum hydroxide (Nephrox) are antacids and do not affect the amount of gastric acid secreted.

3. Psyllium (Fiberall) is a bulk-forming laxative and does not affect the amount of gastric acid secreted.

Pregnancy Category: B

Client Need: Physiological Integrity

5 - 2

④ Laxatives are contraindicated for clients with bowel obstruction. Laxatives promote peristalsis and bowel evacuation. In the event of a bowel obstruction, injury could occur with forceful peristaltic activity.

1, 2, and 3. Narcotic analgesics, antibiotics, and antianxiety drugs would not be contraindicated unless the client was allergic to them.

Pregnancy Category: NR (varies with specific laxative)

Client Need: Safe, Effective Care Environment

5 - 3

③ You will anticipate a prescription for ursodiol (Actigall). Where surgery is precluded and a client has gallstones less than 20 mm in diameter, the medication ursodiol may be prescribed. Ursodiol dissolves gallstones.

1. Simethicone (Mylanta) is administered to treat flatulence associated with gastric bloating. Simethicone is not capable of dissolving gallstones.

2. Magaldrate (Riopan) is an antacid and is not capable of dissolving gallstones.

4. Pancreatin is a digestive enzyme normally administered to treat exocrine pancreatic secretion insufficiency. It is not capable of dissolving gallstones.

Pregnancy Category: B

Client Need: Physiological Integrity

5 - 4

① **Psyllium (Metamucil) is a bulk-forming laxative. Psyllium expands as it absorbs water and increases the bulk of stools. This process encourages peristalsis.**

2. Docusate sodium (Colace) is a stool softener, not a bulk-forming laxative.

3. Loperamide (Imodium) is an antidiarrheal agent, not a bulk-forming laxative.

4. Cimetidine (Tagamet) is an antiulcer medication, not a bulk-forming laxative.

Pregnancy Category: NR
Client Need: Physiological Integrity

5 - 5

② **Aluminum hydroxide (Amphojel) treats hyperphosphatemia. Damaged kidneys are not excreting phosphates. The aluminum salt in Amphojel binds with these phosphates and excretes them via the large intestine.**

1. While the development of ulcers may be a possibility, this is not the primary reason for prescribing Amphojel.

3. Indigestion is not anticipated as a consequence of dialysis.

4. Clients receiving dialysis need excretion of phosphates rather than neutralization of acid.

Pregnancy Category: C
Client Need: Psychosocial Integrity

5 - 6

③ **Loperamide (Imodium) may be prescribed to treat diarrhea. Imodium is an antidiarrheal agent whose impact on stooling results from its inhibition of peristaltic activity.**

1. Dimenhydrinate (Dramamine) is administered to treat motion sickness and has no impact on stooling.

2. Metoclopramide (Reglan) is an antiemetic and has no impact on stooling.

4. Lactulose (Cephulac) is a laxative and would compound the problem.

Pregnancy Category: B
Client Need: Health Promotion/Maintenance

5 - 7

(2) **Constipation is a common side effect of aluminum hydroxide. Clients are usually given stool softeners to prevent constipation. Renal osteodystrophy is a condition characterized by impaired renal function with elevated serum phosphate. Aluminum hydroxide is an antacid and antilithic (prevents stone formation) that binds with phosphate, which is then excreted in the stool.**

1, 3, and 4. Diarrhea, flatulence, and vomiting are not common side effects of aluminum hydroxide.

Pregnancy Category: C

Client Need: Physiological Integrity

5 - 8

(4) **Sucralfate (Carafate) forms a paste that protects ulcers. Carafate is an antiulcer agent that reacts with gastric acid to form a paste that adheres to the surface of ulcers. It is usually taken before meals and at bedtime.**

1. Carafate is an antiulcer agent, not an antacid.

2. Carafate slows absorption of other drugs since it acts as a barrier.

3. Carafate does not block histamine receptor sites.

Pregnancy Category: B

Client Need: Health Promotion/Maintenance

5 - 9

(1) **Ranitidine (Zantac) may cause confusion. Other adverse reactions and side effects of Zantac include reversible leukopenia and pancytopenia and cardiac arrhythmias. Ranitidine (Zantac) is a histamine antagonist and antiulcer medication that inhibits histamine reception and has numerous systemic side effects.**

2. Acetaminophen (Tylenol) is an analgesic antipyretic that has minimal systemic side effects. The assessed allergic reactions of acetaminophen do not include confusion.

3. Sucralfate (Carafate) is an antiulcer enzyme inhibitor that may cause dizziness, sleepiness, and vertigo. However, confusion is not among its side effects.

4. Dihydroxyaluminum sodium carbonate (Rolaids) is an antacid. Assessed allergic reactions do not include confusion.

Pregnancy Category: B

Client Need: Safe, Effective Care Environment

5 - 1 0

③ **Paregoric (camphorated tincture of opium) is a narcotic and may cause respiratory depression. Paregoric is a controlled substance containing morphine.**

1. Paregoric is an antidiarrheal agent.

2. Paregoric is a controlled substance. It contains a narcotic and dependency may occur. It should not be taken indefinitely on a daily basis.

4. Paregoric contains morphine and should not be taken by those with morphine allergy.

Pregnancy Category: B (D for prolonged use at term)

Client Need: Safe, Effective Care Environment

5 - 1 1

④ **Metoclopramide (Reglan) is an antiemetic. Reglan increases sphincter tone in the gastrointestinal tract, thereby reducing nausea and vomiting.**

1. Reglan is an antiemetic and has no effect on pain.

2. Reglan is an antiemetic and has no effect on respiration.

3. Reglan is an antiemetic, not a thrombolytic (an agent that breaks up thrombi).

Pregnancy Category: B

Client Need: Health Promotion/Maintenance

5 - 1 2

② **Docusate sodium (Colace) is a stool softener. Colace softens the stool by pulling water into it. This process also reduces surface tension in the bowel.**

1. Magnesium hydroxide (milk of magnesia) is a laxative, not a stool softener.

3 and 4. Loperamide (Imodium) and bismuth subsalicylate (Pepto-Bismol) are antidiarrheals, not stool softeners.

Pregnancy Category: C

Client Need: Health Promotion/Maintenance

5 - 1 3

① H₂ blockers, or histamine blockers, inhibit the formation of stomach acid. This results in a decrease in the volume of stomach acid and a decrease in the reflux of acidic contents up the esophagus. H₂ blockers include cimetidine (Tagamet) and ranitidine (Zantac).

2 and 3. Both calcium channel blockers and beta blockers are used in the treatment of cardiac disease or hypertension.

4.   There is no class of drugs referred to as potassium blockers.

Pregnancy Category: Varies with specific drug

Client Need: Physiological Integrity

5 - 1 4

③ Ranitidine (Zantac) would be given to treat Curling's ulcers. Curling's ulcers are duodenal ulcers that may occur in clients who have experienced severe burn trauma. They are not uncommon and are treated with H₂ blockers such as cimetidine and ranitidine.

1.   Lanoxin is a cardiac glycoside antiarrhythmic and is not used in the treatment of Curling's ulcers.

2.   Erythromycin (Erythrocin) is an anti-infective and is not used in the treatment of Curling's ulcers.

4.   Ganciclovir (Cytovene) is an antiviral and is not used in the treatment of Curling's ulcers.

Pregnancy Category: B

Client Need: Physiological Integrity

5 - 1 5

③ Clients taking diphenoxylate and atropine (Lomotil) will be monitored for tachycardia. Atropine is an anticholinergic drug that at low dosages is drying to mucous membranes but at high dosages will block vagal stimulation and therefore increase the heart rate.

1.   Atropine may cause an increase in heart rate (tachycardia), not a decrease in heart rate (bradycardia).

2.   Atropine may cause dry mouth, not excessive salivation.

4.   Atropine may cause urinary retention, not urinary incontinence.

Pregnancy Category: C

Client Need: Physiological Integrity

Practice Test 6

Hematologic Agents

OVERVIEW

Hematologic agents are administered as prophylaxis and treatment for various thromboembolytic conditions. They also increase the amount of hemoglobin in the blood, control bleeding, and lyse thrombi.

Hematologic agents include:

- Anticoagulants
- Blood derivatives
- Hematinics
- Thrombolytic enzymes

ANTICOAGULANTS

Anticoagulants are used to prevent and treat blood clot (thrombi) extension and formation. Anticoagulants include oral preparations such as warfarin and injectable preparations such as heparin. Anticoagulants do not dissolve blood clots.

Conditions treated with anticoagulants include:

- Cerebral accident
- Bleeding episodes associated with hemophilia
- Malabsorption syndrome
- Pulmonary embolism

BLOOD DERIVATIVES

Blood derivatives are the components (constituents) that make up whole blood.

Blood derivatives include:

- Albumin
- Antihemophilic factor
- Anti-inhibitor coagulant complex
- Factor IX complex
- Factor IX human
- Plasma protein fractions

Conditions treated with blood derivatives include:

- Hemophilia A (Factor VIII deficiency)
- Hemophilia B (Factor IX deficiency)
- Hypovolemic shock

HEMATINICS

Hematinics are drugs or foods used to increase the number of red blood cells, the amount of hemoglobin in the red blood cells, or both.

Conditions treated with hematinics include:

- Megaloblastic anemia
- Pernicious anemia

THROMBOLYTIC ENZYMES

Thrombolytics break down fibrin blood clots by converting plasminogen (a protein found in many body tissues and fluids) to plasmin (fibrolysin). Plasmin then breaks down the fibrin, which lyses (dissolves) blood clots.

Conditions treated with thrombolytic enzymes include:

- Acute myocardial infarction
- Deep vein thrombosis
- Obstructed arteriovenous cannulae
- Pulmonary emboli

Practice Test 6

Questions

6 - 1

Your client will be discharged from the hospital with a prescription for the liquid iron preparation ferrous sulfate. You will teach the client to:

1. pour the iron preparation into milk prior to drinking.
2. swish and swallow the iron preparation.
3. observe for clay-colored stools.
4. use a straw to drink the iron preparation.

6 - 2

Your client is experiencing thrombocytopenia. Which of the following over-the-counter (OTC) medications should be avoided?

1. simethicone (Mylicon)
2. sucralfate (Carafate)
3. acetaminophen (Tylenol)
4. aspirin (acetylsalicylic acid)

6 - 3

A client is receiving a blood transfusion and asks, "Can I get AIDS from a blood transfusion?" You reply:

1. "Acquired immunodeficiency syndrome is not transmitted in blood."
2. "There is a 50% chance of contracting acquired immunodeficiency syndrome from a blood transfusion."
3. "No one has ever contracted acquired immunodeficiency syndrome from a blood transfusion."
4. "All donated blood is now tested for human immunodeficiency virus antibodies."

6 - 4

Your client has intermittent atrial fibrillation and is receiving warfarin. Upon discharge from the hospital, your teaching will include:

1. "Use aspirin sparingly."
2. "Double warfarin dosage if a day is missed."
3. "Report nosebleeds or hematuria."
4. "Expect dark, tarry-looking stools."

6 - 5

A client was taken to the special procedures laboratory, where streptokinase was injected intravenously. You know the action of this drug will:

1. promote hemostasis.
2. suppress myocardial excitability.
3. inhibit the formation of blood clots.
4. lyse blood clots.

6 - 6

A 9-year-old client has hemophilia A. Which of the following will be given prior to surgery to control bleeding?

1. Lovenox
2. albumin 5%
3. iron sorbitol
4. Factor VIII concentrates

6 - 7

Your client is to be discharged on warfarin (Coumadin) following an episode of thrombophlebitis. Discharge teaching will include instructions to:

1. avoid crossing the legs.
2. wear pants with an elastic waistband.
3. use straight razors for shaving.
4. use birth control pills to prevent pregnancy.

6 - 8

Your client is receiving heparin 1000 units per hour via continuous drip. The client's activated partial thromboplastin time (APTT) is 120 seconds. What action is indicated?

1. Administer protamine sulfate stat.
2. Administer the heparin drip as prescribed.
3. Increase the drip and notify the physician of the activated partial thromboplastin time (APTT).
4. Stop the drip and notify the physician of the activated partial thromboplastin time (APTT).

6 - 9

Your client is to receive heparin 5000 units subcutaneously twice daily. To administer this drug, you will:

1. inject it into the lower abdominal wall.
2. gently massage the site following the injection.
3. insert the needle at a 45-degree angle.
4. Use a 21-gauge needle.

6 - 1 0

A client is experiencing hemorrhagic shock and is to receive a fluid volume expander. Which medication would be indicated?

1. albumin 25%
2. Factor IX complex
3. urokinase
4. Hyperstat IV

6 - 1 1

A client is experiencing lymphedema and a deep vein thrombus is suspected. Which medication would be indicated to prevent further thrombus formation?

1. furosemide (Lasix)
2. cefotaxime (Claforan)
3. heparin
4. lidocaine (Xylocaine)

6 - 1 2

You receive the admission prescriptions on a client with an ischemic cerebral vascular accident. These prescriptions include the administration of heparin sodium 1000 units per hour by continuous infusion. Regarding the administration of this drug, you know that:

1. this medication may also be given orally.
2. toxicity of this medication is treated with vitamin K.
3. this is a peripheral vasodilatory medication.
4. this medication may cause fatal hemorrhage.

6 - 1 3

Your client is receiving alteplase (Activase) to treat an acute inferior myocardial infarction. You know the purpose of this medication is to:

1. dilate coronary arteries and arterioles.
2. lyse any thrombi obstructing the coronary arteries.
3. control life-threatening ventricular arrhythmias.
4. treat hypertensive crisis.

6 - 1 4

A client is to receive iron dextran (DexFerrum). Which of the following instructions will you give this client?

1. "This medication will make your stools very pale."
2. "Avoid all green vegetables."
3. "Take the iron supplement with orange juice."
4. "Iron may not be given by injection."

Practice Test 6

Answers, Rationales, and Explanations

6 - 1

④ **Clients should be taught to take oral liquid iron preparations through a straw. Because liquid iron preparations may stain the teeth and gums, it is recommended that a straw be used to avoid contact with the liquid.**

1. Iron should not be taken with milk because milk decreases iron absorption.

2. Swishing and swallowing liquid iron preparations may stain teeth and gums.

3. Iron preparations may affect stool color (darken the stool green or black).

Pregnancy Category: A
Client Need: Safe, Effective Care Environment

6 - 2

④ **Aspirin (acetylsalicylic acid) should not be administered to clients with thrombocytopenia (a decrease in number of platelets in circulation). Aspirin affects platelet aggregation and prolongs clotting time. Persons with thrombocytopenia have very low platelet counts and therefore impaired clotting.**

1. Simethicone (Mylicon) is an antiflatulant that relieves painful excessive gas in the gastrointestinal tract and does not affect thrombocytopenia.

2. Sucralfate (Carafate) is an antiulcer agent that reacts with gastric acid to form a paste that adheres to the ulcer surface. This drug does not affect thrombocytopenia.

3. Acetaminophen (Tylenol) is a nonopioid analgesic antipyretic and does not affect thrombocytopenia.

Pregnancy Category: D
Client Need: Health Promotion/Maintenance

6 - 3

④ **All donated blood is tested for human immunodeficiency virus antibodies. Clients can potentially contract acquired immunodeficiency syndrome (AIDS) from receiving blood infected with the human immunodeficiency virus.**

1. Acquired immunodeficiency syndrome is spread by contaminated blood and other body fluids; also by needles and breast milk.

2 and 3. People did contract the disease by blood transfusions in the early1980s. Since testing has begun, it is unlikely but still possible to contract the human immunodeficiency virus through blood transfusions. This is especially true if an infected person gives blood during the "window" period. During this period, the blood will not show positive for the human immunodeficiency antibodies.

Pregnancy Category: NR
Client Need: Health Promotion/Maintenance

6 - 4

③ **Clients receiving warfarin (Coumadin) should report nosebleeds and hematuria (blood in the urine). Warfarin is an anticoagulant. Bleeding may be a toxic side effect of warfarin and therefore should be reported.**

1. Aspirin is an antiplatelet and may increase the risk of bleeding. Aspirin should not be taken during administration of warfarin.

2. Doubling a dosage of warfarin may interfere with the maintenance of prothrombin time.

4. Dark, tarry-looking stools are not expected. However, they may indicate a gastrointestinal bleed, which is a reportable toxic side effect of warfarin.

Pregnancy Category: X

Client Need: Health Promotion/Maintenance

6 - 5

④ **Streptokinase lyses (breaks up) blood clots. Thrombolytic agents such as streptokinase activate the fibrinolytic process to lyse blood clots.**

1. Drugs such as Amicar, not streptokinase, promote hemostasis (stop bleeding) and are used in the management of hemorrhage.

2. Antiarrhythmic drugs such as lidocaine and Pronestyl decrease the excitability of the myocardium. They do not affect clotting.

3. Anticoagulants such as heparin and Coumadin inhibit the formation of blood clots, but do not lyse blood clots.

Pregnancy Category: C

Client Need: Physiological Integrity

6 - 6

④ **Factor VIII concentrates will be given prior to surgery to control bleeding. Hemophilia A and B are bleeding disorders. Hemophilia A is due to lack of Factor VIII (a clotting factor). Factor VIII concentrates are given to promote clotting, thereby preventing hemorrhage.**

1. Lovenox is an anticoagulant and is avoided by clients with hemophilia.

2. Albumin 5% is normally administered to treat hypovolemic shock. It does not control bleeding.

3. Iron sorbitol is normally administered to treat iron deficiency anemia. It does not control bleeding.

Pregnancy Category: C

Client Need: Physiological Integrity

6 - 7

(1) **Clients with thrombophlebitis should avoid crossing their legs because it places weight on the popliteal space and decreases venous return to the heart.**

2. Clients with thrombophlebitis should be instructed that constrictive garments like girdles and pants with elastic waistbands are contraindicated because they restrict circulation and decrease venous return.

3. Warfarin (Coumadin) is an anticoagulant. Clients should use only an electric razor for shaving during Coumadin therapy because of bleeding tendencies.

4. Birth control pills are contraindicated with a history of thrombophlebitis since they increase the risk of clots.

Pregnancy Category: D

Client Need: Health Promotion/Maintenance

6 - 8

(4) **The heparin drip should be stopped and the physician notified of the activated partial thromboplastin time (APTT). A normal activated partial thromboplastin time (APTT) is 30 to 45 seconds. During anticoagulant therapy, activated partial thromboplastin time (APTT) should be between 60 to 100 seconds. An APTT of 120 seconds is too long and hemorrhage could occur.**

1. The antidote for heparin (protamine sulfate) is not necessary at this time.

2. The heparin drip should not be left as prescribed because hemorrhage is likely with an APTT of 120 seconds.

3. Increasing the heparin drip will place the client at probable risk for hemorrhage.

Pregnancy Category: X

Client Need: Safe, Effective Care Environment

6 - 9

(1) **You will administer the heparin into the lower abdominal wall (fat pad) about 2 inches beneath the umbilicus and between the right and left iliac crest. This is the site of choice for deep subcutaneous injections of heparin. This area does not have muscular activity and therefore reduces the risk of local capillary bleeding.**

2. Massaging the site where heparin has been injected is not advisable because it can rupture small blood vessels and cause bruising.

3. When injecting heparin, the needle should be inserted at a 90-degree angle to avoid local bleeding and irritation.

4. A small 25- or 26-gauge needle should be used. A 21-gauge needle is too large and can cause trauma to tissue. Do not aspirate, because this may also cause bleeding into the tissue.

Pregnancy Category: X

Client Need: Safe, Effective Care Environment

6 - 1 0

① Albumin 25% would be indicated for a client in hemorrhagic shock. Because of this medication's molecular size, a shift occurs from the extravascular space to the intravascular space. This shift will increase vascular fluid volume and help increase blood pressure.

2. Factor IX complex is administered to treat hemophilia B or anticoagulant overdosage. It does not directly affect vascular fluid volume.

3. Urokinase (Abbokinase) is a thrombolytic enzyme used to treat massive pulmonary embolisms and does not increase vascular fluid volume.

4. Hyperstat IV is given to treat hypertensive crisis. It is contraindicated for clients in shock.

Pregnancy Category: C

Client Need: Physiological Integrity

6 - 1 1

③ Heparin is indicated to prevent further thrombus formation. Heparin is an anticoagulant whose impact on fibrinogen conversion helps prevent clot formation.

1. Furosemide (Lasix) is a diuretic and does not affect thrombus formation.

2. Cefotaxime (Claforan) is a cephalosporin antibiotic and does not affect thrombus formation.

4. Lidocaine is a ventricular antiarrhythmic and does not affect thrombus formation.

Pregnancy Category: C

Client Need: Health Promotion/Maintenance

6 - 1 2

④ Heparin sodium is an anticoagulant whose inhibition of fibrin formation affects the clotting of blood. Because of this, toxic levels may cause potentially fatal bleeding from nearly any vascular site.

1. Heparin is given only parenterally.

2. Toxic levels of heparin are treated with protamine sulfate, not vitamin K.

3. Heparin is not a vasodilatory drug but an anticoagulant.

Pregnancy Category: C

Client Need: Safe, Effective Care Environment

6 - 1 3

② **Alteplase (Activase) is administered to lyse any thrombi obstructing the coronary arteries. Alteplase (Activase) is a thrombolytic enzyme that lyses (dissolves) thrombi. It is administered for the treatment of acute myocardial infarction.**

1. Antianginals such as nitroglycerin (Nitrostat), diltiazem hydrochloride (Cardizem), nifedipine (Procardia), and propranolol hydrochloride (Inderal) dilate coronary arteries.

3. Antiarrhythmics such as procainamide hydrochloride (Pronestyl) control life-threatening ventricular arrhythmias.

4. Antihypertensives such as methyldopate hydrochloride (Aldomet) are administered to treat hypertensive crisis.

Pregnancy Category: C
Client Need: Physiological Integrity

6 - 1 4

③ **You will teach clients taking iron supplements to take them with vitamin C. Vitamin C enhances the absorption of iron. Citrus juices are typically high in vitamin C and will help enhance the absorption of the iron supplement.**

1. Iron supplements are notorious for darkening the stool.

2. A well-balanced diet should not be discouraged and green vegetables should be included.

4. Iron dextran (DexFerrum) may be given parenterally.

Pregnancy Category: C
Client Need: Health Promotion/Maintenance

Practice Test 7

Hormonal Agents

OVERVIEW

Hormonal agents treat, prevent, and inhibit conditions that interfere with the function of the endocrine glands, the hormones they secrete, and the organs they innervate.

Hormonal agents include:

- Androgens and anabolic steroids
- Antidiabetic agents and glucagon
- Corticosteroids
- Estrogens and progestins
- Gonadotropins
- Parathyroid-like substances
- Pituitary hormones
- Thyroid hormones and thyroid hormone antagonists

ANDROGENS AND ANABOLIC STEROIDS

ANDROGENS promote masculinization. The male hormones, testerone and its derivatives, are known as androgens and are secreted under the influence of the pituitary gland. Androgens aid in the development and maintenance of male sex characteristics. Androgens also facilitate the tissue-building process.

Conditions treated with androgens include:

- Delayed puberty
- Hypogonadism (abnormally decreased gonadal function)

ANABOLIC STEROIDS are synthetic drugs chemically related to androgens. They promote tissue processes.

Conditions treated with anabolic steroids include:

- Metastatic breast cancer in women
- Postmenopausal and senile osteoporosis

ANTIDIABETIC AGENTS AND GLUCAGON

Antidiabetic agents and glucagons (a polypeptide hormone that increases blood glucose) are administered to treat diabetes mellitus. The six major categories of antidiabetics are:

(1) Insulin
(2) Sulfonylureas
(3) Alpha-glucosidase inhibitors
(4) Biquanides
(5) Thiazolinediones
(6) Meglitinide insulin

(1) Insulin

Insulin is a protein normally secreted by the beta cells of the isles of Langerhans in the pancreas. Insulin is essential for the correct metabolism of blood glucose and for proper maintenance of blood glucose levels. Without the right secretions of insulin, carbohydrates and fats are not properly metabolized and hyperglycemia and glycosuria occur.

Conditions treated with insulin include:

- Diabetes mellitus
- Diabetic ketoacidosis

(2) Sulfonylureas

Sulfonylureas are oral hypoglycemic agents used to control blood glucose in adult-onset noninsulin-dependent diabetes mellitus (NIDDM), when diet alone is not adequate.

Conditions treated with sulfonylureas include:

- Type 2 noninsulin-dependent diabetes mellitus (NIDDM)

(3) Alpha-Glucosidase Inhibitors

Alpha-glucosidase inhibitors influence the activity of enzymes involved in the metabolism of carbohydrates. As a result, blood sugar levels rise more gradually and sudden increases and decreases are avoided.

Conditions treated with alpha-glucosidase inhibitors include:

- Type 2 noninsulin-dependent diabetes mellitus (NIDDM)

(4) Biquanides

Biquanides help decrease blood sugar levels by decreasing productivity of glucose in the liver. Biquanides also prevent weight loss at the onset of use and help normalize blood fat and cholesterol levels.

Conditions treated with biquanides include:

- Type 2 noninsulin-dependent diabetes mellitus (NIDDM)

(5) Thiazolinediones

Thiazolinediones help reduce insulin resistance (help increase insulin sensitivity).

Conditions treated with thiazolinediones include:

- Type 2 noninsulin-dependent diabetes mellitus (NIDDM)

(6) Meglitinide Insulin

Meglitinide is another insulin designed to treat postprandial (after a meal) hyperglycemia. It increases insulin release more quickly than the sulfonylureas. It is glucose-dependent and decreases as the client's blood glucose level drops. Because of its short half-life, the potential for accumulation is minimal.

Conditions treated with meglitinide include:

- Type 2 noninsulin-dependent diabetes mellitus (NIDDM)

CORTICOSTEROIDS

Corticosteroids are hormones (steroids) secreted directly into the bloodstream by the adrenal cortex (outer portion of the adrenal glands). There are three types of these steroid hormones: glucocorticoids, mineralocorticoids, and androgens. **GLUCOCORTICOIDS** influence the metabolism of sugars, fats, and proteins within body cells and also have a potent anti-inflammatory effect. **MINERALOCORTICOIDS** regulate mineral salts (electrolytes). Maintaining a normal balance of salts and water in the tissues and blood is essential for a healthy, functioning body. **ANDROGENS** are male and female hormones that maintain secondary sex characters. (These hormones are also produced in the ovaries and the testes.)

Conditions treated with corticosteroids include:

- Addison's disease
- Adrenal insufficiency
- Feminization
  (female secondary characteristics in a man)

- Hypopituitarism
- Rheumatoid arthritis
- Virilism
  (male secondary sex characteristics in a woman)

ESTROGENS AND PROGESTINS

The estrogens and progestins (progesterone) are the two endogenous female hormones. They are secreted under the influence of the anterior pituitary gland. The three estrogenic hormones are known as estradiol, estrone, and estriol. The **ESTROGENS** develop and maintain the female reproductive system as well as the primary and secondary sex characteristics. **PROGESTIN** (progesterone) is responsible for changes in the uterine endometrium, the preparation for implantation of the blastocyst, development of the maternal placenta, and development of the mammary glands.

Conditions treated with estrogens and progestins include:

- Abnormal uterine bleeding
- Primary ovarian failure
- Prostate cancer

GONADOTROPINS

Gonads are the embryonic sex glands before differentiation into the male testis or the female ovary. Follicle-stimulating hormones (FSH) and luteinizing hormones (LH) are known as gonadotropins because they influence the organs of reproduction (the gonads) in both sexes. In males and females, FSH and LH influence the secretion of sex hormones, the development of secondary sex characteristics, and the reproductive cycle.

Conditions treated with gonadotropins include:

- Failure to produce ova and/or failure to ovulate
- Failure to produce sperm
- Failure of the testes to descend

PARATHYROID-LIKE SUBSTANCES

The parathyroid gland consists of four small endocrine glands found on the posterior side of the thyroid. Overactivity (hyperparathyroidism) and underactivity (hypoparathyroidism) are the usual causes for the various conditions associated with the parathyroid gland.

Conditions treated with parathyroid-like substances include:

- Hyperparathyroidism
- Kidney stones (hypercalcemia)
- Paget's disease (osteitis deformans)
- Hypoparathyroidism
- Hypocalcemia (tetany)
- Hypocalcemia in clients on chronic dialysis

PITUITARY HORMONES

The pituitary is a pea-sized gland found at the base of the brain in a small pocket-like cavity called the sella turcica. There are two lobes of the pituitary gland, the anterior lobe (adenohypophysis) and the posterior lobe (neurohypophysis).

The **ANTERIOR PITUITARY** secretes hormones that influence the growth of bone tissue, the thyroid gland and its secretions, the adrenal cortex and its secretions, and the secretion of hormones associated with the ovaries in females and the testes in males.

The **POSTERIOR PITUITARY** secretes hormones that influence the reabsorption of water by the kidney tubules, increase the blood pressure by constricting arterioles, maintain labor during childbirth, and cause production of milk from the mammary glands.

Conditions treated with pituitary hormones include:

- Growth failure in children
- Temporary polyuria and polydipsia associated with pituitary trauma

THYROID HORMONES AND THYROID HORMONE ANTAGONISTS

Natural thyroid hormones are secreted directly into the bloodstream by the thyroid gland, located in the neck, anterior to and partially surrounding the thyroid cartilage and upper rings of the trachea. Underactivity (hypothyroidism) and overactivity (hyperthyroidism) are the usual causes for the various conditions associated with the thyroid gland. Synthetic thyroid hormone medications may be administered to treat conditions of the thyroid gland.

HYPOTHYROIDISM is caused by a deficiency of thyroid hormones, resulting in an abnormally slow body metabolism.

Medications used to treat hypothyroidism include:

- Liothyronine sodium (Cytomel)
- Liotrix (Euthroid)

Conditions treated with thyroid hormones include:

- Congenital hypothyroidism
- Cretinism
- Hypothyroidism
- Myxedema
- Nontoxic goiter

HYPERTHYROIDISM is the condition caused by an excessive secretion of thyroid hormones, which results in an abnormally accelerated basal metabolic rate. THYROID HORMONE antagonists are drugs that counteract the action of the thyroid hormones.

Thyroid hormone antagonists used to treat hyperthyroidism include:

- Methimazole (Tapazole)
- Potassium iodine, saturated solution (SSKI)
- Radioactive iodine (sodium iodide) 131

Conditions treated with thyroid hormone antagonists include:

- Hyperthyroidism
- Thyroid cancer
- Thyrotoxic crisis
- Thyroid hormone antagonists are also used to prepare clients for thyroidectomy.

Practice Test 7

Questions

7 - 1

An emaciated client is to receive NPH insulin 20 units 1 hour before breakfast daily. The nurse administering this medication will know to give the medication:

1. intramuscularly at 90 degrees.
2. subcutaneously at 90 degrees.
3. intramuscularly at 45 degrees.
4. subcutaneously at 45 degrees.

7 - 2

A client is to receive 12 units of Regular insulin and 26 units of NPH insulin subcutaneously, daily. Which procedure is correct?

1. Store all insulin in the refrigerator.
2. Massage the injection site after administration.
3. Draw up the NPH insulin first and then the Regular insulin.
4. Roll the NPH insulin bottle between the palms of the hands prior to drawing it up.

7 - 3

Your client received 35 units of NPH insulin at 7 this morning. If the client were to have a hypoglycemic episode, the most likely time would be:

1. just before lunch (11:30 a.m.).
2. midafternoon (2 to 3 p.m.).
3. just before supper (5 p.m.).
4. at bedtime (about 10 to 11 p.m.).

7 - 4

Your client is to receive glyburide (Glynase Pres Tabs). You know to include in your teaching that:

1. glyburide will increase serum glucose.
2. urinary output may increase.
3. glyburide may be taken throughout pregnancy.
4. the dosage will need to be decreased if corticosteroids are added to the regimen.

7 - 5

A child has had recurrent episodes of nephrotic syndrome. Continuous treatment with corticosteroids is being used to minimize relapses. The nurse will observe the client for:

1. a change in cardiac rate and rhythm.
2. gastrointestinal bleeding.
3. weight loss.
4. a decrease in serum glucose.

7 - 6

A client experiencing an acute exacerbation of multiple sclerosis requests information about prednisone therapy. You explain to the client that prednisone is:

1. an immunosuppressant that reduces acute inflammation.
2. a corticosteroid used to treat acute infection.
3. administered exclusively to treat clients with multiple sclerosis.
4. an anti-inflammatory agent that reduces muscular rigidity.

7 - 7

You know that glucagon is given to combat insulin shock. You also know that another secondary action of this medication is to:

1. decrease the heart rate.
2. increase the heart rate.
3. treat a hypertensive crisis.
4. increase renal perfusion.

7 - 8

A client did not take insulin as scheduled and was admitted to the hospital with a blood glucose level of 500 mg/dl. The physician prescribed insulin intravenously. What form of insulin can be given intravenously?

1. Regular
2. NPH
3. Ultralente
4. Lente

7 - 9

Your client has been taking prednisone for the treatment of lymphoma. During an office visit, you notice increased skin fragility, thinning of extremities, and increased fatty deposits on the face and shoulders, giving a "moon face" appearance to your client. Regarding the administration of prednisone, you will expect:

1. an increase.
2. no change.
3. abrupt cessation.
4. a gradual decrease.

7 - 1 0

A 26-year-old gravida I has Type 1 diabetes. Due to a change in insulin requirements during the first trimester, the nurse would carefully observe the client for signs of:

1. hypoglycemia.
2. ketoacidosis.
3. hyperglycemia.
4. pregnancy-induced hypertension.

7 - 1 1

A client with diabetes is experiencing an exacerbation of chronic obstructive pulmonary disease. The client's medication regimen will include, in addition to insulin twice daily, hydrocortisone (Solu-Cortef) 150 mg intravenously every 6 hours. You anticipate the following:

1. An increase in caloric intake.
2. A decrease in the amount of evening insulin.
3. No change, because these medications have no impact on one another.
4. An increase in the amount of insulin required.

7 - 1 2

A client with chronic obstructive pulmonary disease (COPD) has received glucocorticoid therapy for 2 years. Which statement by the client indicates a need for further teaching?

1. "I take a nap every day after lunch."
2. "I have my blood pressure checked every week."
3. "I have increased my daily salt intake."
4. "I take my medication with breakfast every other day."

7 - 1 3

Your pregnant client is expected to have a preterm infant and has been given betamethasone (Celestone). Which of these outcomes indicates the desired effect of the drug betamethasone (Celestone)?

1. decrease in uterine contractions
2. lecithin/sphingomyelin (L/S) ratio 2:1
3. decrease in discomfort during contractions
4. increase in effectiveness of contractions

7 - 1 4

A client with diabetes awakens from an afternoon nap feeling weak, dizzy, and anxious. The nurse observed that the client's skin is cool and clammy. The client complains of a headache. What action is appropriate at this time?

1. Start an intravenous infusion of normal saline.
2. Administer 1/2 cup of fruit juice.
3. Obtain a blood glucose level stat.
4. Administer insulin as needed (prn) according to the sliding scale.

7 - 1 5

Your diabetic client is to receive Humulin R 10 units and Humulin N 20 units, subcutaneously, daily a.m. To prepare this medication, you will:

1. draw up the Regular insulin first, then the Intermediate, in the same syringe.
2. draw up the Intermediate insulin first, then the Regular, in the same syringe.
3. give two separate injections.
4. withhold this mixture because it is incompatible, and notify the physician.

7 - 1 6

You are informed that one of the clients on your medical-surgical unit has been inadvertently double-dosed with a large amount of insulin. You anticipate the administration of:

1. Humulin R 10 units/hour intravenously.
2. normal saline at 100 cc/hour intravenously.
3. glucagon in normal saline intravenously.
4. glucagon in D5W intravenously.

7 - 1 7

A client is receiving the thyroid hormone replacement levothyroxine and has been scheduled for an I 131 Uptake study. You know the client must discontinue levothyroxine:

1. 2 weeks before the study.
2. 3 weeks before the study.
3. 4 weeks before the study.
4. 5 weeks before the study.

7 - 1 8

During admission assessment, your client tells you, "I take insulin, the long-acting kind." You understand that the client's insulin:

1. is the same as NPH or Intermediate insulin.
2. is now obsolete.
3. lasts up to 8 hours.
4. lasts up to 36 hours.

7 - 1 9

A client taking the birth control pill Ortho-Novum 1/35 asks the nurse, "What should I know about my pills?" The nurse's response will include the fact that:

1. Ortho-Novum 1/35 facilitates transport of the sperm through the fallopian tubes.
2. Ortho-Novum 1/35 is not associated with thromboembolism.
3. oral contraceptives such as Ortho-Novum 1/35 inhibit ovulation.
4. Ortho-Novum 1/35 will not interfere with cigarette smoking.

7 - 2 0

A female 60 years old is experiencing osteoporosis. She is placed on calcitonin-salmon (Calcimar) and estrogen therapy. The client is also instructed to walk 1 to 2 miles daily. This treatment is designed to:

1. reduce the vasomotor instability associated with menopause.
2. reduce calcium resorption and increase calcium laydown in the bones.
3. prevent osteoporosis.
4. prevent the formation of blood clots.

7 - 2 1

A client has a head injury and is to be given dexamethasone (Decadron) 10 mg intravenously stat. The purpose of this medication is to:

1. decrease bleeding.
2. sedate the client.
3. decrease inflammation.
4. provide pain relief.

7 - 2 2

Your client has been on a protracted course of corticosteroid therapy to manage asthma. Which of the following information will you include in the client's teaching plan?

1. Steroid therapy for asthma management will be lifelong.
2. Asthma triggers are irrelevant once steroid therapy has begun.
3. Steroids must be tapered off slowly, not stopped abruptly.
4. Steroid therapy has few side effects.

7-23

A client experiencing diabetic ketoacidosis is to receive 10 units per hour of a Regular insulin infusion. The pharmacy dispensed a bag that contains 100 units of insulin in 250 cc of fluid. At what rate will you deliver this infusion?

1. 2.5 cc per hour
2. 10 cc per hour
3. 25 cc per hour
4. 100 cc per hour

7-24

Your client has Type 2 diabetes mellitus and is taking a long-acting insulin as well as insulin lispro injections (Humalog). You will teach the client to take the Humalog injections:

1. 30 minutes before eating or immediately after eating.
2. 15 minutes before eating or immediately after eating.
3. 45 minutes before eating or 15 minutes after eating.
4. 60 minutes before eating or 20 minutes after eating.

7-25

As an adjunct pressor agent, arterial administration of vasopressin (Pitressin) via an infusion pump has been prescribed for a client experiencing a massive gastrointestinal bleed. You know this medication was prescribed in this situation for its ability to:

1. form a protective adhesive paste.
2. neutralize stomach acid.
3. stimulate smooth muscle contraction.
4. block gastric acid production.

7-26

A client with Type 2 diabetes takes 70/30 insulin before breakfast and dinner. Blood glucose has been elevated and is controlled with sliding scale insulin. When using a sliding scale to control blood glucose levels, the nurse will administer:

1. Regular insulin.
2. 70/30 insulin.
3. NPH insulin.
4. PZI insulin.

7 - 2 7

Your client is taking 0.1 mg of levothyroxine (Synthroid) per day. What teaching does your client need in relation to this medication?

1. Take the medication with meals.
2. Dosages can be self-adjusted based on energy needs.
3. Do not change brands.
4. Expect to lose 10 to 15 pounds within the first 6 months.

7 - 2 8

Birth control medications are made from which of the following?

1. vitamins
2. antihypertensives
3. synthetic steroids
4. calcium channel blockers

Practice Test 7

Answers, Rationales, and Explanations

7 - 1

④ **It is best to administer injectable insulin at 45 degrees when clients are emaciated. The needle is likely to go through the subcutaneous tissue and into the muscle if given to emaciated clients at 90 degrees.**

1 and 3. All injectable insulin should be given into the subcutaneous tissue, not into the muscle.

2. Giving an emaciated client an injection at 90 degrees is not recommended. The needle would probably pass through the subcutaneous tissue and into the muscle.

Pregnancy Category: B

Client Need: Safe, Effective Care Environment

7 - 2

④ **NPH insulin is an intermediate-acting insulin that is in suspension. Insulin in suspension should be rolled between the palms of the hands to thoroughly mix it prior to withdrawing the dosage.**

1. Insulin in use may be left for up to 4 weeks at room temperature unless the room temperature is higher than 85° F or below freezing. Extra insulin may be stored in the refrigerator.

2. After injecting insulin, some pressure should be applied to the site immediately after the needle is withdrawn. Pressure should be maintained for a few seconds thereafter. However, the site should not be massaged. Massaging the site may cause bruising.

3. When mixing an intermediate-acting insulin with Regular insulin, the Regular insulin should always be drawn up first.

Pregnancy Category: B

Client Need: Health Promotion/Maintenance

7 - 3

③ **Hypoglycemia would most likely occur just before supper (5 p.m.). NPH insulin is an intermediate-acting insulin that peaks between 6 and 12 hours.**

1. Just before lunch (11:30 a.m.) is not within the peak time of NPH insulin.

2. Hypoglycemia is not as likely to occur so shortly after eating.

4. At bedtime (about 10 to 11 p.m.) is past the peak range of NPH insulin.

Pregnancy Category: B

Client Need: Health Promotion/Maintenance

7 - 4

② **Urinary output may increase with glyburide administration. Glyburide (Glynase Pres Tabs) has a mild diuretic effect in addition to its hypoglycemic effect. As a result, an increase in urinary output may be noted. Glyburide also has a chronotropic effect (increases the heart's rate and strength of contractability).**

1. Glyburide (Glynase Pres Tabs) is a hypoglycemic and therefore decreases serum glucose.
3. Glyburide (Glynase Pres Tabs) should not be taken during pregnancy or by nursing mothers.
4. The dosage of Glyburide (Glynase Pres Tabs) will probably need to be increased if corticosteroids are to be administered.

Pregnancy Category: B

Client Need: Health Promotion/Maintenance

7 - 5

② **Corticosteroids can cause gastrointestinal bleeding; therefore, a stool analysis for occult blood should be completed.**

1. Corticosteroids do not affect heart rate or rhythm.
3. Corticosteroids are likely to cause weight gain, not weight loss. Corticosteroids can cause growth retardation and increase appetite and fluid retention. A client's height and weight should be obtained as baseline data.
4. Corticosteroids can cause elevated serum glucose, and recurrence of nephrosis would be indicated by albumin in the urine.

Pregnancy Category: C

Client Need: Physiological Integrity

7 - 6

① **Prednisone is an immunosuppressant and glucocorticoid that reduces acute inflammation and minimizes tissue damage. As a result, nerve conduction is improved.**

2. Prednisone is a corticosteroid. However, it is not given to treat infection but to reduce acute inflammation. An antibiotic would be given to treat infection.
3. Prednisone has been used for treating a wide range of inflammatory disorders, not just multiple sclerosis.
4. Prednisone is capable of affecting muscular spasticity, not rigidity. Muscular rigidity is associated with Parkinson's disease, not multiple sclerosis.

Pregnancy Category: C

Client Need: Physiological Integrity

7 - 7

② **Glucagon can increase the heart rate. Glucagon has, in addition to its hyperglycemic effect, a positive chronotropic effect (increases the heart's rate and strength of contractability).**

1. Glucagon tends to increase the heart rate, not decrease the heart rate.
3. Glucagon is not used to treat hypertensive crisis.
4. Glucagon has no direct impact on renal perfusion.

Pregnancy Category: B
Client Need: Physiological Integrity

7 - 8

① **Regular insulin is the only form of insulin that can be given intravenously. Regular insulin is clear (not in suspension) and does not contain any modifying agents. Onset of Regular insulin is 1/2 to 1 hour. It peaks between 2 and 3 hours and lasts 4 to 6 hours.**

2, 3, and 4. NPH, Ultralente, and Lente insulins cannot be given intravenously because they contain modifying agents. They are in suspension and are cloudy.

Pregnancy Category: NR
Client Need: Safe, Effective Care Environment

7 - 9

④ **You will anticipate a gradual decrease in prednisone. Prednisone is a corticosteroid. Skin fragility, thinning of extremities, and fatty deposits on the face and shoulders are signs and symptoms congruent with Cushing's syndrome and are probably due to excess corticosteroid intake. Suddenly withdrawing corticosteroids such as prednisone may precipitate adrenal insufficiency; therefore, a gradual decrease of corticosteroids is essential.**

1 and 2. Skin fragility, thinning of extremities, and fatty deposits on the face and shoulders are congruent with Cushing's syndrome. Increasing or maintaining the present level of prednisone will cause the symptoms to escalate.
3. Abrupt withdrawal from corticosteroids may precipitate signs and symptoms of adrenal insufficiency (anorexia, nausea, fatigue, weakness, hypotension, dyspnea, and hypoglycemia).

Pregnancy Category: C
Client Need: Physiological Integrity

7 - 1 0

① The client should be observed for signs of hypoglycemia. There is a decreased need for insulin in the first trimester of pregnant women who take insulin for diabetes. Levels of human placental lactogen (HPL), an insulin antagonist, are low and the developing fetus uses more glucose and glycogen. Nausea and vomiting during this time are also factors in the development of hypoglycemia.

2. Ketoacidosis accompanies hyperglycemia, not hypoglycemia.

3. The nurse will observe for signs of hypoglycemia, not hyperglycemia.

4. Pregnancy-induced hypertension (PIH) is not a factor in the first trimester. It usually occurs in the last trimester and is not associated with diabetes.

Pregnancy Category: B

Client Need: Physiological Integrity

7 - 1 1

④ The client will require an increase in insulin. Hyperglycemia often occurs in diabetics receiving Solu-Cortef due to Solu-Cortef's tendency to stimulate nutritional metabolism and gluconeogenesis (the formation of glycogen).

1. An increase in caloric intake is not anticipated. Diabetics receiving Solu-Cortef tend to have increased serum glucose levels.

2. To compensate for the increased serum glucose levels, diabetics receiving Solu-Cortef will need to increase their insulin dosage, not decrease it.

3. Hyperglycemia often occurs in diabetics receiving Solu-Cortef; as a result, an increase in the insulin dosage may be required.

Pregnancy Category: NR

Client Need: Physiological Integrity

7 - 1 2

③ Increasing salt intake should be discouraged. Glucocorticoid medications promote sodium and fluid retention. A sodium-restricted diet is recommended to prevent edema.

1. "I take a nap every day after lunch." This would be helpful since clients with chronic obstructive pulmonary disease (COPD) tire easily.

2. "I have my blood pressure checked every week." This is a good policy since glucocorticoids promote sodium and fluid retention and thereby increase blood pressure.

4. "I take my medication with breakfast every other day." This is a good policy since this will reduce gastric irritation. Taking the lowest dose possible of glucocorticoids and taking them only every other day will reduce the incidence of cushingoid appearance.

Pregnancy Category: C

Client Need: Health Promotion/Maintenance

7 - 1 3

② Obtaining a lecithin/sphingomyelin ratio of 2:1 would indicate the desired effect of betamethasone (Celestone). Celestone is a glucocorticoid given to pregnant women 24 to 48 hours before birth of a preterm infant (at least 34 weeks before gestation) to facilitate pulmonary maturation in the infant. The lung maturity of preterm infants can be assessed by checking the ration of two surfactant components, lecithin and sphingomyelin (substances in the lung that lower surface tension and are critical for alveolar stability).

1. Celestone is not a smooth muscle relaxant and has no impact on uterine contractions.

3. Celestone is not an analgesic and does not relieve pain.

4. Celestone is not an oxytocic agent and does not affect contractions.

Pregnancy Category: C
Client Need: Health Promotion/Maintenance

7 - 1 4

② Initially it is appropriate to administer 1/2 cup of fruit juice. Weakness, dizziness, and anxiety are symptoms of hypoglycemia. Sugar needs to be given immediately. If the nurse is not sure whether a client is exhibiting signs of hypoglycemia or hyperglycemia, it is better to treat for hypoglycemia to avoid the brain damage that can occur from a prolonged hypoglycemic episode.

1. An intravenous infusion of normal saline would not provide any needed glucose. It would only provide an access for administration of intravenous glucose. The oral sugar should be given while the client can still swallow.

3. It is important to obtain a blood glucose level. However, sugar needs to be administered while awaiting the results.

4. Administering insulin as needed (prn) according to the sliding scale would be appropriate for hyperglycemia, not hypoglycemia. Giving insulin to a hypoglycemic client would potentiate a further decrease in serum glucose.

Pregnancy Category: B
Client Need: Health Promotion/Maintenance

7 - 1 5

① When administering Regular and Intermediate insulin, the Regular insulin is to be drawn up first to avoid getting any Intermediate insulin in the Regular insulin vial. Reversing the process can inactivate the Regular insulin.

2. The Intermediate insulin should not be drawn up first because there is a risk of contaminating the Regular insulin with the Intermediate. The Regular insulin should be drawn up first.

3. Giving two injections will cause your client to receive twice as many needle sticks.

4. Regular and Intermediate insulins are compatible and appropriate mixtures. However, they need to be drawn up in the proper sequence (Regular first, Intermediate second).

Pregnancy Category: B
Client Need: Physiological Integrity

7 - 1 6

④ **You will anticipate the intravenous administration of glucagon in D5W. Glucagon is given to combat insulin shock (hypoglycemic reactions due to overdose of insulin) because it stimulates hepagluconeogenesis (the liver's formation of glucose).**

1. The client already has an excess of insulin. Therefore, Humulin R insulin would not be administered.
2. Administering normal saline at 100 cc per hour intravenously would not help to raise the serum glucose.
3. Glucagon will precipitate in normal saline solution. It may only be mixed with D5W.

Pregnancy Category: B
Client Need: Physiological Integrity

7 - 1 7

③ **The levothyroxine should be discontinued 4 weeks before the I 131 Uptake study is performed. The I 131 Uptake study requires the use of radioactive iodine. To eliminate incorrect results, all interfering factors, such as the administration of levothyroxine, should be withdrawn prior to the study.**

1 and 2. If the I 131 Uptake study is scheduled only 2 to 3 weeks after the levothyroxine has been withdrawn, the results of the study will be invalid.
4. Levothyroxine should be withdrawn 4 weeks before the I 131 Uptake study. It is not necessary to wait longer than 4 weeks.

Pregnancy Category: A
Client Need: Health Promotion/Maintenance

7 - 1 8

④ **The effect of long-acting insulin lasts up to 36 hours. Long-acting insulin, for example Ultralente, is referred to as "peakless" because it has a long sustained effect as opposed to well-defined peaks of action. The onset of long-acting insulin is 6 to 8 hours and the duration is 36 hours.**

1. NPH or Intermediate insulin is not the same as long-acting insulin.
2. Long-acting insulin is an available insulin.
3. Long-acting insulin lasts up to 36 hours, not 8 hours.

Pregnancy Category: B
Client Need: Health Promotion/Maintenance

7 - 1 9

③ **Oral contraceptives such as Ortho-Novum 1/35 inhibit ovulation.**

1. Ortho-Novum 1/35 prevents the transport of the ovum through the fallopian tubes.

2. Thromboembolism is a life-threatening adverse reaction that is associated with oral contraceptives such as Ortho-Novum 1/35.

4. Smoking while taking oral contraceptives will increase the risk of adverse cardiovascular effects.

Pregnancy Category: X
Client Need: Health Promotion/Maintenance

7 - 2 0

② **Calcitonin-salmon (Calcimar), estrogen replacement, and weight-bearing exercises increase calcium laydown in bones. Calcium supplements, along with estrogen replacement and walking exercises, improve bone stability by increasing available calcium for deposit in the bones and encouraging calcium laydown in response to weight-bearing. Estrogen opposes bone resorption (release of calcium from the bones) and is presumed to be effective in treating estrogen-deficiency-induced osteoporosis.**

1. The reduction of vasomotor instability ("hot flashes") is not related to the prevention of osteoporosis.

3. Osteoporosis is fairly inevitable with age, but a strong calcium matrix in the bone prolongs the time that a client can be free of osteoporotic fractures.

4. Estrogen enhances the coagulability of blood and is likely to increase the risk of clot formation.

Pregnancy Category: C
Client Need: Health Promotion/Maintenance

7 - 2 1

③ **Dexamethasone (Decadron) decreases inflammation. Dexamethasone is a glucocorticoid anti-inflammatory agent and affects inflammation by altering prostaglandin synthesis.**

1. Dexamethasone may increase, not decrease, prothrombin time. Guaiac-positive stools should be reported.

2. Dexamethasone is not a sedative hypnotic.

4. Dexamethasone is not an analgesic.

Pregnancy Category: C
Client Need: Health Promotion/Maintenance

7 - 2 2

③ **You will teach clients who have been on a protracted (extended) course of corticosteroid therapy to taper off the medication gradually. Exogenous steroid therapy will, after a period of 2 weeks or so, suppress the function of the adrenal glands. As a result, abrupt withdrawal of the corticosteroids can precipitate adrenal crisis. A gradual tapering off of the steroid dose is recommended to avoid this potentially fatal complication.**

1. Corticosteroid therapy for clients with asthma is usually episodic, not lifelong.
2. The treatment for asthma includes avoidance of "triggers" such as the inhalation of house dust, dander, molds, tobacco smoke, and other strong odors.
4. Corticosteroid use may have many side effects, including gastrointestinal upset, restlessness, hyperglycemia, dermal atrophy, and optic disorders.

Pregnancy Category: C
Client Need: Physiological Integrity

7 - 2 3

③ **25 cc per hour will be delivered.**
Formula: 100 units : 250 cc :: 10 units : X
100X = 2500
X = 25 cc

1, 2, and 4 are incorrect rates per hour.

Pregnancy Category: NR
Client Need: Safe, Effective Care Environment

7 - 2 4

② **Insulin lispro injections (Humalog) should be taken within 15 minutes before eating or immediately after eating because of their rapid onset and short duration of action.**

1, 3, and 4. Taking Humalog within 30, 45, or 60 minutes of eating is contraindicated because its rapid onset could produce symptoms of hypoglycemia. Also, taking Humalog 15 to 20 minutes after eating would be too late to cover the effects of eating, since Humalog has a very short duraton of action. Insulin lispro injections (Humalog) have a shorter onset and shorter duration of action than Regular insulin.

Pregnancy Category: NR
Client Need: Health Promotion/Maintenance

7 - 2 5

③ **Vasopressin (Pitressin) is given in this situation because of its ability to decrease blood flow to the gastrointestinal tract by stimulating smooth muscle contraction.**

1. Antiulcer agents such as sucralfate (Carafate) form a paste that protects damaged mucosa associated with ulcers. However, there is no indication that the client's bleeding is due to ulcers.

2. Antacids such as Maalox neutralize stomach acid. However, there is no indication that the client's bleeding is due to ulcers.

4. Drugs such as ranitidine (Zantac) block gastric acid secretions. However, there is no indication that the client's bleeding is due to ulcers.

Pregnancy Category: C
Client Need: Health Promotion/Maintenance

7 - 2 6

① **When using a sliding scale to control blood glucose levels, the nurse will administer Regular insulin subcutaneously. When insulin is given based on a sliding scale, Regular insulin is always used because of its rapid onset and short duration of action. The onset of subcutaneous Regular insulin is 13 to 60 minutes, peak 2 to 4 hours, and duration 5 to 7 hours.**

2. 70/30 insulin is a premixed dose of 70% NPH intermediate-acting insulin and 30% Regular insulin. This combination is undesirable for short-term management of hyperglycemia because of the intermediate-acting insulin. The onset of intermediate-acting insulin is 1 to 4 hours, peak 6 to 12 hours, and duration 18 to 28 hours.

3. Due to its delayed onset and prolonged duration of action, NPH insulin is not suitable for short-term treatment of elevated blood sugar.

4. PZI is a long-acting insulin. Only short-acting insulin (Regular) should be used in sliding scale insulin regimens. Regular insulin will rapidly lower elevated blood glucose.

Pregnancy Category: C
Client Need: Physiological Integrity

7 - 2 7

③ **The client should be taught not to change brands of levothyroxine (Synthroid) since preparations may vary. It is important that consistent and appropriate thyroid levels be maintained. Taking the medication in the morning is recommended to prevent insomnia.**

1. Synthroid does not have to be taken with meals. It is, however, recommended that it be taken at the same time each day to establish consistency.

2. The dosage of Synthroid should not be self-adjusted. Dosages should be adjusted based on serum laboratory values and under the direction of a health-care provider.

4. Clients taking Synthroid may experience weight loss as a result of increased basal metabolic rate, but weight loss may not occur in all clients.

Pregnancy Category: A
Client Need: Safe, Effective Care Environment

7 - 2 8

③ **Birth control pills are made from synthetic steroids. Birth control pills are effective because of their impact on ovulation. A combination of synthetic estrogen and progestin exerts its contraceptive effect by inhibiting ova release.**

1, 2, and 4. Vitamins, antihypertensives, and calcium channel blockers do not have a contraceptive effect.

Pregnancy Category: Varies with specific medication
Client Need: Health Promotion/Maintenance

Practice Test 8

Immunomodulation Agents

OVERVIEW

Immunomodulation (immunoregulation) refers to the effects of different chemical mediators, hormones, medications, or the immune system on foreign antigens. Immunomodulating agents (working through the body's immune system) will prevent, neutralize, or eliminate the effects of these foreign antigens.

Immunomodulating agents include:

- Antitoxins and antivenins
- Biological response modifiers
- Immune serums
- Immunosuppressants
- Vaccines and toxoids

ANTITOXINS AND ANTIVENINS

ANTITOXINS neutralize poisons, especially those generated by bacteria. Antitoxins produce antibodies in response to specific biologic toxins. Antitoxins are administered prophylactically and for therapeutic purposes.

Conditions treated with antitoxins include:

- Diphtheria
- Gas-gangrene
- Tetanus

ANTIVENINS are serums that contain antitoxins specifically for animal or insect venoms. Antivenins are created from immunized animal serums and are administered to treat clients who have been poisoned by animal or insect venom.

Conditions treated with antivenins include:

- Poisonous spider bites
- Snakebites

BIOLOGICAL RESPONSE MODIFIERS

Biological response modifiers are a group of therapeutic interventions that modify the host response to various conditions or diseases. Biological response modifiers include cytokine, monoclonal antibodies, and vaccines that alter the interaction between clients and their tumors. Biological response modifiers promote antitumor mechanisms found naturally in the immune system.

Conditions treated with biological response modifiers include:

- Chronic hepatitis B
- Metastatic renal cell carcinoma
- Multiple sclerosis (to reduce exacerbations)

IMMUNE SERUMS

Serum from an animal that has been rendered immune to a pathogenic organism can be used to treat a person who has the disease caused by that pathogenic organism. Immune serums contain antibodies for specific antigens.

Conditions treated with immune serums include:

- Tetanus, in clients who have not been immunized with tetanus toxoid but have been exposed to the tetanus pathogen
- Pertussis (whooping cough), as both prophylaxis and treatment

IMMUNOSUPPRESSANTS

Immunosuppressants prevent the formation of immune responses—that is, they suppress the body's natural immune response to antigens.

Conditions treated with immunosuppressants include:

- Organ rejection (heart, kidney, liver, pancreas) as prophylaxis

VACCINES AND TOXOIDS

A VACCINE is a suspension of an infectious agent or some part of an infectious agent administered to create a resistance to that infection. Vaccines are grouped into classes:

(1) Vaccines containing live attenuated (weakened) infectious organisms, such as the vaccine to prevent poliomyelitis.

(2) Vaccines containing infectious agents that can be destroyed by physical or chemical means.

(3) Vaccines containing soluble toxins of microorganisms; i.e., toxoids used in the prevention of diphtheria and tetanus.

(4) Vaccines containing substances extracted from infectious agents; i.e., the capsular polysaccharides extracted from pneumococci.

Conditions treated with vaccines include:

- Mumps
- Poliomyelitis
- Rabies
- Rubella
- Smallpox

TOXOIDS are toxins that have been treated to destroy their toxicity but remain capable of inducing the formation of antibodies by injection. They are sometimes called anatoxins.

Conditions treated with toxoids include:

- Diphtheria
- Tetanus

Practice Test 8

Questions

8 - 1

An example of an injection that provides active immunity would be the:

1. black widow spider antivenin.
2. mumps virus vaccine.
3. rattlesnake antivenom.
4. diphtheria antitoxin.

8 - 2

A client with acquired immunodeficiency syndrome (AIDS) has Kaposi's sarcoma. The physician has prescribed interferon alfa-2b (Intron A) 30 million units, 3 times a week. After the initial treatment, the client states that a friend has leftover interferon alfa-2a (Roferon-A) and asks if it can be substituted. The nurse will tell the client that:

1. the two are interchangeable and the client can use it.
2. different brands of interferon may not be equivalent and may require different dosages.
3. one brand cannot be substituted for another due to differences in chemical components.
4. it is not wise to use old drugs since their potency may be questionable.

8 - 3

Of the following allergies, which would constitute a contraindication for receiving the live rubella and mumps vaccines?

1. aspirin
2. penicillin
3. shellfish
4. eggs

8 - 4

You are advising a mother about immunization for her child. The record shows that her child completed the primary tetanus immunizations 3 years ago. You would advise the mother on a booster of tetanus toxoid if the child:

1. sustained long scratches on a bare leg.
2. had an abscessed tooth.
3. walked in the woods and sustained a cut from a piece of glass.
4. was hospitalized with gastroenteritis.

8 - 5

Your client has had a kidney transplant and is back in the hospital for a different procedure. Which medication will you administer daily in order to maintain a constant blood level and prevent organ rejection?

1. acetaminophen
2. cyclosporine
3. ceftazidime
4. loracarbef

8 - 6

After having received an intradermal injection of a specific antigen, your client develops a large wheal around the injection site. This indicates:

1. poor injection technique.
2. immunity to that antigen.
3. sensitivity to that antigen.
4. impending anaphylaxis.

8 - 7

A client is to begin immunotherapy for allergies. Which is the most accurate description of this process?

1. "You will receive a booster and then your allergy will be under control."
2. "You need a series of injections, which you can get any time it's convenient over the next month."
3. "A series of injections will be given on a regular schedule."
4. "These injections are effective for all known allergies."

8 - 8

A gravida I, 30 weeks gestation, is Rh-negative. Her husband is Rh-positive. As you speak to the client about RhoGam, she expresses concern for the baby she is now carrying. Your reply is based on your knowledge that:

1. RhoGam will kill any antibodies formed.
2. this baby will be Rh-negative.
3. the baby can be treated with blood transfusions at birth.
4. antibodies are not produced until exposure to the antigen.

8 - 9

Immunization against diseases such as diphtheria, tetanus, and pertussis is administered when an infant is approximately 2 months of age. The rationale for waiting until the infant is approximately 2 months of age is that by then, the:

1. vitamin K factor will have stabilized.
2. immune system can respond.
3. digestive system will be more developed.
4. nervous system will be more developed.

8 - 1 0

A client with lung cancer has been receiving chemotherapy. The colony-stimulating factor filgrastim (Neupogen) is to be administered. This drug will:

1. stimulate the appetite.
2. prevent hair loss.
3. combat nausea associated with chemotherapy.
4. increase the white blood cell count.

8 - 1 1

Your client is ready for a kidney transplant and will receive azathioprine ((Imuran) 5 mg/kg po daily. You know the purpose of this drug is to:

1. reduce the potential for postoperative infection.
2. maintain normal body temperature.
3. suppress the client's immune system.
4. increase perfusion to the transplanted kidney.

8 - 1 2

Your client is receiving an initial dosage of the immunosuppressant tacrolimus (Prograf). To prevent the potential for toxic blood levels of this medication, you will teach the client to avoid taking the drug with:

1. orange juice.
2. grapefruit juice.
3. tomato juice.
4. apple juice.

8 - 1 3

To prepare an IV administration of the immunosuppressant basiliximab (Simulect), you will:

1. reconstitute the powder with 10 cc of sterile water.
2. dilute the reconstituted solution in 50 ml of normal saline.
3. shake the IV bag to mix the solution thoroughly.
4. allow the solution to sit at room temperature for 10 to 15 minutes before administering.

8 - 1 4

Your client will be traveling to an area where cholera is endemic. To protect the client, you encourage:

1. the cholera vaccine.
2. gamma globulin injections.
3. the use of water purification tablets.
4. boiling all water vigorously for 15 minutes before drinking.

8 - 1 5

A client comes to an emergency clinic after having been bitten by a dog suspected of having rabies. After thoroughly cleansing the wound with soap and water, you anticipate the administration of:

1. rabies vaccine, adsorbed.
2. rabies vaccine (HDCV) (Imovax Rabies).
3. rabies immune globulin, human (Imogam Rabies).
4. tetanus toxoid immune booster.

Practice Test 8

Answers, Rationales, and Explanations

8 - 1

② The mumps virus vaccine provides active immunity. The mumps vaccine contains attenuated mumps virus, which, when introduced into the body, stimulates antibody production. This immune process is referred to as "active" because antibody production is stimulated.

1 and 3. Antivenins contain antitoxins specific for the animal or insect; e.g., black widow spider antivenin/rattlesnake antivenom. These antivenins and antivenoms act as an antidote but they do not provide immunity from exposure.

4. The diphtheria antitoxin binds with circulating toxins and prevents the spread of the disease. An antitoxin does not facilitate the creation of antibodies.

Pregnancy Category: C

Client Need: Health Promotion/Maintenance

8 - 2

② Different brands of interferon may not be equivalent and may require different dosages. Interferon alfa-2b (Intron A) is an antineoplastic prescribed to treat clients with acquired immunodeficiency syndrome (AIDS).

1. Different brands of interferon cannot be interchanged due to equivalency and dosage differences.

3. The difference is in the equivalency and dosages of various brands of interferon alfa-2b, not in the chemical composition.

4. There is no indication that the drug is old and has questionable potency.

Pregnancy Category: C

Client Need: Health Promotion/Maintenance

8 - 3

④ An allergy to eggs would constitute a contraindication to receiving the live rubella and mumps vaccines. Live rubella and mumps vaccines contain infective dosages of virus, many of which are grown in chicken embryos, or eggs. Egg allergy would therefore be a relative contraindication, or at least a caution, to receiving these vaccines.

1, 2, and 3. There is no evidence that allergy to aspirin, penicillin, or shellfish will precipitate an allergic reaction to the rubella and mumps vaccines.

Pregnancy Category: C

Client Need: Safe, Effective Care Environment

8 - 4

③ **You would recommend a booster of tetanus toxoid if a child sustained a cut from a piece of glass while walking in the woods. The woods are an environment where tetanus spores are more prevalent; especially a rural area near herbivorous animals, soil, garden mold, and manure. Tetanus (lockjaw) is characterized by convulsive contractions of all voluntary muscles and affects both peripheral and cranial nerves. Pain is relieved by Demerol or codeine. Antibiotics are given for secondary infection.**

1. Sustaining scratches does not indicate an exposure to the tetanus bacillus. A booster of tetanus toxoid is not indicated.

2. Having an abscessed tooth does not expose an individual to the tetanus bacillus.

4. Experiencing gastroenteritis does not expose an individual to the tetanus bacillus.

Pregnancy Category: C

Client Need: Health Promotion/Maintenance

8 - 5

② **Cyclosporine will be administered to prevent organ rejection. Cyclosporine is an immunosuppressant drug that is generally taken daily, on schedule, to treat or prevent organ rejection. Its impact on T lymphocytes makes it a crucial medication for those at risk for organ rejection.**

1. Acetaminophen is an analgesic and antipyretic. It does not treat or prevent organ rejection.

3 and 4. Ceftazidime (Tazidime) and loracarbef (Lorabid) are cephalosporins and are not useful in preventing organ rejection.

Pregnancy Category: C

Client Need: Health Promotion/Maintenance

8 - 6

③ **A large wheal around the injection site of a specific antigen indicates a sensitivity to that antigen. Intradermal antigen injections are useful in identifying allergies because a positive reaction, or wheal, usually is a result of a localized antigen-antibody response.**

1. The injected antigen to which the client is sensitive is expected to form a wheal or some localized reaction and is therefore not indicative of poor injection technique.

2. The development of a large wheal would indicate sensitivity to the antigen injected, not immunity.

4. Anaphylaxis, although always a risk for any person with severe allergy, is very rare with intradermal tests.

Pregnancy Category: Varies with specific antigen

Client Need: Physiological Integrity

8 - 7

③ **Immunotherapy for allergies is given in a series of injections on a regular schedule. The process of boosting the immune system depends on a gradual introduction of the offending antigen into the body's system. Increasing the quantity of the offending antigen on a regular schedule will be continued until maintenance levels are reached.**

1. The first booster is just one injection in a series of injections that will follow before a maintenance level will be determined.

2. Injections must be administered at specific times in order to determine the most effective maintenance dose, not just when it is convenient for the client.

4. There is no single injection that is effective for all allergies. It is necessary only to establish a maintenance level to the specific allergies of any given person, not to all known allergies.

Pregnancy Category: Varies with specific injections
Client Need: Health Promotion/Maintenance

8 - 8

④ **Antibodies are not produced by the mother until she is exposed to antigens (the Rh-positive blood of a fetus). A potentially life-threatening condition for an Rh-positive fetus arises when an Rh-negative mother carries an Rh-positive fetus. Following the delivery of the first Rh-positive baby, when the placenta detaches, some of the baby's Rh blood cells (which are antigens to the Rh-negative mother) may escape into the mother's bloodstream. Exposure to the Rh-positive antigens causes the mother to produce antibodies against Rh-positive blood. Those antibodies cross the placenta barrier during subsequent pregnancies and destroy blood cells of any Rh-positive fetus she may carry. To prevent the production of these antibodies, Rh-negative mothers are given RhoGam within 72 hours of every delivery of an Rh-positive baby.**

1. RhoGam does not kill antibodies. It prevents the formation of antibodies. Therefore, RhoGam must be given within the first 72 hours following the delivery, abortion, or miscarriage of an Rh-positive fetus by an Rh-negative mother.

2. When an Rh-negative woman and an Rh-positive man conceive an embryo, that embryo is most probably going to be Rh-positive.

3. The first baby is not usually affected, since the mother has not been sensitized by any antigens from a previous Rh-positive fetus.

Pregnancy Category: C
Client Need: Psychosocial Integrity

8 - 9

② **Immunizations are not begun until an infant is approximately 2 months of age and the immune system is mature enough to respond. Before 2 months of age, the infant is protected by natural passive immunity (the transfer of a mother's antibodies to her fetus in utero).**

1. Vitamin K factor is associated with prothrombin formation and blood clotting and has no impact on immunizations.
3. The digestive system is not associated with immunizations.
4. The nervous system is not associated with immunizations.

Pregnancy Category: C
Client Need: Health Promotion/Maintenance

8 - 1 0

④ **Filgrastim (Neupogen) will stimulate the increase of white blood cell formation and decrease the incidence of infection. Neupogen is a genetically engineered colony-stimulating factor that stimulates the proliferation and maturation of blood cells. Neupogen is especially useful for clients whose chemotherapy increases their risk of developing neutropenia (an abnormally small number of neutrophils).**

1. Filgrastim does not stimulate the appetite.
2. Filgrastim does not prevent hair loss.
3. Filgrastim does not combat nausea associated with chemotherapy.

Pregnancy Category: C
Client Need: Physiological Integrity

8 - 1 1

③ **The purpose of the drug azathioprine (Imuran) is to suppress the client's immune system. The major postoperative complication following a kidney transplantation is graft rejection. A graft rejection is an immunologic attack against the transplanted organ. Antirejection therapy includes drugs such as azathioprine that suppress the immune system and block the body's normal immune response.**

1. Azathioprine is an immunosuppressant, not an anti-infective. Immunosuppressants may actually mask infection following surgery.
2. Azathioprine is an immunosuppressant, not an antipyretic (an agent that reduces fever).
4. Azathioprine does not increase perfusion to the kidneys.

Pregnancy Category: D
Client Need: Health Promotion/Maintenance

8 - 1 2

② **You will teach the client to avoid taking tacrolimus (Prograf) with grapefruit juice. Blood drug levels will be increased if grapefruit juice is taken concomitantly.**

1, 3, and 4. Orange, tomato, or apple juice will not increase the drug blood level of tacrolimus (Prograf). Since any food inhibits the absorption of tacrolimus (Prograf), it is recommended that it be taken on an empty stomach.

Pregnancy Category: C
Client Need: Health Promotion/Maintenance

8 - 1 3

② **The reconstituted solution of basiliximab should have been diluted in 50 ml of normal saline or dextrose 5% for infusion. No other drugs should be added or infused simultaneously through the same IV line.**

1. Basiliximab powder should be reconstituted in 50 cc of sterile water, not 10 cc.

3. When mixing the basiliximab solution, the bag should be carefully inverted to prevent the formation of foam and air bubbles. The solution should not be shaken.

4. The reconstituted solution of basiliximab should be infused immediately.

Pregnancy Category: B
Client Need: Safe, Effective Care Environment

8 - 1 4

① **You will encourage clients traveling in areas where cholera is endemic to receive the cholera vaccine. The cholera vaccine is given to adults, and children over 10 years of age, in 2 injections 1 week to 1 month apart. The vaccine contains killed Vibrio cholerae.**

2. Gamma globulin provides a generalized passive immunity by increasing a person's antibody titer. Gamma globulin does not protect against the specific organism that causes cholera (Vibrio cholerae).

3. Water purification tablets are not the most convenient or reliable form of protection against cholera. Water treated with tablets must stand for 30 to 60 minutes before the water can be drunk.

4. If there is a reason to believe that drinking water is contaminated, it should be boiled vigorously for a minimum of 30 minutes.

Pregnancy Category: C
Client Need: Health Promotion/Maintenance

8 - 1 5

③ **You will anticipate administering the rabies immune globulin, human (Imogam Rabies) to anyone bitten by an animal suspected of having rabies. This injection will provide passive immunity to rabies. The rabies immune globulin, human (Imogam Rabies) should not be confused with rabies vaccines, which are killed microorganisms that produce active immunity.**

1 and 2. Rabies vaccine adsorbed and rabies vaccine (HDCV) (Imovax Rabies) are both administered as a pre-exposure prophylaxis rabies immunization for people in high-risk groups, such as veterinarians. They produce active immunity.

Practice Test 9

Autonomic Nervous System Agents

OVERVIEW

The autonomic nervous system is composed of the sympathetic and parasympathetic nervous systems. Autonomic nervous system agents are administered to treat, prevent, and inhibit conditions associated with these two systems.

Autonomic nervous system agents include:

- Adrenergics (sympathomimetics)
- Adrenergic blockers (sympatholytics)
- Anticholinergics (parasympatholytics)
- Cholinergics (parasympathomimetics)
- Neuromuscular blockers
- Skeletal muscle relaxants

ADRENERGICS (SYMPATHOMIMETICS)

Adrenergics (sympathomimetics) are nerve fibers that, when stimulated, release epinephrine at their endings. Adrenergics generally produce one or more of the following reactions:

- Wakefulness, rapid reaction to stimuli, quickened reflexes
- Constriction of blood vessels, decrease in gastric motility
- Increase in heart rate
- Increased use of glucose along with release of fatty acids from the adipose tissues

Conditions treated with adrenergics include:

- Cardiac decompensation (adrenergics increase cardiac output)
- Shock (adrenergics restore blood pressure in acute hypotensive states)
- Adrenergics are also administered to increase blood perfusion to vital organs; i.e., kidneys.

ADRENERGIC BLOCKERS (SYMPATHOLYTICS)

Adrenergic blockers oppose or inhibit adrenergic nerve function. They can cause antagonistic effects of serotonin $5HT_2$ receptors and inhibit reuptake of norepinephrine.

Conditions treated with adrenergic blockers include:

- Vascular headaches, to prevent or abort
- Migraine headaches, to prevent or abort

ANTICHOLINERGICS (PARASYMPATHOLYTICS)

Anticholinergics (parasympatholytics) mimic the action of the sympathetic nervous system. The sympathetic nervous system coordinates actions that are used to cope with stress. Some effects of sympathetic stimulation include thick, odoriferous secretions, increased heart rate, dilated bronchi, and increased mental activity.

Conditions treated with anticholinergics (parasympatholytics) include:

- Peptic ulcers, as adjunct therapy
- Allergic rhinitis
- Renal colic
- Spastic states

CHOLINERGICS (PARASYMPATHOMIMETICS)

Cholinergics mimic the activity of the parasympathetic nervous system. The parasympathetic nerves are involuntary autonomic nerves that help regulate body functions. The parasympathetic nervous system is associated with conservation and restoration of energy stores. Some effects of parasympathetic stimulation include constriction of pupils, contraction of smooth muscle in the alimentary canal, constriction of bronchioles, slowing of the heart rate, and increased secretion by all the glands (except the sweat glands).

Conditions treated with cholinergics (parasympathomimetics) include:

- Acute painful musculoskeletal conditions
- Cholinergics are also administered as an antidote for nondepolarizing neuromuscular blockers.
- Acute postoperative/postpartum nonobstructive (functional) urine retention
- Myasthenia gravis

NEUROMUSCULAR BLOCKERS

Neuromuscular blockers provide skeletal muscle relaxation by antagonizing (interrupting) the effects of acetylcholine, which in turn blocks neuromuscular transmission.

Neuromuscular blockers include:

- Mivacurium chloride (Mivacron)
- Pancuronium bromide (Pavulon)
- Succinylcholine chloride (Anectine)

Neuromuscular blockers are administered to:

- Facilitate endotracheal intubation
- Facilitate mechanical ventilation
- Provide muscle relaxation during surgery

SKELETAL MUSCLE RELAXANTS

Skeletal muscle relaxants are administered to relieve acute muscle pain. Although the action of skeletal muscle relaxants is not fully understood, they are thought to relieve pain by their sedative effects and their ability to reduce transmission of nerve impulses from the spinal cord to the skeletal muscles.

Skeletal muscle relaxants include:

- Diazepam (Valium)
- Cyclobenzaprine (Flexeril)
- Methocarbamol (Robaxin)

Conditions treated with skeletal muscle relaxants include:

- Muscle spasms
- Acute painful musculoskeletal conditions

Practice Test 9

Questions

9 - 1

A client scheduled for surgery is given atropine sulfate 0.5 mg parenterally preoperatively. What indications of the drug's effectiveness might the nurse expect?

1. increased heart rate and dryness of mouth
2. bradycardia and pupillary constriction
3. increased bowel sounds and increased salivation
4. decreased respirations and decreased heart rate

9 - 2

Your client is exhibiting signs of acute renal failure. Which of the following infusions will increase renal perfusion?

1. lidocaine at 2 mg per minute
2. nitroglycerin at 5 mcg per minute
3. dopamine at 35 mcg/kg of body weight per minute
4. dopamine at 2 mcg/kg of body weight per minute

9 - 3

Your client is receiving Thorazine 50 mg tablets by mouth, 4 times a day. The client frequently complains of dry mouth. You will anticipate a prescription for:

1. Urecholine.
2. Cogentin.
3. Emcyt.
4. Artane.

9 - 4

A client with severe epistaxis may be treated with gauze pads soaked in:

1. desoximetasone (Topicort).
2. benzoyl peroxide (Benoxyl).
3. phenylephrine (Neo-Synephrine).
4. nystatin (Mycostatin).

9 - 5

Which of the following medications is most appropriate in the treatment of muscle spasms?

1. acetaminophen (Tylenol)
2. promethazine (Phenergan)
3. cefprozil (Cefzil)
4. cyclobenzaprine (Flexeril)

9 - 6

A well-meaning family member gave your client a sulfa antibiotic tablet. Three hours later the client arrives at the Emergency Department with a blood pressure of 60/38 mmHg. For which medication do you anticipate a prescription?

1. nitroglycerin gr 1/150 sublingual
2. dopamine infusion
3. ranitidine (Zantac)
4. gentamicin (Garamycin)

9 - 7

A client with multiple sclerosis reports increased spasticity of the affected extremities. Baclofen (Lioresal) has been prescribed to reduce spasticity. The nurse explains to the client that side effects of baclofen include:

1. fluid retention.
2. insomnia.
3. hypertension.
4. drowsiness.

9 - 8

What is a major concern for the nurse caring for an intubated trauma client receiving succinylcholine (Anectine)?

1. assessing dry mouth and giving good mouth care
2. monitoring the respiratory rate carefully
3. assessing the effectiveness of the drug by pinching the client's skin.
4. providing adequate analgesia and psychological support

9 - 9

Postoperatively, a client developed a paralytic ileus. Which of the following drugs would the nurse administer to treat this condition?

1. anticholinergics
2. cholinergics
3. beta-adrenergic blocking agents
4. adrenergics

9 - 10

A client is experiencing severe lower back muscle pain. Which medication may be prescribed?

1. torsemide (Demadex)
2. fludarabine phosphate (Fludara)
3. diltiazem (Cardizem)
4. cyclobenzaprine (Flexeril)

Practice Test 9

Answers, Rationales, and Explanations

9 - 1

(1) The nurse can expect increased heart rate, dryness of mouth, and also pupil dilation when atropine sulfate is given. Atropine is an antimuscarinic drug (parasympatholytic/anticholinergic). Increased heart rate, dryness of mouth, and pupillary dilation are among antimuscarinic effects.

2. Bradycardia and pupil constriction are among the effects of muscarinics (parasympathomimetics) and are therefore not associated with the effects of atropine.

3. Increased bowel sounds and increased salivation are among the effects of muscarinics (parasympathomimetics) and are therefore not associated with the effects of atropine.

4. Decreased respirations and decreased heart rate are among the effects of muscarinics (parasympathomimetics) and are not associated with the effects of atropine.

Pregnancy Category: C

Client Need: Physiological Integrity

9 - 2

(4) Dopamine can increase renal perfusion. Dopamine (Dopastat, Intropin) is a sympathomimetic medication that is dosage dependent. At low dosages (less than 10 micrograms per kilogram of body weight per minute), it predominantly affects beta-receptors, producing a positive inotropic effect (influencing the force of muscular contractility) and renal dilation, which in turn increases renal perfusion.

1. Lidocaine is an antiarrhythmic and does not affect renal perfusion.

2. Nitroglycerin is an antianginal and does not affect renal perfusion.

3. Dopamine at 35 micrograms per kilogram of body weight per minute is an extremely high dosage and would cause vasoconstriction and perhaps decreased renal perfusion.

Pregnancy Category: C

Client Need: Health Promotion/Maintenance

9 - 3

(1) Urecholine is a cholinergic that may be prescribed to decrease dry mouth associated with the administration of major tranquilizers such as Thorazine.

2. Cogentin is an antiparkinson medication that prevents or reduces extrapyramidal side effects seen with the administration of major tranquilizers. Dry mouth is a side effect of Cogentin.

3. Emcyt is an antineoplastic agent prescribed as a palliative treatment for advanced metastatic prostate cancer. It does not affect salivation.

4. Artane is an antiparkinson medication prescribed to prevent or reduce extrapyramidal side effects seen with the administration of major tranquilizers. Dry mouth is a side effect of Artane.

Pregnancy Category: C

Client Need: Physiological Integrity

9 - 4

③ **Phenylephrine (Neo-Synephrine) -soaked gauze pads can help treat epistaxis (nosebleeds). Phenylephrine (Neo-Synephrine) is a sympathomimetic drug that stimulates the sympathetic nervous system. Applied locally, its sympathetic effect tends to constrict local blood vessels, thereby decreasing bleeding.**

1. Desoximetasone (Topicort) is a steroid and has no impact on bleeding.

2. Benzoyl peroxide (Benoxyl) is an antiacne medicine and has no impact on bleeding.

4. Nystatin (Mycostatin) is an antifungal and has no impact on bleeding.

Pregnancy Category: C

Client Need: Health Promotion/Maintenance

9 - 5

④ **Cyclobenzaprine (Flexeril) is prescribed for the treatment of muscle spasms. Flexeril is a skeletal muscle relaxant that affects neuronal activity. Because of this, it is an appropriate choice in the treatment of muscle spasms.**

1. Acetaminophen (Tylenol) is an antipyretic analgesic and has no impact on muscle spasms.

2. Promethazine (Phenergan) is an antiemetic and has no impact on muscle spasms.

3. Cefprozil (Cefzil) is a cephalosporin antibiotic and has no impact on muscle spasms.

Pregnancy Category: B

Client Need: Physiological Integrity

9 - 6

② **A prescription for dopamine is anticipated. Allergic reactions may be manifested by hypotension due to vascular bed changes in an anaphylaxis-type reaction. Dopamine, administered in large doses (10 mcg/kg/min), is a vasopressor that can cause renal vasoconstriction, which increases blood pressure and cardiac output and improves renal flow.**

1. Nitroglycerin is a vasodilator that would further lower blood pressure.

3. Ranitidine (Zantac) is an antiulcer medication and would not affect blood pressure.

4. Gentamicin (Garamycin) is an anti-infective and would not affect blood pressure.

Pregnancy Category: C

Client Need: Physiological Integrity

9 - 7

④ **Side effects of baclofen (Lioresal) include drowsiness. Drowsiness is the most frequently reported side effect of Lioresal. Clients who are taking this drug should be cautioned about operating a moving vehicle. Lioresal reduces spasticity by relaxing skeletal muscles.**

1, 2, and 3. Baclofen (Lioresal) does not cause fluid retention, insomnia, or hypertension.

Pregnancy Category: C

Client Need: Safe, Effective Care Environment

9 - 8

④ **Providing adequate analgesia and psychological support are essential for clients who are intubated. Succinylcholine (Anectine) is a neuromuscular blocking agent (a curare-like drug). Since curare-like drugs produce skeletal relaxation or paralysis but do not alter consciousness or awareness of and perception of pain, it is essential that adequate analgesia and psychological support be given.**

1. Assessing for dry mouth and providing good mouth care would be appropriate for any intubated client. It is more important to assess for increased respiratory secretions and suction.
2. Monitoring the respiratory rate is not a concern since the respiratory rate is set on the respirator.
3. The use of a peripheral nerve stimulator to assess response to medication is less painful than pinching the client's skin.

Pregnancy Category: C
Client Need: Psychosocial Integrity

9 - 9

② **Cholinergic medications such as neostigmine stimulate gastrointestinal motility and may be prescribed for the management of paralytic ileus.**

1. Anticholinergics inhibit the action of acetylcholine and cause a decrease in gastrointestinal motility. These types of medications would be prohibited.
3. Beta-adrenergic blocking agents act similarly to the cholinergics but are slower.
4. Adrenergics reduce peristalsis and would be contraindicated in the management of a paralytic ileus.

Pregnancy Category: C
Client Need: Psychosocial Integrity

9 - 1 0

④ **Cyclobenzaprine (Flexeril) may be prescribed for lower back pain. Cyclobenzaprine (Flexeril) is a skeletal muscle relaxant whose action is not clearly understood, but it does relieve muscle spasms.**

1. Torsemide (Demadex) is a loop diuretic and has no impact on muscle pain.
2. Fludarabine phosphate (Fludara) is an antimetabolite and has no impact on muscle pain.
3. Diltiazem (Cardizem) is an antianginal antiarrhythmic and has no impact on skeletal muscle pain.

Pregnancy Category: B
Client Need: Physiological Integrity

Practice Test 10

Central Nervous System Agents

OVERVIEW

Central nervous system agents affect the functioning of nervous tissue. Many of these agents penetrate the blood-brain barrier and exert their effects directly on the brain and spinal cord.

Central nervous system agents include:

- Antianxiety agents
- Anticonvulsives
- Antidepressants
- Antiparkinsonians
- Antipsychotics
- Central nervous system stimulants
- Narcotics and opioid analgesics
- Nonnarcotic analgesics and antipyretics
- Nonsteroidal anti-inflammatory substances
- Sedative hypnotics

ANTIANXIETY AGENTS

Antianxiety agents are used in the short-term treatment of anxiety. Long-term use of antianxiety agents is not recommended because of the potential for drug dependency associated with serious withdrawal symptoms. Some antianxiety drugs are controlled substances.

Antianxiety agents include:

- Alprazolam (Xanax)
- Diazepam (Valium)
- Midazolam hydrochloride (Versed)

Conditions treated with antianxiety agents include:

- Acute alcohol withdrawal
- Seizure disorders, as adjunct therapy
- Mild to moderate anxiety
- Panic attacks
- Antianxiety agents may also be administered before endoscopic procedures to reduce client anxiety.

ANTICONVULSIVES

Anticonvulsives manage convulsions and seizures. Most anticonvulsives are administered in the treatment of specific types of seizure, such as generalized tonic-clonic seizures, partial seizures, and status epilepticus.

Anticonvulsives include:

- Phenobarbital (Solfoton)
- Phenobarbital sodium (sodium luminal)
- Phenytoin (Dilantin)

Conditions treated with anticonvulsives include:

- Epilepsy
- Febrile seizures
- Generalized tonic-clonic seizures
- Seizures associated with preeclampsia or eclampsia

ANTIDEPRESSANTS

Antidepressants are psychotherapeutic substances used in the management of various types of depression as well as in depression associated with anxiety. Antidepressants fall into two major divisions:

(1) monoamine oxidase inhibitors (MAOIs) (2) tricyclic antidepressants

MONOAMINE OXIDASE INHIBITORS (MAOIs) include:

- Fluoxetine (Prozac)
- Phenelzine sulfate (Nardil)

TRICYCLIC ANTIDEPRESSANTS include:

- Amitriptyline (Elavil)
- Clomipramine hydrochloride (Anafranil)
- Doxepin (Sinequan)

Conditions treated with antidepressants include:

- Depression
- Obsessive-compulsive disorders

ANTIPARKINSONIANS

Antiparkinsonians treat the symptoms of parkinsonism (paralysis agitans); i.e., tremors, muscle rigidity and weakness, masklike face, difficulty chewing and swallowing, and a shuffling gait. Antiparkinsonians also treat many of the symptoms of extrapyramidal disorders.

Antiparkinsonians include:

- Carbidopa (Lodosyn)
- Levodopa (Larodopa)

Conditions treated with antiparkinsonians include:

- Drug-induced extrapyramidal disorders; i.e., tremors, chorea, athetosis (irregular twisting of hands), and dystonia
- Parkinsonism

ANTIPSYCHOTICS

Antipsychotics are used in the management of various psychotic conditions. A few antipsychotics have specific uses; for example, lithium carbonate is used to treat manic-depressive psychosis.

Antipsychotics include:

- Haloperidol (Haldol)
- Thioridazine (Mellaril)

Conditions treated with antipsychotics include:

- Behavioral problems associated with chronic organic mental syndrome
- Nonpsychotic behavioral disorders
- Psychotic disorders; i.e., schizophrenia
- Motor and phonic tics in clients with Tourette syndrome

CENTRAL NERVOUS SYSTEM STIMULANTS

Central nervous system (CNS) agents temporarily increase the functional activity of the brain and spinal cord along with the nerves and organs that control voluntary and involuntary acts.

CNS stimulants include:

- Amphetamines
- Anorexiants
- Analeptics

AMPHETAMINES stimulate the central nervous system. Prolonged use of amphetamines may cause drug dependency. Amphetamines are administered to treat conditions such as narcolepsy and obesity.

ANALEPTICS stimulate the central nervous system. They are administered most frequently to treat clients who have been poisoned or have depressed the central nervous system with drugs such as barbiturates.

ANOREXIANTS are substances that suppress the appetite by stimulating the central nervous system. These substances are administered primarily to treat obesity as a short-term adjunct.

CNS stimulants include:

- Amphetamine sulfate
- Doxapram hydrochloride (Dopram)
- Dextroamphetamine sulfate (Dexedrine)
- Methylphenidate (Ritalin)

Conditions treated with CNS stimulants include:

- Exogenous obesity (obesity due to overeating), as adjunct therapy
- Attention Deficit Disorder with hyperactivity
- Narcolepsy (uncontrolled bouts of sleep)

CNS stimulants are also administered to stimulate the respiratory system postanesthesia.

NARCOTICS AND OPIOID ANALGESICS

Narcotics are capable of depressing the central nervous system. They relieve pain and produce sleep. Opioid analgesics are narcotics derived from opium (poppy plants). Narcotics and opioid analgesics are controlled substances.

Narcotics and opioid analgesics include:

- Codeine (codeine sulfate)
- Morphine sulfate (Roxanol)
- Meperidine hydrochloride (Demerol)

Conditions treated with narcotics and opioids include:

- Moderate to severe pain

NONNARCOTIC ANALGESICS AND ANTIPYRETICS

Nonnarcotic analgesics relieve pain. Unlike narcotic analgesics, they do not cause physical dependency. There are two groups of nonnarcotic analgesics:

(1) salicylates (various forms of a white crystalline acid derived from phenol), including aspirin and substances related to aspirin

(2) nonsalicylates, including ibuprofen and indomethacin

Nonnarcotic analgesics and antipyretics include:

- Acetaminophen (Tylenol)
- Aspirin (ASA)

Conditions treated with nonnarcotic analgesics and antipyretics include:

- Elevated body temperature
- Rheumatoid arthritis
- Mild to moderate pain
- Rheumatic fever

NONSTEROIDAL ANTI-INFLAMMATORY SUBSTANCES

The nonsteroidal anti-inflammatory substances (NSAIDs) are prostaglandin inhibitors. They have, to varying degrees, analgesic, antipyretic, and anti-inflammatory effects. Nonsteroidal anti-inflammatory substances are most effectively used to relieve pain and inflammation.

Nonsteroidal anti-inflammatory substances include:

- Ibuprofen (Motrin)
- Tolmetin sodium (Tolectin)
- Indomethacin (Indocin)

Conditions treated with nonsteroidal anti-inflammatory substances include:

- Acute painful shoulder
- Rheumatoid and osteoarthritis
- Primary dysmenorrhea

SEDATIVE HYPNOTICS

Sedatives produce a soothing, tranquilizing effect. Some are controlled substances. Sedative hypnotics fall into three divisions: general, nervous, and vascular.

Sedative hypnotics include:

- Chloral hydrate (Noctec)
- Secobarbital sodium (Seconal)
- Pentobarbital (Nembutal)

Conditions treated with sedative hypnotics include:

- Insomnia
- Sedative hypnotics are also administered for preoperative sedation and sedation in general.

Practice Test 10

Questions

1 0 - 1

A client is experiencing acute tendinitis and is to receive naproxen sodium. Which of the following instructions would be the most appropriate to give this client?

1. "Make sure you take this medicine on an empty stomach."
2. "This medication is a narcotic and may cause drowsiness."
3. "Take ibuprofen if you continue to experience discomfort."
4. "Eat a meal prior to taking this medication."

1 0 - 2

Which of the following medications would be used in the treatment of mood disorders?

1. fluoxetine (Prozac)
2. ranitidine (Zantac)
3. atenolol (Tenormin)
4. digoxin (Lanoxin)

1 0 - 3

A client has ingested too many "diet pills" containing amphetamines. You will monitor the client for:

1. hypotension.
2. sedation.
3. tachyarrhythmias.
4. euphoria.

1 0 - 4

Which of the following analgesics would the nurse anticipate administering to a client experiencing renal calculi?

1. acetaminophen (Tylenol) 325 mg po
2. meperidine (Demerol) 50 mg IM
3. naproxen (Naprosyn) 500 mg po
4. promethazine (Phenergan) 25 mg IM

1 0 - 5

Which analgesic should be questioned on the plan of care for a school-age child with sickle-cell disease having a vaso-occlusive crisis?

1. acetaminophen (Tylenol) with codeine
2. propoxyphene, aspirin, caffeine (Darvon compound 65)
3. oxycodone and acetaminophen (Tylox)
4. morphine (Astramorph)

1 0 - 6

You are administering Elavil 25 mg tablets qid to a client experiencing depression. You will teach the client that the therapeutic benefits of Elavil will be expected within:

1. 1 week.
2. 7 to 10 days.
3. 2 to 4 weeks.
4. 5 to 6 weeks.

1 0 - 7

Which of the following medications would be used in the treatment of tonic-clonic seizures?

1. captopril (Capoten)
2. ranitidine (Zantac)
3. digoxin (Lanoxin)
4. divalproex sodium (Depakote)

1 0 - 8

Fentanyl (Duragesic) 25-microgram transdermal patches are to be applied daily for a client experiencing chronic pain. You will:

1. expect full analgesia within 1 hour.
2. question the dosage of the drug.
3. anticipate hypertensive and tachypneic side effects.
4. apply the patch to the same area consistently.

10 - 9

A client who has been taking Stelazine is brought to the Emergency Department. Assessment reveals: Drooping head, protruding tongue, and involuntary chewing movements. You suspect:

1. akathisia.
2. dyskinesia.
3. waxy flexibility.
4. pseudoparkinsonism.

10 - 10

A client experiencing mania is to begin lithium therapy. Regarding the administration of lithium, you know that:

1. the first lithium level is to be drawn 1 month after the regimen has begun.
2. lithium may only be given intravenously and only in a clinical setting.
3. therapeutic lithium levels are between 2 and 7 mEq/l.
4. 1000 mg per day by mouth is an average dose of lithium.

10 - 11

You will administer the analgesic Demerol to a client in labor. Which nursing intervention will prevent neonatal respiratory depression?

1. Administer Demerol during the latent phase.
2. Administer Demerol during the active phase.
3. Administer Demerol and naloxone in the transition phase.
4. Administer Narcan to the neonate immediately following delivery.

10 - 12

Your client has just received electroconvulsive therapy. Which of the following medications would you anticipate administering post treatment?

1. Anectine
2. Brevital
3. atropine
4. aspirin

1 0 - 1 3

A client has complained of difficulty sleeping since admission to the hospital. Chloral hydrate liquid 7 1/2 gr at bedtime is prescribed. The available chloral hydrate is 10 gr per fluid dram. How many milliliters will the nurse administer?

1. 2 ml
2. 3 ml
3. 4 ml
4. 5 ml

1 0 - 1 4

The nurse is instructing a client with Parkinson's disease about the medication levodopa (L-Dopa). In order to maximize the efficacy of levodopa, the nurse will instruct the client to take the medication:

1. before meals and major activities.
2. before bedtime, to reduce daytime sedation.
3. only when symptoms are bothersome.
4. after meals, to reduce gastrointestinal irritation.

1 0 - 1 5

A parent arrives in the Emergency Department with a toddler, stating, "My child ate a whole bottle of Tylenol." In addition to serum acetaminophen levels, what laboratory work will be requested?

1. thyroid studies
2. serum potassium studies
3. renal studies
4. liver studies

1 0 - 1 6

Your 82-year-old client is experiencing a major depression. The client also has angle-closure glaucoma. You would anticipate a prescription for which one of the following tricyclic antidepressants?

1. amitriptyline (Elavil)
2. perphenazine/amitriptyline (Etrafon)
3. protriptyline (Vivactil)
4. desipramine (Pertofrane)

10-17

Which one of the following medications is associated with the treatment of delirium tremens?

1. Stelazine
2. Antabuse
3. Librium
4. Prolixin

10-18

A client is receiving tranylcypromine sulfate (Parnate) 10 mg tablet by mouth, 3 times a day. Which of the following would be appropriate to include in the diet?

1. tomatoes, pears, and cabbage
2. coffee and chocolate
3. bananas, raisins, and cheddar cheese
4. corned beef and fava beans

10-19

To avoid the side effects of the anticholinergic medication Artane, you will teach clients to:

1. take the medication 30 minutes before meals.
2. consume a high-fiber diet and have adequate fluid intake.
3. void every 2 hours during the day.
4. have a handkerchief available to cope with drooling.

10-20

Your client is scheduled for a dilatation and curettage. The evening before surgery, the physician prescribes secobarbital (Seconal) hour of sleep. In addition to promoting sleep, you understand that this medication is given to:

1. reduce the level of anxiety.
2. lessen bronchial secretions.
3. decrease the muscle tone of the uterus.
4. minimize the need for postoperative analgesia.

Practice Test 10

Answers, Rationales, and Explanations

10 - 1

④ **Clients receiving nonsteroidal anti-inflammatory medications such as naproxen (Naprosyn, Anaprox) should eat a meal prior to taking the medications because of their irritating effects on the stomach.**

1. Nonsteroidal anti-inflammatory medications should not be taken on an empty stomach because of their irritating effects on the gastric mucosa.

2. Naproxen is not a narcotic and does not have any sedative effects.

3. Ibuprofen is in the same drug classification as naproxen and should not be taken simultaneously.

Pregnancy Category: B

Client Need: Physiological Integrity

10 - 2

① **Fluoxetine (Prozac) is used to treat mood disorders. Fluoxetine (Prozac) belongs to a category of drugs called selective serotonin reuptake inhibitors (SSRIs). Because serotonin levels have been found to affect mood, this category of drugs is prescribed to treat mood disorders such as depression.**

2. Ranitidine (Zantac) is an antiulcer agent and does not affect mood.

3. Atenolol (Tenormin) is an antihypertensive agent and does not affect mood.

4. Digoxin (Lanoxin) is a cardiac glycoside (increases the force of cardiac contraction) and does not affect mood.

Pregnancy Category: B

Client Need: Physiological Integrity

10 - 3

③ **Clients taking amphetamines should be monitored carefully for tachyarrhythmias. Amphetamines are central nervous system (CNS) stimulants whose side effects include tachyarrhythmias, nervousness, sleeplessness, and loss of appetite.**

1 and 2. Hypotension and sedation are associated with sedatives and hypnotics, not stimulants like amphetamines.

4. Euphoria may occur. However, it is not a common side effect of amphetamines.

Pregnancy Category: Varies with specific amphetamine

Client Need: Health Promotion/Maintenance

10-4

② **The nurse will anticipate administering meperidine (Demerol) to clients experiencing renal calculi. Meperidine (Demerol) is a narcotic analgesic that may be given IM, IV, or po. Its potent analgesic properties would be appropriate for a client experiencing renal calculi, which are very painful.**

1. The comparatively mild analgesic effects of acetaminophen (Tylenol) would be ineffective for controlling the level of pain associated with renal calculi.

3. The anti-inflammatory and analgesic properties of naproxen (Naprosyn) would be ineffective for controlling the pain associated with renal calculi.

4. Promethazine (Phenergan) is an antiemetic, not an analgesic. It may be prescribed to potentiate an analgesic.

Pregnancy Category: B; D if used for prolonged periods in large doses at term

Client Need: Health Promotion/Maintenance

10-5

② **Aspirin should be questioned if prescribed for children or teenage clients. Aspirin is not usually prescribed for children or teenagers because of its association with Reye's syndrome.**

1. Acetaminophen (Tylenol) with codeine would not be questioned because of the severe pain caused by vaso-occlusive crisis.

3. Oxycodone and acetaminophen would not be questioned because of the severe pain caused by vaso-occlusive crisis.

4. Morphine (Astramorph) could be prescribed because of the severe pain caused by vaso-occlusive crisis.

Pregnancy Category: C; D (in third trimester)

Client Need: Safe, Effective Care Environment

10-6

③ **The therapeutic benefits of amitriptylin hydrochloride (Elavil) should be expected within 2 to 4 weeks of administration. Elavil is a tricyclic antidepressant (TCA) administered to relieve symptoms of depression.**

1. In addition to the therapeutic benefits of Elavil (relief from symptoms of depression), clients may also benefit from the sedative effects of the medication within the first week of medication.

2. It is not usual for the therapeutic benefits of Elavil to be experienced within 7 to 10 days of the drug's administration.

4. The therapeutic benefits should be evident before the fifth to sixth week of its administration.

Pregnancy Category: NR

Client Need: Psychosocial Integrity

1 0 - 7

④ **Divalproex sodium (Depakote) is an anticonvulsant whose impact on neural transmission makes it very effective in the treatment of tonic-clonic seizures (grand mal).**

1. Captopril (Capoten) is an antihypertensive and has no impact on convulsions.
2. Ranitidine (Zantac) is an antiulcer medication and has no impact on convulsions.
3. Digoxin (Lanoxin) is a cardiac glycoside and has no impact on convulsions.

Pregnancy Category: D
Client Need: Physiological Integrity

1 0 - 8

② **You will question the dosage. Fentanyl transdermal (Duragesic) should not be applied daily. Fentanyl transdermal is a narcotic opioid analgesic. The patches are applied every 72 hours. The medication is slowly absorbed into the system and the full analgesic effect is not reached until after 24 hours.**

1. The full analgesic effect of fentanyl transdermal (Duragesic) is not reached until approximately 24 hours after the first application.
3. Like other opioids, fentanyl transdermal (Duragesic) may cause hypotension and respiratory distress, not hypertension and tachypnea.
4. The application site of fentanyl transdermal (Duragesic) should be alternated in order to avoid irritation of the skin.

Pregnancy Category: C
Client Need: Physiological Integrity

1 0 - 9

② **Dyskinesia will be suspected. Dyskinesia is among the side effects of Stelazine administration. Dyskinesia includes the following symptoms: Lack of control over voluntary movements; e.g., protruding tongue, drooping head, chewing motions, stiffness of neck, and dysphagia (inability to swallow or difficulty in swallowing).**

1. Akathisia presents as motor restlessness with an inability to be still. It is a common side effect of neuroleptic (antipsychotic) medications.
3. Clients who maintain certain postures for hours are said to have waxy flexibility. The alteration in behavior is associated with untreated schizophrenia.
4. Pseudoparkinsonism includes masklike facial expressions, tremors, and drooling.

Pregnancy Category: NR
Client Need: Physiological Integrity

10-10

④ **An average dose of lithium is 1000 mg daily. The usual dose is 300 mg, 3 to 4 times daily by mouth.**

1. Lithium levels are generally monitored daily when the regimen is first begun, not 1 month into the regimen.
2. Lithium's route is by mouth and is usually taken by clients at home, not in a clinical setting.
3. Lithium levels between 2 and 7 mEq/L are toxic. Therapeutic lithium levels range from 0.5 to 1.5 mEq/l.

Pregnancy Category: D

Client Need: Psychosocial Integrity

10-11

② **Neonatal respiratory depression can be prevented by administering Demerol during the active phase. There is time for the medication to exit the mother's system before delivery.**

1. Giving the Demerol during the latency phase is too early and may slow labor.
3. It is too late for Demerol and naloxone (Narcan) administration when the client is in the transition phase. During transition, cervical dilation is already 8 to 10 cm.
4. The focus is to prevent respiratory depression of the neonate, not treat it after it occurs. Narcan is a treatment for respiratory depression, not a preventive.

Pregnancy Category: D

Client Need: Safe, Effective Care Environment

10-12

④ **Aspirin (acetylsalicylic acid) is frequently given to relieve headaches following elctro-convulsive therapy.**

1. Succinylcholine (Anectine) is a neuromuscular blocking agent administered immediately prior to electroconvulsive therapy. It produces skeletal paralysis, which reduces the possibility of fractures.
2. Methohexital (Brevital) is a quick-acting anesthetic administered immediately prior to electro-convulsive therapy.
3. Atropine prevents aspiration by decreasing respiratory secretions.

Pregnancy Category: D

Client Need: Physiological Integrity

10-13

② The nurse will administer 3 ml. Chloral hydrate is a sedative/hypnotic prescribed to facilitate sleep and decrease anxiety in the preoperative client.

Formula: 1 fluid dram = 4 cc

10 : 4 :: 7.5 : X

10X = 30

X = 3 ml

1, 3, and 4 are incorrect calculations.

Pregnancy Category: C

Client Need: Safe, Effective Care Environment

10-14

① The nurse will instruct the client to take the medication levodopa (L-Dopa) before meals and major activities. When levodopa (L-Dopa) is taken prior to meals or other activities of the day, the drug tends to facilitate the client's mobility and promotes functional capacity. Levodopa is a precursor of dopamine, a neurotransmitter in the central nervous system.

2. Levodopa does cause drowsiness. However, it is necessary that it be taken at frequent intervals to maintain a therapeutic level, not just before bedtime.

3. Levodopa must be taken on a regular basis in order to be effective, not just when symptoms are bothersome.

4. Levodopa may cause gastrointestinal irritation, which can be minimized by taking small amounts of food prior to administration.

Pregnancy Category: NR

Client Need: Physiological Integrity

10-15

④ Liver studies are usually requested for persons who have ingested large amounts of acetaminophen. Acetaminophen (Tylenol) is a common analgesic and antipyretic. Toxic levels of this over-the-counter (OTC) drug may cause severe liver damage.

1. Tylenol has no impact on the thyroid gland.

2. Tylenol does not affect serum potassium levels.

3. There is no indication that toxic levels of Tylenol cause renal damage.

Pregnancy Category: B

Client Need: Safe, Effective Care Environment

10-16

④ **A prescription for desipramine (Pertofrane) would be anticipated. Pertofrane is an antidepressant with only slight anticholinergic side effects (minimal dilation of pupils and drying of eyes). It would interfere the least in clients with glaucoma.**

1 and 3. Amitriptyline (Elavil) and protriptyline (Vivactil) are tricyclic antidepressants with significant anticholinergic properties (they would act as mydriatics, dilating the pupils and drying the eyes). They should not be administered to clients with glaucoma.

2. Perphenazine/amitriptyline (Etrafon) is an antipsychotic and has no impact on glaucoma.

Pregnancy Category: C

Client Need: Physiological Integrity

10-17

③ **Chlordiazepoxide (Librium) is associated with the treatment of delirium tremens. Librium is a sedative/hypnotic used in the treatment of anxiety as well as for symptoms of alcohol withdrawal, such as delirium tremens.**

1. Stelazine is a major tranquilizer. It is a phenothiazine derivative used in the treatment of psychotic disorders or used short-term for nonpsychotic anxiety. It has no impact on delirium tremens.

2. Antabuse is used as an aversive therapy in the management of impulsive drinking (alcoholism). Antabuse produces a sensitivity to alcohol that causes nausea, vomiting, hypertension, and profuse perspiration. It is not prescribed to treat delirium tremens.

4. Prolixin is a phenothiazine derivative used to manage symptoms of psychotic disorders. Many clients receive this medication intramuscularly on an outpatient basis monthly. It is not prescribed to treat delirium tremens.

Pregnancy Category: NR

Client Need: Physiological Integrity

10-18

① **Tomatoes, pears, and cabbage are appropriate foods to include in the diet of clients receiving monoamine oxidase (MAO) inhibitors, inasmuch as these foods do not contain tyramine. Examples of MAO inhibitors include Parnate, Marplan, and Nardil.**

2. Foods containing caffeine, such as coffee, chocolate, tea, and cola drinks, are discouraged since they stimulate the release of vasopressors norepinephrine and epinephrine.

3 and 4. Bananas, raisins, cheddar cheese, corned beef, and fava beans contain tyramine and are restricted. Clients receiving MAO inhibitors should not consume foods containing tyramine because they may precipitate a hypertensive crisis.

Pregnancy Category: C

Client Need: Safe, Effective Care Environment

10-19

(2) **You will teach clients to consume a high-fiber diet and maintain an adequate fluid intake because constipation can be a problem for clients taking an anticholinergic medication.**

1. Taking Artane 30 minutes before meals will not prevent the nausea associated with this medication. However, taking Artane with meals can help prevent nausea.

3. Urinary hesitancy can be treated by voiding when the urge occurs, which may be before or after 2 hours.

4. Dry mouth, not drooling, is associated with anticholinergic medications such as Artane.

Pregnancy Category: NR
Client Need: Safe, Effective Care Environment

10-20

(1) **Secobarbital (Seconal) reduces the level of anxiety in clients who are scheduled for surgery through its sedative/hypnotic effects.**

2. Medications like atropine (not Seconal) reduce bronchial secretions, suppress salivation and perspiration, and reduce incidence of laryngospasm.

3. Seconal has no impact on the muscle tone of the uterus. Tocolytic medications like ritodrine hydrochloride and terbutaline sulfate are administered to prevent or delay preterm labor. They reduce the intensity and frequency of uterine contractions and lengthen the gestation period.

4. Seconal is not used to minimize the need for postoperative analgesia because it is a short-acting barbiturate. When administered before surgery, it will have very little effect postoperatively.

Pregnancy Category: C
Client Need: Psychosocial Integrity

Practice Test 11

Nutritional Agents

OVERVIEW

Nutritional agents treat, prevent, and inhibit various vitamin and mineral deficiencies. They are also administered as supplements in metabolic disorders.

Nutritional agents include:

- Calories
- Minerals
- Vitamins

CALORIES

A calorie is a unit of heat. In connection with nutrition, calories (Kilocalories) refer to the energy content of food (that is, the fuel or energy value of the food).

Conditions treated with calories include:

- Anorexia
- Marasmic kwashiorkor (severe calorie and protein deficiency)

MINERALS

Minerals are inorganic elements or compounds occurring in nature. Minerals are necessary constituents of all body cells. They form the largest part of the hard portions of the body, such as bone, nails, and teeth. Minerals regulate the permeability of cell membranes and capillaries, the excitability of muscle and nerve tissue, osmotic pressure, equilibrium, acid-base balance, and blood volume. They are also constituents of secretions from glands. Some of the principal minerals include calcium, iodine, phosphorus, potassium, and sodium.

Conditions treated with minerals include:

- Muscle cramps (treated with sodium)
- Muscle weakness, changes in electrocardiogram (treated with potassium)
- Retarded growth, weakness (treated with phosphorus)
- Rickets, tetany, brittle bones (treated with calcium)
- Simple goiter (treated with iodine)

VITAMINS

Vitamins are essential for normal growth and good nutrition. Most vitamins are acquired from outside sources, such as food, because they cannot be manufactured by the body. There are vitamins, however, that can be manufactured by the body; they are vitamins A and K. Vitamins are found in two main groupings: the water-soluble vitamins (vitamin C and the B complex vitamins B_1, B_2, B_3, B_5, B_6, B_{12}) and the fat-soluble vitamins (vitamins A, D, E, K).

Conditions treated with water-soluble vitamins include:

- Anemia (treated with vitamin B_{12})
- Beriberi (treated with vitamin B)
- Scurvy (treated with vitamin C)
- Wounds (treated with vitamin C)

Conditions treated with fat-soluble vitamins include:

- Hypoprothrombinemia (lack of blood-clotting Factor II, treated with vitamin K)
- Night blindness (treated with vitamin A)
- Rickets/osteomalacia (treated with vitamin D)

Practice Test 11

Questions

11-1

Your client is diagnosed with pernicious anemia, as evidenced by low vitamin B_{12} levels. How will the B_{12} be replaced?

1. 1 tablet by mouth daily
2. 1 tablet by mouth weekly
3. 100 µg (mcg) intramuscularly 1 time only
4. 100 µg (mcg) intramuscularly every month

11-2

A newborn has phenylketonuria and will require a special diet to control phenylalanine levels. The parents should avoid giving the newborn foods containing:

1. saccharin.
2. cyclamate.
3. cobalamin concentrate.
4. aspartame.

11-3

A pregnant client is diagnosed with severe preeclampsia. Which medication do you anticipate administering?

1. potassium chloride
2. Kayexalate
3. magnesium sulfate
4. dopamine

11-4

Which of the following vitamins should be monitored for clients taking warfarin (Coumadin)?

1. vitamin A
2. vitamin C
3. vitamin E
4. vitamin K

1 1 - 5

A child is being treated for iron-deficiency anemia. The parents will be taught about the administration of oral iron medication. Teaching has been most effective if the parents state they will:

1. give the medication with a snack of crackers and peanut butter.
2. give the medication diluted in apple juice.
3. give the medication on an empty stomach 3 times a day.
4. temporarily reduce the dosage if the stools become very dark in color.

1 1 - 6

A client has experienced a gunshot wound and is bleeding profusely. Which of the following is most appropriate to administer?

1. oxygen
2. aminophylline
3. digoxin
4. heparin

1 1 - 7

A client is experiencing the effects of folic acid deficiency. For which vitamin do you anticipate a prescription?

1. vitamin C
2. vitamin K
3. vitamin B_3
4. vitamin B_9

1 1 - 8

A 6-year-old client is receiving intravenous dextrose 5% in water via microdrip infusion set. The set delivers 60 drops per milliliter. To infuse at 75 cc per hour, the nurse will adjust the rate of flow to deliver:

1. 12 drops per minute.
2. 18 drops per minute.
3. 60 drops per minute.
4. 75 drops per minute.

1 1 - 9

The vitamin that acts as an antilipemic is:

1. A.
2. B$_3$.
3. C.
4. K.

1 1 - 1 0

Which of the following common over-the-counter (OTC) medications might be taken by a person with osteoporosis?

1. acetaminophen (Tylenol)
2. diphenhydramine (Benadryl)
3. calcium carbonate (Tums)
4. dihydroxyaluminum sodium carbonate (Rolaids)

1 1 - 1 1

A client with anemia presents at the Emergency Department with chest pain. For which medication do you anticipate a prescription?

1. benzonatate (Tessalon)
2. sucralfate (Carafate)
3. oxygen by nasal cannula
4. 4 liters of normal saline intravenously

1 1 - 1 2

A client with osteoporosis is taking a calcium supplement. Which vitamin might be taken concurrently?

1. A
2. B$_3$
3. D
4. K

1 1 - 1 3

A client has pregnancy-induced hypertension (PIH) and is to receive magnesium sulfate. This drug is given for which pharmacologic effect?

1. cathartic
2. antihypertensive
3. antiemetic
4. anticonvulsive

11-14

A client is experiencing essential hypertension. Which dietary intervention would be most helpful in lowering the client's blood pressure?

1. restricting potassium intake
2. increasing calcium intake
3. increasing fluid intake
4. restricting sodium intake

11-15

A client newly diagnosed with congestive heart failure should have which of the following foods removed from the serving tray?

1. fruit salads
2. breads
3. high-protein foods such as meat or peanut butter
4. pickles, ketchup, and mustard

11-16

A client is experiencing manifestations of vitamin A deficiency. Which of the following foods would you plan to include in the diet?

1. carrots
2. onions
3. white potatoes
4. hot peppers

11-17

After a phlebotomy, you will teach the client to avoid foods such as:

1. pork.
2. fruits.
3. liver.
4. milk and milk products.

1 1 - 1 8

Which of the following drugs would be most useful in the prevention of osteoporosis?

1. potassium
2. calcium (Os-Cal)
3. phytonadione (vitamin K_1)
4. ascorbic acid (vitamin C)

1 1 - 1 9

Your client has a zinc deficiency. You expect your assessment to reveal:

1. sparse hair growth; soft, misshapen nails; and dry, scaling skin.
2. abnormal bleeding tendencies.
3. muscle weakness.
4. mouth soreness and gastrointestinal distress.

Practice Test 11

Answers, Rationales, and Explanations

11 - 1

④ 100 μg (mcg) of **B$_{12}$** administered intramuscularly once a month is the anticipated treatment for clients with pernicious anemia. Pernicious anemia occurs as a result of an inability to absorb dietary vitamin **B$_{12}$**, which is due to an intrinsic factor deficit. As a result, vitamin **B$_{12}$** injections must be given for life, not just once.

1 and 2. Vitamin B$_{12}$ by mouth is not absorbed by clients with pernicious anemia due to lack of an intrinsic factor deficit.

3.   Injections of vitamin B$_{12}$ are administered for life, not just once.

Pregnancy Category: C
Client Need: Physiological Integrity

11 - 2

④ **Aspartame is high in phenylalanine and should be avoided. Aspartame is the generic name for the artificial sweeteners Equal and Nutrasweet. Both are composed of two amino acids, phenylalanine and aspartic acid. Individuals with phenylketonuria (PKU) are unable to metabolize the amino acid phenylalanine. High levels of phenylalanine can cause mental retardation if clients are not placed on a low-phenylalanine diet.**

1.   Saccharin (an artificial sweetener) is not contraindicated for clients with phenylketonuria because it does not contain phenylalanine.

2.   Cyclamate (an artificial sweetener) is not contraindicated for clients with phenylketonuria because it does not contain phenylalanine.

3.   Cobalamin concentrate (vitamin B$_{12}$) is a medication that contains 500 mg of cobalamin per gram. It is prescribed for the treatment of vitamin B$_{12}$ deficiency and is not contraindicated for clients with phenylketonuria.

Pregnancy Category: Not Known
Client Need: Safe, Effective Care Environment

11 - 3

③ **Clients with preeclampsia may have the medication magnesium sulfate prescribed. Prevention of seizures in the preeclamptic client is a major concern. Magnesium sulfate's anticonvulsant effect is thought to be due to its impact on acetylcholine release. Because of this, it is used in both treatment and prevention of seizures associated with preeclampsia.**

1.   Potassium chloride is an electrolyte replacer and has no impact on seizure prevention or treatment.

2.   Kayexalate is used in the treatment of hyperkalemia (elevated potassium levels) and has no impact on seizure prevention or treatment.

4.   Dopamine is used in the treatment of hypotension and has no impact on seizure prevention or treatment.

Pregnancy Category: A
Client Need: Health Promotion/Maintenance

1 1 - 4

④ **Persons taking warfarin (Coumadin) must monitor their vitamin K intake to avoid impairing the medication's anticoagulant effect. Vitamin K affects blood coagulation because it stimulates the production of prothrombin, which helps form blood clots.**

1 and 2. There is no indication that vitamins A or C interfere with the administration of the antico-agulant Coumadin.

3. Vitamin E protects red blood cell membranes against hemolysis, but it has no impact on coagulation.

Pregnancy Category: X

Client Need: Safe, Effective Care Environment

1 1 - 5

③ **Oral iron is usually administered 3 times a day, between meals (on an empty stomach). An acid environment enhances absorption, as does ascorbic acid (vitamin C). Citrus juice would be a good fluid with which to swallow the medication.**

1. Iron is best absorbed if given on an empty stomach rather than with a snack.

2. More effective ways to decrease staining of teeth from liquid iron is to administer it via a straw or dropper and to clean the teeth immediately after administration.

4. A therapeutic dosage will often turn the stools a dark greenish color. The dosage should not be decreased if this occurs.

Pregnancy Category: A

Client Need: Physiological Integrity

1 1 - 6

① **It is appropriate to administer supplemental oxygen to persons who are bleeding pro-fusely. Oxygen is transported to the body's tissues by hemoglobin. When blood is lost, the oxygen-carrying capacity diminishes.**

2. Aminophylline is a bronchodilator and has no impact on oxygen saturation.

3. Digoxin is a cardiac glycoside and has no impact on oxygen saturation.

4. Heparin is an anticoagulant, which in fact may worsen bleeding. It has no impact on oxygen saturation.

Pregnancy Category: NR

Client Need: Safe, Effective Care Environment

11-7

④ **A prescription for folic acid (vitamin B₉) would be anticipated for clients with folic acid deficiency. Folic acid is a water-soluble vitamin and one of the B-complex vitamins. A deficiency may cause a type of anemia. Supplements may be given intramuscularly, intravenously, subcutaneously, or by mouth.**

1. Ascorbic acid (vitamin C) deficiency, not folic acid deficiency, causes scurvy, a condition marked by weakness, anemia, spongy gums, and a tendency for mucous membrane hemorrhage.

2. Phytonadione (vitamin K) deficiency, not folic acid deficiency, acts primarily on the clotting of blood.

3. Niacin (vitamin B₃) deficiency, not folic acid deficiency, causes a condition known as pellagra. The skin turns dark and flakes off as if burned by the sun.

Pregnancy Category: A
Client Need: Health Promotion/Maintenance

11-8

④ **The nurse will adjust the rate of flow to deliver 75 drops per minute.**

1, 2, and 3 are incorrect calculations.

Formula:

$$\text{Drops per minute} = \frac{\text{total volume to infuse} \times \text{drop factor}}{\text{total time of infusion in minutes}}$$

$$\text{Drops per minute} = \frac{75 \times 60}{60} = \frac{4500}{60} = 75$$

Pregnancy Category: C
Client Need: Safe, Effective Care Environment

11-9

② **Vitamin B₃ (also known as niacin or nicotinic acid) is an antilipemic. It directly stimulates the metabolism of lipids and depresses the synthesis of other fatty proteins. Meat, poultry, and fish are the source of approximately 50% of the niacin consumed by Americans. Other sources high in niacin include enriched breads and cereals. Green leafy vegetables are also rich sources of niacin.**

1. Vitamin A is a fat-soluble vitamin that promotes good night vision, healthy mucous membranes, and skin, and the growth of body tissues. It is not an antilipemic.

3. Vitamin C is an antioxidant necessary in maintaining the integrity of blood vessels. An inadequate amount of vitamin C causes scurvy. Fruits and vegetables supply rich amounts of vitamin C. Vitamin C is not an antilipemic.

4. Vitamin K acts primarily in the clotting of blood. Significant sources of vitamin K include liver, green leafy vegetables, and milk. Vitamin K is not an antilipemic.

Pregnancy Category: C
Client Need: Health Promotion/Maintenance

11-10

③ **A person with osteoporosis might take calcium carbonate (Tums) as a calcium supplement. Osteoporosis is characterized by reduced bone mass. Bone mass is in part due to maintenance of adequate dietary calcium. A calcium supplement such as Tums might be taken to maintain adequate serum calcium levels.**

1. Acetaminophen (Tylenol) is an analgesic antipyretic and has no impact on osteoporosis.

2. Diphenhydramine (Benadryl) is an antihistamine and has no impact on osteoporosis.

4. Dihydroxyaluminum sodium carbonate (Rolaids) is an antacid and has no impact on osteoporosis.

Pregnancy Category: C

Client Need: Health Promotion/Maintenance

11-11

③ **You would anticipate a prescription for oxygen by nasal cannula. Anemic persons have a decreased oxygen-carrying capacity due to their decreased hemoglobin. As a result, their oxygen content is low. Supplemental oxygen would be indicated if ischemia (insufficient blood supply to the heart) is evidenced as chest pain.**

1. Benzonatate (Tessalon) is an antitussive (prevents or relieves coughing) and has no impact on anemia.

2. Sucralfate (Carafate) is an antiulcer drug and has no impact on anemia.

4. Four liters of normal saline administered intravenously is a very large amount of fluid and is usually indicated for volume depletion, not chest pain.

Pregnancy Category: NR

Client Need: Physiological Integrity

11-12

③ **Vitamin D should be taken concurrently with calcium supplements in the treatment of osteoporosis. Calcium absorption and bone density are dependent on vitamin D because vitamin D promotes calcium absorption.**

1. Vitamin A is a fat-soluble vitamin that is necessary for good night vision, but it has no impact on calcium absorption.

2. Vitamin B_3 is a water-soluble vitamin. A deficiency of this vitamin causes pellagra. Vitamin B_3 has no impact on calcium absorption.

4. Vitamin K is a fat-soluble vitamin needed for clotting of blood. It has no impact on calcium absorption.

Pregnancy Category: C

Client Need: Health Promotion/Maintenance

11-13

④ **Magnesium sulfate will be administered for its anticonvulsive effect. Magnesium sulfate decreases central nervous system (CNS) activity. Even though magnesium sulfate will decrease blood pressure as a side effect, it is given as an anticonvulsant. Apresoline might be prescribed to lower blood pressure when magnesium sulfate is being taken.**

1. Magnesium sulfate is not a cathartic. A cathartic is a laxative, such as milk of magnesia.
2. Magnesium sulfate is not an antihypertensive. An antihypertensive such as Apresoline lowers blood pressure.
3. Magnesium sulfate is not an antiemetic. An antiemetic such as Dramamine is used to prevent or treat nausea.

Pregnancy Category: A
Client Need: Physiological Integrity

11-14

④ **Moderate sodium restriction of less than 2500 mg daily is considered to be an acceptable treatment for clients experiencing essential hypertension. Sodium increases circulating volume by causing the kidneys to reabsorb water. This increase in circulating volume increases blood pressure.**

1. Potassium intake should not be restricted unless a client is experiencing hyperkalemia.
2. Calcium intake does not have a marked effect on blood pressure.
3. Increasing fluid intake may increase circulating fluid volume and increase blood pressure.

Pregnancy Category: Not Known
Client Need: Physiological Integrity

11-15

④ **Persons who experience congestive heart failure are typically put on a moderate-sodium diet, usually no more than 2000 mg/day. Foods that are high in sodium are to be avoided, such as salty snacks, canned soups, processed meats, and condiments (ketchup and mustard).**

1, 2, and 3. Neither fruit salads, breads, nor meats are particularly high in sodium.

Pregnancy Category: Not Known
Client Need: Health Promotion/Maintenance

11-16

① You will teach the client to include carrots in the diet. Other foods high in vitamin A include: Spinach, apricots, sweet potatoes, and cantaloupe. Signs and symptoms of vitamin A deficiency include: Night blindness (which can lead to permanent blindness, or xerophthalmia), hardening of the skin, partial loss of senses such as taste and smell, vulnerability to respiratory infections, and faulty development of bones and teeth.

2, 3, and 4. Onions, white potatoes, and hot peppers are not high in vitamin A.

Pregnancy Category: C

Client Need: Health Promotion/Maintenance

11-17

③ You will teach the client to avoid "blood-building" foods such as legumes, liver, clams, and oysters following a phlebotomy (removing blood from the body through a vein). Foods that provide a high iron intake will counteract the effects of the phlebotomy.

1. Pork is not high in iron and would not be contraindicated.
2. Fruits are not high in iron and would not be contraindicated.
4. Milk and milk products are not high in iron and would not be contraindicated.

Pregnancy Category: C

Client Need: Health Promotion/Maintenance

11-18

② Calcium (Os-Cal) is useful in preventing osteoporosis. Osteoporosis is a skeletal disorder characterized by bone mass reduction. One of the major causes of osteoporosis is inadequate calcium intake. Calcium is needed to form and strengthen bone. Vitamin D promotes the absorption of calcium and phosphorus.

1. Potassium is a mineral and principal cation in intracellular fluid. It aids in regulation of osmotic pressure and acid-base balance. It does not, however, have a direct impact on bone mass.
3. Phytonadione (vitamin K_1) is required for synthesis of blood coagulation Factors II, VII, IX, and X but has no impact on bone mass.
4. Ascorbic acid (vitamin C) is prescribed in the management of scurvy and some gastrointestinal diseases. Vitamin C has no impact on bone mass.

Pregnancy Category: C

Client Need: Health Promotion/Maintenance

11-19

①   **Signs and symptoms of zinc deficiency include: Sparse hair growth; soft, misshapen nails; and dry, scaling skin. Zinc deficiency usually occurs from excessive intake of foods that bind zinc and prevent its absorption.**

2.   A deficiency in vitamin K is associated with abnormal bleeding tendencies.

3.   A deficiency in vitamin E is associated with muscle weakness and intermittent claudication.

3.   A niacin deficiency is associated with mouth soreness and gastrointestinal distress.

Pregnancy Category: C
Client Need: Physiological Integrity

Practice Test 12

Ophthalmic, Otic, and Nasal Agents

OVERVIEW

Ophthalmic, otic, and nasal agents treat, prevent, and inhibit conditions affecting the eyes, ears, and nose.

Ophthalmic, otic, and nasal agents include:

- Miotics
- Mydriatics
- Nasal agents
- Ophthalmic anti-infectives
- Ophthalmic anti-inflammatories
- Ophthalmic vasoconstrictors
- Otics

MIOTICS

Miotics cause the pupil to contract (constrict).

Miotic substances include:

- Carbachol (intraocular) (Miostat)
- Pilocarpine (Piloptic)

Conditions treated with miotics include:

- Primary open-angle glaucoma
- Miotics are also administered to create pupillary miosis (contraction) in ocular surgery.

MYDRIATICS

Mydriatics dilate the pupil. In certain diseases of the eye, the pupil must be dilated during treatment to prevent adhesions of the pupils.

Mydriatics include:

- Atropine sulfate (Atropine-1)
- Cyclopentolate hydrochloride (Mydrilate)
- Epinephrine hydrochloride (Glaucon)

Conditions treated with mydriatics include:

- Cycloplegia (paralysis of ciliary muscles)
- Open-angle glaucoma

NASAL AGENTS

Nasal agents are administered to treat various conditions of the nose.

Nasal agents include:

- Beclomethasone dipropionate (Beconase)
- Fluticasone propionate (Flonase)
- Oxymetazoline hydrochloride (Afrin)
- Phenylephrine hydrochloride (Neo-Synephrine)

Conditions treated with nasal agents include:

- Nasal congestion
- Nosebleed
- Seasonal and perennial allergic rhinitis

OPHTHALMIC ANTI-INFECTIVES

Ophthalmic anti-infectives are administered to treat or prevent infections in the eyes.

Ophthalmic anti-infectives include:

- Bacitracin (AK-Tracin)
- Silver nitrate solution
- Erythromycin ointment

Conditions treated with ophthalmic anti-infectives include:

- Conjunctivitis
- Corneitis
- Corneal ulcers
- Ophthalmia neonatorum, as prophylaxis

OPHTHALMIC ANTI-INFLAMMATORIES

Ophthalmic anti-inflammatories are administered to treat tissue reactions to various types of injury to the eyes caused by surgery, allergy, and foreign objects.

Ophthalmic anti-inflammatories include:

- Dexamethasone (Maxidex)
- Fluorometholone (Flarex)
- Diclofenac sodium (Voltaren Ophthalmic)

Conditions treated with ophthalmic anti-inflammatories include:

- Corneal injury from burns, chemicals, and penetration of foreign objects
- Inflammatory allergic conditions of conjunctiva, cornea, and sclera
- Inflammatory conditions of the eyelids
- Postoperative inflammation following removal of a cataract

OPHTHALMIC VASOCONSTRICTORS

Ophthalmic vasoconstrictors constrict blood vessels and the pupil of the eye.

Ophthalmic vasoconstrictors include:

- Naphazoline hydrochloride (Allerest)
- Tetrahydrozoline hydrochloride (Collyrium)
- Oxymetazoline hydrochloride (Visine)

Conditions treated with ophthalmic vasoconstrictors include:

- Allergies
- Ocular congestion, irritation, itching
- Minor eye irritations

OTICS

Otics are administered to treat various conditions of the ear.

Otics include:

- Boric acid solution (Ear-dry)
- Carbamide peroxide (Murine Ear)

Conditions treated with otics include:

- External ear canal infection
- Impacted cerumen (earwax)

Practice Test 12

Questions

1 2 - 1

Which of the following medications will the nurse administer for the prophylactic eye care of a newborn?

1. saline
2. tetracycline
3. vitamin K
4. silver nitrate

1 2 - 2

A client is receiving 2 drops of ophthalmic anti-infective tobramycin (Tobrex) every 8 hours to treat an infection in the right eye. You will observe the client for:

1. overgrowth of nonsusceptible organisms.
2. ototoxicity.
3. nephrotoxicity.
4. seizures.

1 2 - 3

Which of the following medications would be administered to dilate the pupils prior to an ophthalmoscopic procedure?

1. Prostigmin
2. atropine
3. Antilirium
4. Mestinon

1 2 - 4

A client was prescribed Isopto Atropine 1% ophthalmic solution, 1 drop 3 times a day for acute iritis. Discharge instructions for this client will include the following:

1. "Rest the eyedropper tip lightly on the inner canthus during instillation."
2. "Call the physician immediately for any occurrence of dry mouth."
3. "Avoid hazardous activities until blurring subsides."
4. "Headaches, eye pain, and continued blurring are common and expected side effects."

1 2 - 5

A client will undergo a mastoidectomy due to chronic otitis media. Hydrogen peroxide solution will be used for postauricular care. The primary purpose for this treatment is to:

1. kill bacteria at the postoperative site.
2. soften the tissue at the suture site.
3. cleanse the postoperative site.
4. minimize the potential for infection.

1 2 - 6

A client experiencing rhinitis is to receive beclomethasone dipropionate (Beconase). The drug will be sprayed in each nostril tid. To administer this drug, you will teach the client to:

1. tilt the head slightly backward and insert the nozzle into the nostril.
2. rotate the medication gently between the palms of the hands prior to administration.
3. blow the nose to clear the nasal passages prior to administration.
4. keep both nostrils open while instilling the medication.

1 2 - 7

A client with acquired immunodeficiency syndrome (AIDS) has contracted an opportunistic infection of the eyes (cytomegalovirus/CMV). You anticipate the administration of ganciclovir (Cytovene). You will teach the client that this drug:

1. causes birth defects.
2. may be administered as an intravenous bolus.
3. may be given initially q 12 hours for 7 to 14 days.
4. is unlikely to cause nausea or vomiting.

1 2 - 8

Which of the following drugs should not be administered to clients with asthma?

1. nystatin (Mycostatin) vaginal inserts
2. desoximetasone (Topicort) ointment
3. pilocarpine (Carpine) ophthalmic solution
4. nitroglycerin (Transderm-Nitro) 2 mg/24-hour patch

Practice Test 12

Answers, Rationales, and Explanations

1 2 - 1

② Tetracycline and erythromycin are administered prophylactically to prevent ophthalmia neonatorum. Ophthalmia neonatorum is a general term referring to any conjunctival infection of the newborn. Prophylaxis of gonorrhea and/or chlamydia in the newborn is accomplished by administration of tetracycline (1%) ointment or erythromycin (0.5%) drops immediately after birth.

1. Saline is not an anti-infective or antibiotic and cannot prevent infections due to the gonococcus or chlamydia organisms.

3. Vitamin K is associated with the normal clotting of blood, not with prevention of infection.

4. Silver nitrate has been replaced as the drug of choice to prevent ophthalmia neonatorum because it is not effective against chlamydia.

Pregnancy Category: Tetracycline, NR; erythromycin, B
Client Need: Health Promotion/Maintenance

1 2 - 2

① Clients receiving the ophthalmic anti-infective tobramycin (Tobrex) should be observed for overgrowth of nonsusceptible organisms, including fungi.

2. Ototoxicity is an adverse reaction to the intravenous/intramuscular preparations of tobramycin, not the ophthalmic form.

3. Nephrotoxicity is an adverse reaction to the intravenous/intramuscular preparations of tobramycin, not the ophthalmic form.

4. Seizures are an adverse reaction to the intravenous/intramuscular preparations of tobramycin, not the ophthalmic form.

Pregnancy Category: B
Client Need: Safe, Effective Care Environment

1 2 - 3

② Atropine dilates the pupils. Atropine is an anticholinergic drug whose impact on the adrenergic system causes pupillary dilatation. Its temporary effect makes it one of the drugs of choice prior to ophthalmoscopic procedures.

1, 3, and 4. Neostigmine bromide (Prostigmin), physostigmine salicylate (Antilirium), and pyridostigmine (Mestinon) are all cholinergics (parasympathomimetics) and cause the pupils of the eyes to constrict (are miotics).

Pregnancy Category: C
Client Need: Physiological Integrity

12-4

③ **Clients using atropine ophthalmic solutions will be taught to avoid hazardous activities until blurring subsides. Atropine causes mydriasis (dilatation of the pupil), and blurring can occur. To provide safety, clients should be warned to avoid activities such as operating machinery or driving.**

1. Touching the inner canthus with the tip of the dropper contaminates the dropper and the medication.

2. Dry mouth is an expected effect of atropine and clients should be advised to use candies or gum to relieve this symptom.

4. Headaches and eye pain are symptoms of glaucoma, a complication of atropine administration, and should be reported. If not corrected, permanent blindness may occur.

Pregnancy Category: C
Client Need: Health Promotion/Maintenance

12-5

④ **The purpose of hydrogen peroxide in this situation is to minimize the potential for infection. Hydrogen peroxide can kill bacteria and it is also an excellent cleansing agent that loosens adherent deposits and detritus (degenerative matter).**

1. Hydrogen peroxide can kill bacteria (is a germicidal). However, its use in this situation is associated with its ability to minimize infection by maintaining a clean postoperative site.

2. Hydrogen peroxide is not a lubricant and will not soften the tissue at the suture site.

3. Hydrogen peroxide can keep the postoperative site clean. However, the ultimate purpose for keeping the site clean is to minimize the potential for infection.

Pregnancy Category: Not Known
Client Need: Health Promotion/Maintenance

12-6

③ **The client will be taught to blow the nose and clear the nasal passages to ensure that the medication (beclomethasone dipropionate) can be absorbed properly; otherwise, the medication will not come in contact with the mucous membranes of the nose and be absorbed into the bloodstream.**

1. The client should tilt the head slightly forward to insert the nozzle into the nostril. This technique allows the medication to adhere to the nasal membranes as opposed to having the medication become lost down the throat when the head is tilted backward.

2. The container of beclomethasone dipropionate should be shaken well before use. This technique allows the suspension to be evenly distributed when sprayed.

4. When instilling spray into a nostril, the other nostril should be closed. The client should inspire gently when spraying medication into the nose.

Pregnancy Category: C
Client Need: Physiological Integrity

1 2 - 7

① Ganciclovir (Cytovene) causes birth defects. Female clients taking this drug should be taught to use effective birth control methods during treatment. Male clients should be taught to use barrier contraception during therapy and for a minimum of 90 days following treatment.

2. Ganciclovir (Cytovene) should not be given as an intravenous bolus. It should be administered over a minimum of 1 hour. Infusions that are too rapid may result in increased toxicity. An infusion pump should be used.

3. The client receiving ganciclovir (Cytovene) normally receives 5 mg/kg intravenously every 12 hours for 14 to 21 days initially.

4. Nausea, vomiting, diarrhea, anorexia, abdominal discomfort, flatulence, and dyspepsia are common adverse reactions to ganciclovir (Cytovene).

Pregnancy Category: C
Client Need: Physiological Integrity

1 2 - 8

③ Pilocarpine (Carpine) ophthalmic solution is contraindicated for clients with asthma. Pilocarpine is a miotic (causes pupils to contract) used in the treatment of glaucoma. It is a cholinergic medication that is systemically absorbed and may cause bronchospasm or bronchoconstriction.

1. Nystatin (Mycostatin) vaginal inserts do not cause bronchospasm or bronchoconstriction and are not contraindicated for clients with asthma. This medication is administered for the treatment of local and intestinal candida infections.

2. Desoximetasone (Topicort) ointment does not cause bronchospasm or bronchoconstriction and is not contraindicated for clients with asthma. This medication is a topical glucocorticoid used to manage a variety of allergic immunologic reactions.

4. Nitroglycerin (Transderm-Nitro) is used in the long-term prophylactic management of angina pectoris. It does not cause bronchospasm or bronchoconstriction.

Pregnancy Category: B
Client Need: Safe, Effective Care Environment

Practice Test 13

Respiratory Tract Agents

OVERVIEW

Respiratory tract agents treat, prevent, and inhibit conditions associated with ventilation, perfusion, and diffusion that interfere with the interchange of gases between clients and the air they breathe.

Respiratory tract agents include:

- Antihistamines
- Antitussives
- Bronchodilators
- Mucolytics and expectorants

ANTIHISTAMINES

Histamine is present in various tissues of the body. Histamine acts on the vascular system by producing dilation of the arterioles and increased permeability of capillaries and venules. Antihistamines are administered to counteract the effects of histamine. Antihistamines block almost all the effects of histamine by competing with it at the histamine receptor sites. Antihistamines constrict vessels.

Antihistamines include:

- Cetirizine hydrochloride (Zyrtec)
- Clemastine fumarate (Tavist)
- Diphenhydramine hydrochloride (Benadryl)

Conditions treated with antihistamines include:

- Chronic idiopathic urticaria
- Motion sickness
- Seasonal allergic rhinitis

ANTITUSSIVES

Antitussives are used to relieve coughing. CENTRALLY ACTING ANTITUSSIVES depress the cough center located in the medulla. PERIPHERALLY ACTING ANTITUSSIVES anesthetize receptors in the respiratory passages.

Centrally acting antitussives include:

- Codeine
- Dextromethorphan

Peripherally acting antitussives include:

- Benzonatate (Tessalon)

Conditions treated with antitussives include:

- Nonproductive cough
- Coughing, for symptomatic relief

BRONCHODILATORS

Bronchodilators dilate (open) the bronchus. There are two divisions of bronchodilators:

(1) Sympathomimetics, which dilate the bronchus by their beta-adrenergic activity.

(2) Xanthine derivatives, which dilate the bronchus by directly relaxing the smooth muscle of the bronchus.

Sympathomimetic bronchodilators include:

- Albuterol (Ventolin)
- Terbutaline (Bricanyl)

Xanthine-derivative bronchodilators include:

- Aminophylline (Truphylline)
- Epinephrine hydrochloride (Adrenalin Chloride)
- Theophylline (Theolair liquid)

Conditions treated with bronchodilators include:

- Anaphylaxis
- Bronchial asthma
- Bronchospasm

MUCOLYTICS AND EXPECTORANTS

MUCOLYTICS loosen secretions in the respiratory tract. EXPECTORANTS assist the client in coughing up thick, tenacious mucus from the respiratory tract.

Mucolytics include:

- Acetylcysteine (Mucomyst)

Expectorants include:

- Guaifenesin (Robitussin)

Conditions treated with mucolytics and expectorants include:

- Thick secretions in clients with pneumonia, as adjunct therapy
- Chronic asthma
- Cough due to cold or minor bronchial irritation
- Respiratory conditions associated with dry, unproductive cough

Practice Test 13

Questions

1 3 - 1

A client with asthma will be taught how to use an inhaler containing beclomethasone (Beclovent). Included in your teaching will be the instruction to:

1. rinse the mouth with water after each use of the inhaler.
2. use during an asthma attack for immediate relief.
3. use as needed (prn).
4. keep the inhaler chilled.

1 3 - 2

For which group of drugs might a person experiencing rhinitis seek a prescription?

1. analgesics
2. antipyretics
3. antihistamines
4. anti-infectives

1 3 - 3

A client arrives in the Emergency Department stating, "I've broken out all over. I guess it was something I ate." You anticipate a prescription for:

1. diphenhydramine (Benadryl) 250 mg by mouth.
2. diphenoxylate and atropine sulfate (Lomotil) 5 mg by mouth.
3. diphenhydramine (Benadryl) 25 mg by mouth.
4. phenytoin (Dilantin) 100 mg by mouth.

1 3 - 4

Which of the following is often seen in over-the-counter (OTC) preparations for the relief of nasal congestion?

1. epinephrine (Bronkaid and Primatene)
2. Dextromethorphan (Pertussin)
3. acetylcysteine and guaifenesin
4. phenylpropanolamine (PPA)

1 3 - 5

Your client has been taking theophylline-SR (Theolair-SR) but has grown weaker. The client states, "I can no longer swallow pills." Which is the best action to take?

1. Crush the medication and mix it with applesauce for administration.
2. Allow the client to chew the medication and "chase" it with juice.
3. Withhold the medication.
4. Consult with the physician concerning a liquid dosage of the medication.

1 3 - 6

A client is to receive the first dosage in a series of allergy injections. Which of the following medications should be available?

1. amoxicillin
2. verapamil (Calan)
3. ipratropium bromide (Atrovent)
4. epinephrine 1:1000

1 3 - 7

An acquaintance is experiencing wheezing and shortness of breath following a bee sting. You tell your acquaintance that:

1. intentional exposure to bee stings will build up immunity.
2. wheezing and shortness of breath are not caused by bee stings.
3. this type of allergic reaction can only happen once.
4. carrying a bee-sting kit containing epinephrine is advisable.

1 3 - 8

A client with asthma had a new inhalant prescribed, ipratropium (Atrovent). You instruct the client to report which common side effect?

1. drowsiness
2. hypertension
3. bradycardia
4. palpitations

1 3 - 9

A client was admitted to the hospital with shortness of breath and wheezing. The client was placed on the B-adrenergic agonist drug Albuterol. What expected effect on the respiratory system will you assess?

1. vasodilation
2. vasoconstriction
3. bronchodilation
4. bronchoconstriction

1 3 - 1 0

A client is experiencing chronic obstructive pulmonary disease (COPD). After undergoing a cholecystectomy, the client complains of incisional pain. Arterial blood gases over the past 3 years show: pH 7.40, pCO_2 65, PO_2 60. O_2 saturation in room air is 90%. What dosage of oxygen will you administer?

1. 100% facemask
2. 50% facemask
3. 1 to 2 l/min by nasal cannula
4. 10 l/min by nasal cannula

1 3 - 1 1

Which of the following medications is a bronchodilator and may be prescribed, along with other medications, to treat pneumonia?

1. beclomethasone (Vanceril)
2. albuterol (Ventolin)
3. ampicillin (Omnipen)
4. acetaminophen (Tylenol)

1 3 - 1 2

A client with diabetes is experiencing an asthma attack and is placed on epinephrine (Primatene). You will teach the client that:

1. blood pressure may become elevated, leading to danger of stroke.
2. less insulin will be required, or oral hypoglycemic agents may be needed.
3. pupil constriction may occur, leading to decreased vision.
4. bradycardia commonly occurs with the medication.

1 3 - 1 3

Which of the following medications should be available for a client scheduled for an intravenous pyelogram (IVP)?

1. potassium chloride (K-Dur)
2. epinephrine (Adrenalin)
3. fludarabine (Fludara)
4. acyclovir (Zovirax)

1 3 - 1 4

A client with cystic fibrosis has been placed on the drug dorinase alfa (Pulmozyme). You know this drug improves pulmonary function by:

1. decreasing viscosity of pulmonary secretions.
2. direct vasodilatation of pulmonary and systemic vascular beds.
3. reducing inflammatory changes in the airway.
4. inhibiting the enzyme responsible for the production of pulmonary secretions.

1 3 - 1 5

Cetirizine hydrochloride (Zyrtec) has been prescribed for a client experiencing perennial allergic rhinitis. Which comment by the client tells you he has understood what you taught him about this medication?

1. "Even if I have to take this drug 3 times a day, it will be worth it."
2. "I can use ice chips or hard candy to relieve dry mouth."
3. "I'm glad this drug won't keep me from driving a school bus."
4. "I can still take the Nubain the doctor gave me for my low back pain."

1 3 - 1 6

A client with chronic obstructive pulmonary disease is receiving 1 gm of aminophylline in 1000 cc of 5% dextrose in water at 20 cc/hour. Laboratory results indicate that the client's serum aminophylline level is 25 mcg/ml. You will:

1. notify the physician.
2. increase the rate of the infusion to 24 cc/hour.
3. put 1 g of aminophylline in 500 cc of dextrose 5% and decrease the rate to 10 cc/hour.
4. continue the infusion.

1 3 - 1 7

To prevent a febrile reaction to a blood trans-fusion, you will anticipate a prescription for:

1. diphenhydramine.
2. theophylline.
3. terbutaline sulfate.
4. epinephrine.

1 3 - 1 8

Isoetharine hydrochloride (Bronkosol) is prescribed for a 19-year-old who is wheezing on expiration. The nurse will observe for which of the following side effects of this medication?

1. pallor and dyspnea
2. bradycardia and diplopia
3. diarrhea and elevated blood pressure
4. tachycardia and headache

1 3 - 1 9

A client is using a Primatene Mist inhaler. The nurse will anticipate which of the following assessment findings?

1. hypotension
2. bradycardia
3. drowsiness
4. tachycardia

1 3 - 2 0

Following the flu, your client says, "I have this nonproductive cough that I can't seem to get rid of." You anticipate a prescription for the cough suppressant:

1. triprolidine hydrochloride.
2. dextromethorphan hydrochloride.
3. terbutaline sulfate.
4. epinephrine bitartrate.

1 3 - 2 1

Your client is receiving the expectorant guaifenesin (extended-release) capsule 600 mg daily. You understand the purpose of this drug is to:

1. prevent or relieve coughing.
2. suppress the cough reflex.
3. liquefy thick, tenacious sputum.
4. produce local anesthesia to the throat.

Practice Test 13

Answers, Rationales, and Explanations

1 3 - 1

① **Rinsing the mouth after each use helps prevent oral fungal infections, which are a common side effect of beclomethasone (Beclovent), a long-acting glucocorticoid.**

2. Beclomethasone (Beclovent) is not intended for use during an attack of asthma. The medication is for prophylactic use only.

3. To be effective, the dosages of beclomethasone (Beclovent) must be on a schedule, not prn.

4. Beclomethasone (Beclovent) is to be delivered at room temperature, not chilled.

Pregnancy Category: C
Client Need: Health Promotion/Maintenance

1 3 - 2

③ **Antihistamines are useful in treating rhinitis. Rhinitis (inflammation of the nasal mucosa) is an allergic reaction to airborne pollens. Antihistamines, because of their ability to block histamine reception, are the treatment of choice for allergies of this type.**

1. Analgesics are prescribed to relieve pain and do not treat the symptoms of allergic reactions caused by histamine release.

2. Antipyretics are agents that relieve or reduce fever. They are not effective in the treatment of allergic reactions.

4. Anti-infectives inhibit growth of or kill microorganisms and are not effective in the treatment of allergic reactions.

Pregnancy Category: Varies with each medication
Client Need: Health Promotion/Maintenance

1 3 - 3

③ **A prescription for diphenhydramine (Benadryl) 25 mg by mouth is anticipated. Benadryl is an antihistamine used in the treatment of allergic reactions. Initial dosage is generally 25 mg to 50 mg by mouth.**

1. Diphenhydramine 250 mg is an excessive dosage.

2. Diphenoxylate and atropine sulfate (Lomotil) are antidiarrheal agents.

4. Phenytoin (Dilantin) is an anticonvulsant.

Pregnancy Category: B
Client Need: Physiological Integrity

13 - 4

④ **Phenylpropanolamine (PPA) is a decongestant that is found in most over-the-counter (OTC) preparations used for relief of nasal congestion.**

1. Bronkaid and Primatene (epinephrine) are bronchodilators and may be prescribed for bronchospasms. These drugs do not relieve nasal congestion.

2. Dextromethorphan (Pertussin) is an antitussive (relieves coughing) and does not treat nasal congestion.

3. Acetylcysteine and guaifenesin are expectorants (they promote ejection of mucus from the lungs) and do not relieve nasal congestion.

Pregnancy Category: NR

Client Need: Physiological Integrity

13 - 5

④ **The physician should be consulted concerning a liquid dosage of the medication since the client is unable to swallow pills. Theophylline (Theolair-SR) is a bronchodilator that is available in liquid form and the dosage can be adjusted.**

1 and 2. Crushing or chewing sustained-release medication causes premature release of the medication.

3. The client needs the medication and it should not be withheld.

Pregnancy Category: C

Client Need: Health Promotion/Maintenance

13 - 6

④ **Epinephrine should be available when a client is receiving the first dosage in a series of allergy injections. Although the amount of antigen injected is small, there is always the possibility of an extreme allergic reaction. Epinephrine, due to its stimulant effect on the sympathetic nervous system, is the drug of choice for treating a severe allergic reaction.**

1. Amoxicillin is a penicillin antibiotic and has no impact on allergic reactions.

2. Verapamil (Calan) is an antiarrhythmic and has no impact on allergic reactions.

3. Ipratropium bromide (Atrovent) is normally administered to treat rhinitis and bronchospasm associated with COPD.

Pregnancy Category: C

Client Need: Safe, Effective Care Environment

1 3 - 7

④ Carrying a bee-sting kit is advisable for people allergic to bee stings. The venom of stinging insects can be very allergenic. Commercially prepared bee-sting kits contain epinephrine, which, because of its stimulant effect on the central nervous system, is the treatment of choice for allergic reactions of this type.

1. Persons with allergies should avoid exposure. Immunity will not develop with repeated stings.
2. Bee stings can cause severe allergic reactions. Allergic reactions can intensify over time.
3. Reactions may worsen with repeated exposure to bee stings.

Pregnancy Category: C
Client Need: Health Promotion/Maintenance

1 3 - 8

④ Clients receiving ipratropium (Atrovent) will be taught to report palpitations. Atrovent is an anticholinergic (it blocks parasympathetic nerve fibers) bronchodilator that inhibits some vagal responses. For this reason, palpitations are fairly common.

1, 2, and 3. Drowsiness, hypertension, and bradycardia are not typical side effects of anticholinergic bronchodilators. Nervousness, hypotension, and tachycardia are more common.

Pregnancy Category: B
Client Need: Health Promotion/Maintenance

1 3 - 9

③ B-adrenergic agonist drugs relax smooth muscles of all airways from the trachea to the terminal bronchioles (they cause bronchodilation). They are best administered as inhalants. Side effects of oral administration include tremor, tachycardia, and palapitations.

1 and 2. Vasodilation and vasoconstriction are caused by beta-adrenergic antagonists that block the beta receptors.

4. Bronchoconstriction is also caused by beta-adrenergic antagonists that block the beta receptors.

Pregnancy Category: Varies with specific drug
Client Need: Physiological Integrity

13-10

③ **Low dosages of oxygen (1 to 2 l/min) via nasal cannula should be administered in this situation. Persons with chronic obstructive pulmonary disease (COPD) many times retain carbon dioxide, as is evidenced in this instance with a pCO_2 of 65 (normal pCO_2 is 35 to 45). Persons who retain CO_2 depend on low oxygen levels as their impetus to breathe (referred to as the "hypoxic drive"). Very high oxygen administration would override this drive and cause respiratory failure.**

1. 100% facemask is too high a dosage.
2. 50% facemask is too high a dosage.
4. Ten liters per minute by nasal cannula is too high a dosage. Such high oxygen dosages might override the hypoxic drive, which may be present in a person who chronically retains CO_2.

Pregnancy Category: NR
Client Need: Physiological Integrity

13-11

② **Albuterol (Ventolin) may be prescribed, along with other medications, to treat pneumonia. Albuterol is a bronchodilator and exerts its bronchodilatory effect by relaxing the bronchial muscles.**

1. Beclomethasone (Vanceril) is a steroid inhalant.
3. Ampicillin (Omnipen) is a penicillin antibiotic.
4. Acetaminophen (Tylenol) is an analgesic antipyretic.

Pregnancy Category: C
Client Need: Health Promotion/Maintenance

13-12

① **You will teach the client about elevated blood pressure and the danger of strokes. Clients receiving epinephrine (Primatene) should be taught to assess their blood pressure. Epinephrine (Primatene) is a sympathomimetic drug. Because of its impact on the sympathetic nervous system, vasoconstriction, tachycardia, and hypertension may occur.**

2. Taking epinephrine (Primatene) may lead to a need for increased dosages of insulin/oral hypoglycemics in clients with diabetes.
3. Sympathomimetics such as epinephrine dilate pupils.
4. Sympathomimetics such as epinephrine tend to cause tachyarrhythmias, not bradycardia.

Pregnancy Category: C
Client Need: Health Promotion/Maintenance

13 - 13

② **Epinephrine (Adrenalin) must be available for clients having an intravenous pyelogram (IVP). Epinephrine (Adrenalin) is a bronchodilator and cardiac stimulant administered to manage anaphylaxis due to hypersensitivity to the contrast medium used for intravenous pyelogram (IVP). An intravenous pyelogram is a diagnostic test used to visualize the renal system and assess its function. A radiopaque dye is injected into the client's veins. Because anaphylaxis has sometimes occurred in response to the dye, resuscitation equipment and drugs such as epinephrine must be available.**

1. Potassium chloride (K-Dur) is administered to manage potassium depletion. This client does not demonstrate a need for this medication (K-Dur).

3. Fludarabine (Fludara) is administered to manage Hodgkin's lymphoma and chronic lymphocytic leukemia. This client does not have either of these conditions.

4. Acyclovir (Zovirax) is an antiviral agent. This client does not demonstrate a need for this type of medication.

Pregnancy Category: C

Client Need: Safe, Effective Care Environment

13 - 14

① **Dornase alfa improves pulmonary function for clients with cystic fibrosis by decreasing the viscosity and elasticity of pulmonary secretions.**

2. Clients experiencing primary pulmonary hypertension could benefit from a drug that can directly dilate pulmonary and systemic vascular beds, such as epoprostenol sodium (Flolan), not dornase alfa (Pulmozyme).

3. Dornase alfa (Pulmozyme) does not affect inflammatory changes in the airway. Clients with bronchial asthma could benefit from such a drug.

4. Cystic fibrosis is an inherited disease affecting the exocrine glands. Enzyme activity has not been associated with the cause or symptoms of the disease.

Pregnancy Category: B

Client Need: Physiological Integrity

13 - 15

② **Ice chips and hard candy help relieve dry mouth associated with the administration of cetirizine hydrochloride (Zyrtec).**

1. Cetirizine hydrochloride is usually taken once a day. Onset of action is 20 to 60 minutes, peak 0.5 to 1.5 hours, duration 14 hours.

3. Somnolence is a common adverse reaction to Zyrtec and clients should be warned not to drive or perform hazardous activities if they experience this side effect.

4. Cetirizine hydrochloride (Zyrtec) should not be taken concurrently with alcohol or other CNS depressants such as the narcotic analgesic nalbuphine hydrochloride (Nubain).

Pregnancy Category: B

Client Need: Health Promotion/Maintenance

1 3 - 1 6

① **The physician should be notified if a client's serum aminophylline level is abnormal. The therapeutic range for aminophylline is 10 to 20 mcg/ml.**

2 and 3. Infusing more of the aminophylline by increasing the drops per minute or the concentration will further elevate the serum aminophylline level.

4. The serum aminophylline level is elevated. The infusion should be stopped and the physician notified.

Pregnancy Category: C

Client Need: Health Promotion/Maintenance

1 3 - 1 7

① **A febrile reaction to a blood transfusion may be averted by a prophylactic administration of diphenhydramine (Benadryl).**

2 and 3. Theophylline and terbutaline sulfate are bronchodilators and would not be effective in preventing a febrile reaction to a blood transfusion.

4. Epinephrine would be the drug of choice in the event of anaphylaxis. However, it would not be effective in preventing a febrile reaction to a blood transfusion.

Pregnancy Category: B

Client Need: Safe, Effective Care Environment

1 3 - 1 8

④ **When administering isoetharine hydrochloride (Bronkosol), the nurse will observe for tachycardia and headache. Isoetharine hydrochloride is a sympathomimetic beta-adrenergic drug with selective action of beta-2 stimulation of the bronchial mucosa. Adverse side effects include hypertension, tachycardia, restlessness, headache, tremors, nausea, and vomiting.**

1. Pallor and dyspnea are not side effects of isoetharine hydrochloride (Bronkosol).

2. Bradycardia and diplopia are not side effects of isoetharine hydrochloride (Bronkosol).

3. Diarrhea and elevated blood pressure are not side effects of isoetharine hydrochloride (Bronkosol).

Pregnancy Category: C

Client Need: Physiological Integrity

1 3 - 1 9

④ **Clients using the Primatene Mist inhaler should be assessed for tachycardia. Epinephrine (Primatene Mist) is an alpha and beta receptor stimulator (bronchodilator). This medication also stimulates the sympathetic nervous system and may cause tachycardia, palpitations, hypertension, and morbid (unhealthy) ventricular arrhythmias.**

1. Epinephrine (Primatene Mist) may cause hypertension, not hypotension, because it stimulates the sympathetic nervous system.
2. Epinephrine (Primatene Mist) may cause tachycardia, not bradycardia, because it stimulates the sympathetic nervous system.
3. Epinephrine (Primatene Mist) stimulates the sympathetic nervous system and may cause restlessness, nervousness, and tremors, not drowsiness, because it stimulates the sympathetic nervous system.

Pregnancy Category: C
Client Need: Health Promotion/Maintenance

1 3 - 2 0

② **You anticipate a prescription for the cough suppressant dextromethorphan hydrochloride (Robitussin).**

1, 3, and 4. Triprolidine hydrochloride, terbutaline sulfate (Brethine), and epinephrine bitartrate are all bronchodilators, not cough suppressants.

Pregnancy Category: C
Client Need: Physiological Integrity

1 3 - 2 1

③ **You understand the purpose of guaifenesin extended-release capsules is to liquefy thick, tenacious sputum so that it can be removed from the bronchopulmonary mucous membranes. It is an expectorant.**

1. Guaifenesin is an expectorant, not an antitussive. Antitussives prevent or relieve coughing, not expectorants.
2. Antitussives suppress the cough reflex, not expectorants.
4. Guaifenesin does not produce any anesthesia.

Pregnancy Category: C
Client Need: Physiological Integrity

Practice Test 14

Topical Agents

OVERVIEW

Topical agents treat and inhibit conditions associated with a defined area of the body, such as the skin and hair.

Topical agents include:

- Local anesthetics
- Local anti-infectives
- Scabicides and pediculicides
- Topical corticosteroids

LOCAL ANESTHETICS

Local anesthetics create partial or complete loss of sensation without loss of consciousness. Local anesthetics produce brief effects by slowing down nerve transmission only in the areas where they are applied or injected.

Local anesthetics include:

- Benzocaine (Americaine)
- Lidocaine (Prilocaine)

Conditions treated with local anesthetics include:

- Hemorrhoidal discomfort
- Stitch cuts
- Warts, in surgical removal

LOCAL ANTI-INFECTIVES

Local anti-infectives are administered to treat various infections limited to one place or area on the body. They are normally available as ointments, creams, lotions, gels, pledgets, solutions, shampoos, powders, and sprays.

Local anti-infectives include:

- Butoconazole nitrate (Femstat)
- Gentamicin sulfate (Garamycin)

Conditions treated with local anti-infectives include:

- Superficial burns, abrasions
- Vulvovaginal infections caused by Candida

SCABICIDES AND PEDICULICIDES

SCABICIDES kill mites, especially those associated with scabies (a highly communicable skin disease caused by an arachnid).

Scabicides include:

Lindane (Kwell)

PEDICULICIDES are substances that kill lice.

Pediculicides include:

- Permethrin (Nix)

Conditions treated with scabicides and pediculicides include:

- Parasite infestation (scabies)
- Pediculosis capitis (head lice)
- Pediculosis corporis (body lice)

TOPICAL CORTICOSTEROIDS

Topical corticosteroids interfere with the inflammation and pruritus associated with various conditions. Topical corticosteroids exhibit anti-inflammatory, antipruritic, vasoconstrictive, and antiproliferative activity.

Topical corticosteroids include:

- Hydrocortisone (Cortizone)
- Hydrocortisone acetate (Cortaid)

Conditions treated with topical corticosteroids include:

- Inflammation and pruritus associated with corticosteroid-responsive dermatoses
- Seborrheic dermatitis of the scalp

Practice Test 14

Questions

1 4 - 1

A client diagnosed with herpes genitalis would benefit most from which medication?

1. Zovirax
2. penicillin G
3. Topicort
4. Lidex

1 4 - 2

The parents of a 6-year-old child with pediculosis capitis have received a prescription for permethrin (Nix). You will teach the parents to apply this medication to their child's hair:

1. once a day for 1 week.
2. undiluted to dry hair and work into a lather for 4 to 5 minutes.
3. after washing the hair with a regular shampoo and very warm water.
4. after using a fine-toothed comb to remove nits from the hair shafts.

1 4 - 3

You have provided a client who has head lice with information about lindane (Kwell) shampoo. Which statement made by the client indicates a correct understanding of this medication?

1. "I will need to apply this shampoo daily for 2 weeks."
2. "None of the members of my family will have to use the shampoo."
3. "This shampoo will treat my head lice as well as my dandruff condition."
4. "It is important for me to comb my hair with a fine-toothed comb since the shampoo won't remove all the nits."

1 4 - 4

Your client has a fungal keratitis and will receive natamycin (Natacyn), an antifungal 5% ophthalmic solution. You understand this drug may be administered as often as:

1. 1 drop every 15 minutes for the first 3 to 4 days.
2. 1 drop every 30 minutes for the first 3 to 4 days.
3. 1 drop every hour for the first 3 to 4 days.
4. 1 drop every 2 hours for the first 3 to 4 days.

1 4 - 5

Following the removal of a cataract, your client will receive the drug diclofenac sodium 0.1% (Voltarol). You understand the purpose of this drug in this situation is to:

1. relieve postoperative discomfort.
2. facilitate wound healing.
3. treat postoperative inflammation.
4. minimize visual sensitivity to light.

1 4 - 6

Your client has acute iritis of the right eye. The client is to receive an atropine sulfate ophthalmic solution 2 drops tid to ease the discomfort of photophobia associated with this drug. You will advise the client to:

1. wear protective clothing and avoid exposure to sunlight.
2. place a patch over the affected eye.
3. remain indoors for 30 to 60 minutes following the administration of the solution.
4. wear dark glasses (sunglasses).

1 4 - 7

Your client has a surface bacterial infection of the cornea. You will teach the client how to administer the ophthalmic ointment bacitracin (AK-Tracin). Which statement by the client indicates a correct understanding of your teaching?

1. "I will wash my hands before and after I administer the ointment."
2. "I will make sure to put plenty of ointment in my eye."
3. "I will know the ointment is in the right place if I let the tip of the dispenser touch my eyelid."
4. "After I apply the ointment, I will expect itching and burning."

1 4 - 8

Your client has a candidal infection on both feet. Amphotericin B (Fungizone) 3% cream has been prescribed. You will teach the client how to administer this drug. Which statement by the client suggests that he knows how to apply this medication?

1. "I should not rub or massage the cream into the affected places on my feet."
2. "I will only need to apply a thin coat of the cream to my feet."
3. "I will make sure to clean my feet before I apply the cream."
4. "I should apply an occlusive dressing after applying the cream to my feet."

1 4 - 9

A client with vulvovaginal candidiasis is to receive miconazole nitrate (Monistat 3) 100-mg suppositories. You will teach the client about this medication. Which statement by the client indicates she understands the information you have given to her?

1. "I will make sure that the suppositories are inserted high into my vagina."
2. "I'm glad this medication won't interfere with my vaginal contraceptive diaphragm."
3. "It's nice that I don't need to worry about this medicine staining my clothes."
4. "I will not need to avoid sexual intercourse while using these suppositories."

1 4 - 1 0

A client experiencing chronic anginal attacks is to begin using nitroglycerin (Nitrostat) ointment 2%. Which statement by the client indicates the correct understanding of how to administer this drug?

1. "I will put the ointment on with my fingertips."
2. "I will make sure to rub the ointment in really well."
3. "Once the ointment has been applied, I will cover the area with a plastic film."
4. "It won't make any difference if I put the ointment on a hairy part of my body."

1 4 - 1 1

Your client has psoriasis. When teaching the client about Psoralens long-wave ultraviolet light (PUVA) therapy, you should stress:

1. consulting with the dermatologist.
2. that lesions may fade with treatment.
3. avoiding exposure to the sun.
4. coping with psychosocial aspects.

Practice Test 14

Answers, Rationales, and Explanations

1 4 - 1

(1) **A client with herpes genitalis would benefit from the antiviral medication Acyclovir (Zovirax). Zovirax interferes with the structure and replication of the herpes virus (herpes simplex virus type 2).**

2. Penicillin G is an antibiotic, not an antiviral, and has no impact on herpes.

3 and 4. Desoximetasone (Topicort) and Fluocinonide (Lidex) are topical corticosteroids administered to treat inflammation associated with steroid-response dermatoses. They are not antivirals and would not be useful in treating herpes genitalis.

Pregnancy Category: C
Client Need: Health Promotion/Maintenance

1 4 - 2

(3) **You will teach the parents to treat their child's pediculosis by applying the permethrin (Nix) after the hair has been washed and toweled dry. The medication should remain on the hair for 10 minutes before rinsing off with water. The permethrin (Nix) kills live lice as well as nits (lice eggs).**

1. A one-time treatment is usually all that is necessary.

2. Permethrin (Nix) is applied to the hair after it has been washed and toweled dry. Nix is not a shampoo and does not lather. It should remain on the hair 10 minutes.

4. It is not necessary to remove nits (lice eggs) with a comb. The medication kills live lice as well as the nits (lice eggs).

Pregnancy Category: B
Client Need: Physiological Integrity

1 4 - 3

(4) **Fine-toothed combs (nit combs) are used to remove any nits on the hair shafts. Lindane (Kwell) is used in the treatment of pediculosis (head lice) and scabies (itch mite). When applied to treat head lice, the shampoo kills live lice. However, the nits (the eggs of the lice) may continue to cling to the hair shafts.**

1. Kwell shampoo is applied once to treat head lice. It may be repeated in a week if needed.

2. All family members should be treated with Kwell shampoo because of the highly contagious nature of pediculosis (head lice).

3. Kwell shampoo is a pediculicide (kills lice). It is not indicated in the treatment of eczema, dermatitis, or other skin conditions such as dandruff.

Pregnancy Category: B
Client Need: Safe, Effective Care Environment

14 - 4

③ **It may be necessary to instill the anti-infective antifungal natamycin (Natacyn) 5% solution every hour for the first 3 to 4 days of treatment. Dosage may then be reduced to 1 drop 6 to 8 times daily. Timely administration of the drug is critical, since blindness can result from this infection.**

1, 2, and 4. Drops may be instilled as often as 1 drop every hour for the first 3 to 4 days.

Pregnancy Category: C

Client Need: Physiological Integrity

14 - 5

③ **The purpose of diclofenac sodium 0.1% (Voltarol) following the removal of a cataract is to treat postoperative inflammation. This medication is an ophthalmic anti-inflammatory.**

1. Diclofenac sodium 0.1% (Voltarol) is not an analgesic and has no direct impact on pain. Indirectly, pain is relieved due to its anti-inflammatory effects.

2. Wound healing following the removal of a cataract is not associated with the administration of any drug. Normal body functions bring about the healing.

4. A patch is generally placed over the affected eye to protect it from physical harm. The patch will also prevent any sensitivity the client may have to light following the trauma of surgery.

Pregnancy Category: B

Client Need: Health Promotion/Maintenance

14 - 6

④ **The client should be taught to wear dark glasses. Photophobia (unusual intolerance to light) is an adverse reaction experienced by some clients who are medicated with atropine sulfate ophthalmic solution.**

1. It is not necessary for the client to wear protective clothing since photosensitivity is not associated with the administration of atropine sulfate ophthalmic solution. Photophobia is an adverse side effect.

2. A patch should not be worn. Wearing a patch could further irritate the eyes. Dark glasses are more appropriate inasmuch as they block out the light.

3. It is not necessary to remain indoors after the administration of the medication. Dark glasses will protect the client from the light.

Pregnancy Category: C

Client Need: Physiological Integrity

1 4 - 7

  ① Clients should always wash their hands before and after applying ophthalmic ointments; otherwise, reinfection is likely. In addition to reinfection, the client could introduce new bacteria into the eyes.

  2. The client should be instructed to place only a small amount of ointment in the eye. Also, the client should be told that temporary blurred (hazy) vision is expected.

  3. To prevent contamination, the tip of the dispenser should not touch the client's eye, eyelid, fingers, or other surfaces.

  4. Itching and burning are reportable adverse reactions, not expected outcomes.

Pregnancy Category: C
Client Need: Health Promotion/Maintenance

1 4 - 8

  ③ The client should understand that cleaning the feet before applying the amphotericin B (Fungizone) will facilitate absorption of the drug.

  1. The client should make sure that the amphotericin B (Fungizone) cream is rubbed into the affected areas of the feet thoroughly. Rubbing and massaging the medication into the tissues will facilitate absorption of the drug. Also, skin becomes discolored if the drug is not rubbed in well.

  2. Amphotericin B (Fungizone) should be applied liberally to all affected areas of the feet.

  4. Occlusive dressings are contraindicated and should be avoided. They tend to facilitate the collection of moisture and create a breeding bed for the growth of candidas.

Pregnancy Category: B
Client Need: Physiological Integrity

1 4 - 9

  ① It is important that the Monistat suppositories be inserted high into the vagina so that the medication can reach all affected areas.

  2. Concurrent use of some latex products such as vaginal contraceptive diaphragms and Monistat are not recommended because of possible interaction. Other forms of contraception should be considered during drug therapy.

  3. Clients should be told that the vaginal form of miconazole nitrate (Monistat 3) may stain clothing.

  4. Sexual intercourse should be avoided during the time of vaginal treatment with Monistat.

Pregnancy Category: B
Client Need: Physiological Integrity

1 4 - 1 0

③ **The nitroglycerin (Nitrostat) should be covered with a film to aid in its absorption. Also, it is important that all medication from the previous application be cleaned off before placing new ointment on the client. This will prevent overdosage.**

1. Nitroglycerin (Nitrostat) ointment 2% should be administered using an applicator. If the bare fingertips are used, the drug will be absorbed through the fingers of the client or the nurse.

2. The Nitrostat ointment should not be rubbed in because this will interfere with the rate of absorption.

4. The ointment should be placed on a nonhairy part of the client's body so that absorption can easily take place.

Pregnancy Category: C
Client Need: Physiological Integrity

1 4 - 1 1

③ **Sunlight should be avoided by clients receiving Psoralens long-wave ultraviolet light (PUVA) therapy. Following PUVA therapy, the skin remains photosensitive until the methoxsalen (a lotion that may enhance melanogenesis) is excreted. Sunlight should be avoided for approximately 8 hours after medication has been given; otherwise, there is overexposure.**

1. It is not necessary to consult a dermatologist. You will teach the client about overexposure.

2. It is true that lesions may fade with treatment, but they recur eventually in the same area and new lesions may occur in other places.

4. The client will need emotional support. However, the fact that PUVA therapy involves ultraviolet light suggests the importance of teaching the client about overexposure to the sun.

Pregnancy Category: C
Client Need: Safe, Effective Care Environment

Practice Test 15

Miscellaneous Medications

OVERVIEW

The "miscellaneous" category comprises drugs that are of mixed character. Among the miscellaneous drugs are agents that are uncategorized.

Miscellaneous agents include:

- Antigout substances
- Diagnostic skin tests
- Enzymes
- Gold salts

- Miscellaneous antagonists and antidotes
- Spasmolytics
- Uterine substances

ANTIGOUT SUBSTANCES

Antigout substances are administered to treat the symptoms of gout, which are caused by the deposit of urate crystals in the joints. Antigout substances function in three general ways: They reduce the production of uric acid, reduce inflammation, and increase the excretion of uric acid by the kidneys.

Antigout substances include:

- Allopurinol (Zyloprim)
- Colchicine (Colgout)

- Probenecid (Benemid)

Conditions treated with antigout substances include:

- Gouty arthritis
- Hyperuricemia secondary to malignancies

DIAGNOSTIC SKIN TESTS

Diagnostic skin tests such as the tuberculin purified protein derivative (PPD Mantoux, ST) are used to determine if a client has a specific disease; i.e., tuberculosis.

Diagnostic skin tests include:

- Tuberculin purified protein derivative histoplasmin

Conditions treated with diagnostic skin tests include:

- Histoplasmosis
- Mumps

- Tuberculosis

ENZYMES

Enzymes are complex proteins capable of inducing chemical changes in other substances without being changed themselves. Enzymes act as organic catalysts in initiating or speeding up specific chemical reactions.

Enzymes include:

- Chymopapain (Chymodiactin)
- Hyaluronidase (Wydase)

Conditions treated with enzymes include:

- Inflammatory and infected lesions (in debridement)
- Herniated lumbar disk
- Enzymes are also administered as adjunct therapy to increase absorption and dispersion of injected drugs.

GOLD SALTS

Gold salts are derived from gold (chemical symbol Au).

Gold salts include:

- Auranofin (Ridaura)
- Gold sodium thiomalate (Aurolate)

Conditions treated with gold salts include:

- Rheumatoid arthritis

MISCELLANEOUS ANTAGONISTS AND ANTIDOTES

Antagonists and antidotes are usually administered to counteract the action of something or neutralize poisons or the effects of poisons.

Miscellaneous antagonists include:

- Dimercaprol (BAL in Oil)
- Edetate disodium (Disotate)

Conditions treated with antagonists include:

- Arsenic or gold poisoning
- Hypercalcemic crisis

Miscellaneous antidotes include:

- Activated charcoal
- Digoxin immune Fab (ovine) (Digibind)

Conditions treated with antidotes include:

- Life-threatening intoxication with digitoxin or digoxin
- Overdosage of acetaminophen

SPASMOLYTICS

Spasmolytics are administered to relieve muscle spasms.

Spasmolytics include:

- Flavoxate hydrochloride (Urispas)
- Oxybutynin chloride (Ditropan)

Conditions treated with spasmolytics include:

- Neurogenic bladder
- Dysuria, for symptomatic relief

UTERINE SUBSTANCES

Three types of substances are administered for their effects on the uterus:

(1) Oxytocics

(3) Abortifacients

(2) Uterine relaxants

OXYTOCIC substances stimulate the uterus.

Oxytocic agents include:

- Methylergonovine maleate (Methergine)
- Oxytocin (Pitocin)

Conditions treated with oxytocics include:

- Postpartum uterine bleeding
- Uterine atony

UTERINE RELAXANTS are administered to soothe and relax the muscles of the uterus. They are administered to prevent the potential for abortion and miscarriage.

Uterine relaxants include:

- Terbutaline sulfate (Brethine)
- Magnesium sulfate

Conditions treated with uterine relaxants include:

- Threatened abortion

ABORTIFACIENTS are used to cause or induce an abortion.

Abortifacients include:

- RU 486 (Mifepristone)
- Prostaglandin gel

Conditions treated with abortifacients include:

- Pregnancy, to induce therapeutic abortion
- Pregnancy, to induce elective abortion

Practice Test 15

Questions

1 5 - 1

A client has mistakenly taken twice the pre-scribed dosage of warfarin "for several days." You would anticipate which of the following prescriptions?

1. protamine sulfate
2. heparin
3. Coumadin
4. vitamin K

1 5 - 2

Disulfiram (Antabuse) 500-mg tablets by mouth have been prescribed daily for your client. You will teach the client to avoid:

1. cough syrups.
2. all forms of alcohol.
3. foods containing tyramine.
4. B vitamins.

1 5 - 3

Which route will the nurse expect to use when administering oxytocin (Pitocin) to a woman in labor?

1. oral
2. intramuscular injection
3. intravenous piggyback setup
4. straight-line intravenous infusion

1 5 - 4

A client arrives in the Emergency Department and states, "I took an overdose of Xanax." Which medication is the most appropriate to administer at this time?

1. activated charcoal
2. succimer (Chemet)
3. dimercaprol (BAL in Oil)
4. amoxicillin (Amoxil)

1 5 - 5

Prior to a procedure requiring some sedation, a client is given intravenous diazepam (Valium). Within minutes, the client's respiratory rate is 6 breaths per minute. Which medication do you anticipate administering?

1. naloxone (Narcan)
2. edetate calcium disodium (Calcium EDTA)
3. flumazenil (Romazicon)
4. sodium polystyrene sulfonate (Kayexalate)

1 5 - 6

A client received a tuberculin skin test (Mantoux) 48 hours ago. A 10-mm induration is now present at the injection site. This induration would be indicative of:

1. no clinical evidence of tuberculosis.
2. an active tubercular infection.
3. the immune system reacting to the tubercular bacillus. There may be an active or dormant infection present.
4. a probable infection with miliary tuberculosis if close contact with an infected client has occurred.

1 5 - 7

A client with leukemia is being treated with chemotherapy. The client is also receiving allopurinol (Zyloprim). Which of the following client statements reflects the best understanding of the desired effect of this medication?

1. "Allopurinol will keep me from losing so much hair from chemotherapy."
2. "Allopurinol will prevent nausea and vomiting from the chemotherapy."
3. "Allopurinol will get rid of the trash when the bad cells die."
4. "Allopurinol will prevent ulcers in my mouth and intestine."

1 5 - 8

A client has severe nocturnal heartburn. Which medication would be indicated?

1. docusate sodium (Colace)
2. bisacodyl (Dulcolax)
3. psyllium (Metamucil)
4. cisapride (Propulsid)

1 5 - 9

A child was brought to the Emergency Department following acute poisoning with an iron preparation. The nurse will anticipate a prescription for:

1. physostigmine (Antilirium).
2. acetylcysteine (Mucomyst).
3. deferoxamine (Desferal).
4. succimer (Chemet).

1 5 - 1 0

A pediatric client is admitted to your unit with suspected lead poisoning. Which medication would prevent potential toxicity?

1. flumazenil (Romazicon)
2. edetate calcium disodium (Calcium EDTA)
3. calcium carbonate (Dicarbosil)
4. cefazolin sodium (Kefzol)

1 5 - 1 1

Succimer is administered for which of the following conditions?

1. infection
2. lead poisoning
3. mosquito bite
4. tick bite

15-12

It has been determined that your client has gonorrhea. In addition to 4.8 million units of penicillin G procaine IM, you will anticipate a prescription for probenecid (Benemid) 1 gm po. You understand the probenecid will be given to:

1. minimize any allergic response to the penicillin.
2. facilitate renal tubular secretion of penicillin.
3. increase blood levels of penicillin.
4. reduce the gastrointestinal distress caused by penicillin.

15-13

Your client is experiencing great-toe pain. Serum uric acid levels are elevated to 8 mg/dl. Which of the following medications would you give?

1. penicillin G potassium (Pfizerpen)
2. aspirin (acetylsalicylic acid)
3. acetaminophen (Tylenol)
4. allopurinol (Zyloprim)

15-14

Your client is experiencing apnea as a consequence of anaphylactic shock. Which of the following treatments will be most appropriate?

1. diphenhydramine
2. intubation and 100% oxygen
3. acetaminophen (Tylenol)
4. aminophylline (Truphylline)

15-15

An unconscious client is brought to the Emergency Department. You learn that the client took an overdose of Valium pills. You will anticipate a prescription for the antagonist:

1. activated charcoal.
2. naloxone hydrochloride (Narcan).
3. ipecac syrup.
4. flumazenil (Romazicon).

15 - 16

Which of the following routes of medication administration will the nurse recognize as having the slowest absorption rate?

1. intravenous infusion
2. intramuscular injection
3. subcutaneous injection
4. oral administration

15 - 17

A client recovering from a cholecystectomy has received morphine sulfate in the postanesthesia care unit. When the client was returned to the surgical unit, the vital signs were: Blood pressure 124/64, pulse 64 beats per minute, respirations 8 per minute, temperature 97.4. Which of the following medications will the nurse anticipate administering?

1. atropine sulfate 1.0 mg IV
2. flumazenil (Romazicon) 0.2 mg IV
3. meperidine (Demerol) 50 mg IV
4. naloxone (Narcan) 0.2 mg IV

15 - 18

Which of the following medications might be given postpartum to reduce the risk of hemorrhage after the placenta is delivered?

1. oxytocin (Pitocin)
2. heparin
3. ampicillin (Omnipen)
4. albuterol (Ventolin)

15 - 19

A heparin infusion is being given to a client. The morning's laboratory studies indicate: PTT 246 sec, K+ 4.6 mmol/l, NA+ 136 mmol/l. You anticipate a prescription for:

1. protamine sulfate
2. promethazine
3. procainamide
4. propranolol

Practice Test 15

Answers, Rationales, and Explanations

1 5 - 1

④ **A prescription for vitamin K is anticipated. Vitamin K is the recommended treatment for warfarin (Coumadin) toxicity. Warfarin is an anticoagulant. Warfarin's anticoagulant action is due to its ability to interfere with hepatic synthesis of vitamin K (a clotting factor). When an overdose of warfarin has been taken, vitamin K is administered as an antidote.**

1. Protamine sulfate is an antidote (antiheparin agent) that is recommended for treatment of heparin toxicity.

2. Heparin is another anticoagulant. Administering another anticoagulant would contribute to the potential for hemorrhage.

3. Coumadin is a trade name for warfarin sodium.

Pregnancy Category: X

Client Need: Safe, Effective Care Environment

1 5 - 2

② **Clients must be taught that any consumption of alcohol while taking Antabuse may produce a severe, potentially fatal reaction. Products that contain alcohol include sauces made with wine, aftershave lotions, colognes, liniments, and some cough syrups.**

1. Clients receiving Antabuse should avoid all forms of alcohol. Cough syrups that contain alcohol are only one source of alcohol.

3. Foods containing tyramine are not contraindicated for clients receiving Antabuse. Foods containing tyramine should be avoided by clients taking monoamine oxidase (MAO) inhibitors because a combination of foods containing tyramine and MAO inhibitors can produce a hypertensive crisis. Foods high in tyramine are: Bananas, liver, beer, chocolate, red wine, aged cheese, and avocadoes.

4. B vitamins are likely to be prescribed for clients receiving Antabuse since the clients are alcoholics and may be malnourished.

Pregnancy Category: NR

Client Need: Health Promotion/Maintenance

1 5 - 3

③ **Intravenous piggyback setup is the only acceptable route of administration for oxytocin (Pitocin) during labor. Furthermore, an intravenous pump should be used to carefully regulate the flow. Note: With a piggyback, the nurse can cut off the oxytocin and still have a line open. Also, some women are very sensitive to oxytocin and could have tetanic contractions (continuous contraction of uterine muscles).**

1. Oxytocin may be given orally postpartum to control bleeding but should never be administered orally prior to delivery since it may cause tetanic contractions and uterine rupture.

2. Oxytocin may be given intramuscularly after delivery to control postpartum hemorrhage and promote uterine involution. It should not be administered intramuscularly prior to delivery.

4. Straight-line intravenous infusion would not be safe since the entire infusion would be shut off if complications arose from the oxytocin.

Pregnancy Category: C

Client Need: Safe, Effective Care Environment

1 5 - 4

① **Activated charcoal is an agent that binds with many drugs and helps prevent their absorption from the digestive system. Because of these properties, activated charcoal would help prevent the systemic toxic effects of alprazolam (Xanax) overdose by binding with the drug prior to absorption.**

2. Succimer (Chemet) is a chelating agent that is administered to treat lead poisoning.

3. Dimercaprol (BAL in Oil) is a chelator used to treat arsenic or gold poisoning.

4. Amoxicillin (Amoxil) is a penicillin antibiotic and not an antidote for Xanax overdose.

Pregnancy Category: D

Client Need: Safe, Effective Care Environment

1 5 - 5

③ **A prescription for flumazenil (Romazicon) is anticipated. Flumazenil competes with benzodiazepines at the receptor sites. Because of this action, it is antagonistic to benzodiazepines such as Valium. It is used in the treatment of respiratory depression associated with benzodiazepine toxicity.**

1. Naloxone (Narcan) is used in the treatment of opioid narcotic overdose, not respiratory depression due to Valium administration.

2. Edetate calcium disodium (Calcium EDTA) is a treatment for lead toxicity, not respiratory depression due to Valium administration.

4. Sodium polystyrene sulfonate (Kayexalate) is prescribed to treat hyperkalemia (elevated serum potassium), not respiratory depression due to Valium administration.

Pregnancy Category: C

Client Need: Health Promotion/Maintenance

1 5 - 6

③ **A 10-mm induration indicates a positive reaction to the tuberculin skin test. An active or dormant infection may be present. Further diagnostic studies would need to be scheduled to determine active tuberculosis. A 10-mm induration is significant in persons born in Asia, Africa, and Latin America; underserved low-income populations; residents of long-term care facilities; or in high-risk persons with diabetes, renal failure, or those receiving immunosuppressants.**

1. A 0.4-mm induration is a negative reaction when there is no clinical evidence of tuberculosis.

2. Either an active or dormant infection might be present with a 10-mm induration. Further diagnostic studies would need to be scheduled, such as a chest X ray.

4. A 5- to 9-mm induration would indicate a probable infection if contact with an infected person has occurred.

Pregnancy Category: C
Client Need: Health Promotion/Maintenance

1 5 - 7

③ **Allopurinol is an antigout agent that helps rid the body of purines, which can accumulate as cells die rapidly from chemotherapy. Additional fluids also enhance excretion of purines by the kidneys.**

1. Allopurinol has no effect on alopecia (hair loss). No medications are presently known to prevent alopecia due to chemotherapy.

2. Antiemetic drugs, not antigout drugs, are used to treat nausea and vomiting.

4. Allopurinol is not effective in the treatment of stomatitis (inflammation of the mouth).

Pregnancy Category: C
Client Need: Physiological Integrity

1 5 - 8

④ **Cisapride (Propulsid) reduces the symptoms of "heartburn." It is a gastrointestinal antireflux medication that stimulates activity of the gastrointestinal tract and increases gastric motility.**

1. Docusate sodium (Colace) is a stool softener and has no impact on reflux.

2. Bisacodyl (Dulcolax) is a laxative and has no impact on reflux.

3. Psyllium (Metamucil) is a laxative and has no impact on reflux.

Pregnancy Category: C
Client Need: Physiological Integrity

1 5 - 9

③ **The nurse will anticipate a prescription for deferoxamine (Desferal). This drug is a heavy metal antagonist given to manage acute toxic iron ingestion. Desferal chelates (binds with) unbound iron and excretes it through the urinary system.**

1. Physostigmine (Antilirium) reverses anticholinergic excess, such as atropine overdose, not iron poisoning.

2. Acetylcysteine (Mucomyst) is the antidote for acetaminophen (Tylenol) overdose, not iron poisoning.

4. Succimer (Chemet) is the antidote for lead poisoning, not iron poisoning.

Pregnancy Category: NR

Client Need: Safe, Effective Care Environment

1 5 - 1 0

② **Edetate calcium disodium (Calcium EDTA) can prevent potential lead toxicity. Calcium EDTA is a chelating agent (a drug that bonds with a substance, such as lead, and takes it out of the body) and an antidote for lead poisoning. It binds with lead to form a soluble stable compound that is excreted by the kidneys.**

1. Flumazenil (Romazicon) is a benzodiazepine antagonist used as an antidote to treat minor tranquilizer and antianxiety agent overdose. It has no impact on lead poisoning.

3. Calcium carbonate (Dicarbosil) is an antacid and has no impact on lead poisoning.

4. Cefazolin sodium (Kefzol) is a cephalosporin antibiotic and has no impact on lead poisoning.

Pregnancy Category: NR

Client Need: Health Promotion/Maintenance

1 5 - 1 1

② **Succimer is a heavy metal chelating agent that reduces blood lead levels in children. Three to 4 million children may have blood lead levels high enough to cause neurobehavioral and other adverse health effects. Chelation mobilizes the lead from the blood and soft tissues by enhancing its deposition in bones and its excretion in the urine.**

1, 3, and 4. Succimer is a heavy metal chelating agent and would not be given for infection, mosquito bites, or tick bites.

Pregnancy Category: C

Client Need: Health Promotion/Maintenance

1 5 - 1 2

③ **You understand probenecid has been prescribed because it can increase the blood levels of penicillin. Probenecid is often prescribed as an adjunct to penicillin therapy.**

1. Probenecid is an antigout medication. It is not an antidote (a substance that neutralizes poisons or their effects) or an antagonist (a substance that counteracts a drug).

2. Probenecid inhibits renal tubular secretion of penicillin and is able to increase blood serum levels of penicillin cephalosporins.

4. One of the side effects of probenecid administration is gastrointestinal distress. Also, the penicillin was administered IM, not po.

Pregnancy Category: C

Client Need: Health Promotion/Maintenance

1 5 - 1 3

④ **Allopurinol (Zyloprim) is indicated in the treatment of hyperuricemic gout attacks. Because this medication inhibits the production of uric acid, the uric acid level drops and hyperuricemic gout abates (subsides).**

1. Penicillin G potassium (Pfizerpen) is a penicillin antibiotic and has no impact on uric acid levels.

2 and 3. Aspirin (acetylsalicylic acid) and acetaminophen (Tylenol) are antipyretic analgesics that may provide temporary pain relief but will have no impact on uric acid levels.

Pregnancy Category: C

Client Need: Physiological Integrity

1 5 - 1 4

② **The appropriate treatment at this time would be intubation and 100% oxygen. When a client is apneic due to anaphylactic shock (a generalized allergic hypersensitivity of the body to a foreign protein or drug), oxygen is administered. A client experiencing anaphylaxis and respiratory arrest (apnea) requires artificial positive pressure ventilation via an endotracheal tube with 100% oxygen.**

1. Diphenhydramine (Benadryl) is an antihistamine that is useful in managing allergic reactions (including anaphylaxis). However, because the client is apneic, the most appropriate action would include the administration of oxygen.

3. Acetaminophen (Tylenol) is an antipyretic and analgesic and is not given to manage anaphylaxis or its consequence.

4. Aminophylline (Truphylline) is a bronchodilator that may be administered to manage airway obstruction due to asthma or chronic obstructive pulmonary disease. However, the priority at this time is the administration of oxygen.

Pregnancy Category: NR

Client Need: Physiological Integrity

1 5 - 1 5

④ **You will anticipate a prescription for flumazenil (Romazicon) for a client who has taken an overdose of diazepam (Valium). Flumazenil (Romazicon) is a benzodiazepine antagonist that competitively inhibits the action of benzodiazepines such as Valium.**

1. Activated charcoal is not an antagonist. It is an adsorbent that prevents the absorption of chemicals and drugs through the gastrointestinal tract. It may be prescribed, for example, to a child who accidentally ingested an overdose of aspirin.

2. Naloxone hydrochloride (Narcan) is an antagonist that displaces narcotic analgesics such as Darvon and Talwin, not benzodiazepines such as Valium. It is administered to treat altered levels of consciousness. Overdoses of heroin are typically treated with intravenous Narcan.

3. Ipecac syrup induces vomiting. It may be administered to induce vomiting due to ingestion of poison. Ipecac would not be given to this client because the client is unconscious and could aspirate. Also, ipecac is not an antagonist and would do nothing to reverse respiratory depression.

Pregnancy Category: C
Client Need: Physiological Integrity

1 5 - 1 6

④ **Oral administration of medications has the slower absorption rate because medications must be absorbed through the gastrointestinal tract before entering the circulation.**

1. Administering medications by intravenous infusion provides the fastest absorption rate since they are placed directly into the circulatory system.

2. An intramuscular injection is faster than the oral route but slower than an intravenous infusion. It takes time for medications given into a muscle to be absorbed by the bloodstream.

3. Subcutaneous injections have a faster rate of absorption than the oral route but slower than intravenous infusions and intramuscular injections. There are fewer large blood vessels to absorb medications in the subcutaneous tissue compared to the larger blood beds that serve muscles.

Pregnancy Category: Varies with specific drug
Client Need: Safe, Effective Care Environment

15-17

④ **The nurse will anticipate a prescription for naloxone (Narcan). Naloxone (Narcan) is a narcotic agonist administered to treat oversedation from narcotic analgesics. A respiratory rate < 12/min is a sign of respiratory depression most likely caused by the morphine sulfate administered in the postanesthesia area.**

1. Atropine sulfate may be prescribed to treat bradycardia (heart rate < 60). It is not prescribed to treat respiratory depression.

2. Flumazenil (Romazicon) is a benzodiazepine antagonist and as such may be prescribed for overdoses of medications like diazepam (Valium).

3. Meperidine (Demerol) should not be given. It is a narcotic analgesic and would further depress respiration.

Pregnancy Category: B

Client Need: Physiological Integrity

15-18

① **Oxytocin (Pitocin) might be given postpartum to reduce the risk of hemorrhage after the placenta is delivered. Pitocin controls bleeding by facilitating contraction of the uterine muscle following the expulsion of the placenta.**

2. Heparin is an anticoagulant, which would increase bleeding, and should not be administered.

3. Ampicillin (Omnipen) is an antibiotic and has no impact on contractions.

4. Albuterol (Ventolin) is a bronchodilator and has no impact on contractions.

Pregnancy Category: NR

Client Need: Health Promotion/Maintenance

15-19

① **You anticipate a prescription for protamine sulfate. Protamine sulfate is a heparin antagonist (antidote) that neutralizes the anticoagulant effect of heparin. The effect of protamine sulfate is monitored by activated partial thromboplastin time (APTT). An APTT greater than 100 seconds signifies spontaneous bleeding.**

2. Promethazine hydrochloride is an antiemetic antihistamine agent and has no impact on blood coagulation.

3. Procainamide is an antiarrhythmic and has no impact on blood coagulation.

4. Propranolol is a beta-adrenergic blocking agent and has no impact on blood coagulation.

Pregnancy Category: C

Client Need: Physiological Integrity

Common Abbreviations

ā	before		OD	right eye
ac	before meals		OS	left eye
AD	right ear		os	mouth
ad lib	as needed		oz	ounce
amp	ampule		p̄	after
AS	left ear		po	by mouth
AU	each ear		PR	rectally
bid	twice a day		prn	when needed
cap	capsule		PV	vaginally
cc	cubic centimeter; 1 cc = 1 ml		q	every
D/C	discontinue		qd	every day
dl	deciliter		qh	every hour
dr	dram		qid	four times a day
elix	elixir		qod	every other day
gm	gram		s̄	without
gr	grain		SA	sustained action
h	hour		SC	subcutaneous
hs	hour of sleep		SL	sublingual
IM	intramuscular		Sol	solution
IV	intravenous		SR	sustained release
kg	kilogram		ss	one half
KVO	keep vein open		stat	immediately
L	left		tab	tablet
l	liter		tbs	tablespoon
mg	milligram		tid	three times a day
mEq	milliequivalent		tinct	tincture
ml	milliliter		TPR	total parenteral nutrition
NG	nasogastric		tsp	teaspoon
NPO	nothing by mouth			

Drug Names and Pronunciations, Trade Names, and Classification(s)

{Drug names in parentheses are available in Canada only.}

Acetaminophen [a-seat-a-**mee**-noe-fen]
{Abenol}, Aceta, Actamin, Aminofen, Anacin-3, Apacet, APAP, {Apo-Acetaminophen}, Arthritis Pain Formula Aspirin-Free, Atasol, Banesin, Dapa, Datril, Dolanex, Dorcol Children's Fever and Pain Reducer, {Exdor}, Feverall, Genapap, Genebs, Helenol, Liquiprin, Meda Cap, Myapap, Neopap, Oraphen, Panadol, Panex, Paracetamol, Phenaphen, Redutemp, Ridenol, {Robigesic}, {Rounox}, Snaplets-FR, St. Joseph's Aspirin-Free, Suppap, Tapanol, Tempra, Tenol, Tylenol, Ty-Pap, Ty-Tap, Valadol, Valorin
Classifications:
Nonopioid analgesic, antipyretic

Acetylysteine [a-se-til-**sis**-teen]
Mucomyst, Mucosil
Classification:
Antidote to acetaminophen

Acyclovir [ay-**sye**-kloe-veer]
Zovirax
Classification:
Antiviral

Adenosine [a-**den**-oh-seen]
Adenocard
Classification:
Antiarrhythmic

Albumin [al-**bu**-min]
Classification:
Blood derivative

Albuterol [al-**byoo**-ter-ole]
{Novosalmol}, Proventil, salbutamol, Ventolin
Classification:
Bronchodilator (beta-adrenergic agonist)

Allopurinol [al-oh-**pure**-i-nole]
{Alloprin}, {Apo Allopurinol}, Lopurin, {Novo-purol}, {Purinol}, Zyloprim
Classification:
Antigout agent (xanthene oxidase inhibitor)

Alprazolam [al-**pra**-soe-lam]
{Apo-Alpraz}, {Novo-Alprazol}, {Nu-Alpraz}, Xanax
Classification:
Sedative/hypnotic (benzodiazepine)

Alteplase [**al**-te-plase]
Activase, {Activase rt-PA}, tissue plasminogen activator, t-PA
Classification:
Thrombolytic

Aluminum Hydroxide [a-**loo**-me-num]
AlternaGEL, Alucap, {Alugel}, Aluminet, Alu-tab, Amphojel, Basalgel, Dialume, Nephrox
Classifications:
Antacid, electrolyte modifier (hypophosphatemic)

Aminophylline [am-in-**off**-i-lin]
{Corophyllin}, {Palaron}, Phyllocontin, Truphylline
Classification:
Bronchodilator (phosphodiesterase inhibitor)

Amlodipine besylate [am-**loe**-di-peen] [**bye**-sye-late]
Norvasc
Classifications:
Antihypertensive (calcium channel blocker), antianginal

Amphotericin B [am-foe-**ter**-i-sin]
Fungizone
Classification:
Antifungal

Antihemophilic Factor [an-tee-hee-mee-**fill**-ik]
AHF-M, Factor VIII S.D., Hemofil M, Humate P,
Koate HP, Kogenate, Monoclate P, Profilate OSD,
Recombinate
Classifications:
Hemostatic, blood derivative

Aspirin [**as**-pir-in]
acetylsalicylic acid, {Apo-ASA}, {Apo-Asen},
{Arthrinol}, {Arthrisin}, {Artria S.R}, Aspirgum,
ASA, {Astrin}, Bayer Aspirin, Bayer Timed-
Release Arthritic Pain Formula {Coryphen},
Easprin, Ecotrin, 8-hour Bayer Timed Release,
Empirin, {Entrophen}, Genprin, Halfprin,
{Headstart}, Measurin, Norwich Aspirin,
{Riphen}, {Sal-Adult}, {Sal-Infant}, St. Joseph
Adult Chewable Aspirin, Therapy Bayer,
ZORprin
Classifications:
Nonopioid analgesic, nonsteroidal anti-inflamma-
tory, antipyretic, antiplatelet agent

Atenolol [a-**ten**-oh-lole]
{Apo-Atenolol}, Tenormin
Classifications:
Antihypertensive, beta-adrenergic blocker (selec-
tive), antianginal

Atropine [**a**-troe-peen)
Atropair, Atro-Pen, Atropisol, Isopto-Atropine,
I-Tropine, {Minims Atropine}, Ocu-Tropine
Classifications:
Anticholingeric (antimuscarinic), antiarrhythmic,
ophthalmic (mydriatic)

Beclomethasone [be-kloe-**meth**-a-sone]
Beclovent, Beconase, Beconase AQ Nasal,
Vancenase, Vancenase AQ Nasal, Vanceril
Classification:
Glucocorticoid (long-acting)

Betamethasone Valerate [bay-ta-**meth**-a-sone]
Alphatrex, Betatrex, Valisone, Valnac
Classification:
Corticosteroid

Bethanechol chloride [be-**than**-e-kole]
DuVoid, Myotonochol, Urebeth, Urechloine,
Urolax
Classification:
Cholinergic (direct-acting)

Bisacodyl [bis-a-**koe**-dill]
{Bisacolax}, Bisco-Lax, Carter's Little Pills,
Dacodyl, Deficol, Dulcogen, Dulcolax, Fleet
Laxative, {Laxit}, Theralax
Classification:
Laxative (stimulant)

Botulinum [bot-u-**lee**-num]
Classification:
Antitoxin

Bromocriptine [broe-moe-**krip**-teen]
Parlodel
Classification:
Antiparkinsonian

Bumetanide [byoo-**met**-a-nide]
Bumex
Classification:
Diuretic (loop)

Calcitonin [kal-si-**toe**-nin]
Salmon: Calcimar, Miacalcin. Human: Cibacalcin
Classifications:
Hormone, electrolyte modifier (hypocalcemic)

Calcium carbonate [**kal**-see-um] [**kar**-boh-nate]
Cal Carb-Hd, Calciday, Cal-Sup, Caltrate,
Gencalc, Nephro-calci, Os-Cal, Oysco, Oystcal,
Titrilac, Tums
Classification:
Electrolyte

Carbamazepine [kar-ba-**maz**-e-peen]
{Apo-Carbamazepine}, Epitol, {Mazepine}, {Novo Carbamaz}, Tegretol
Classification:
Anticonvulsant

Carbamide peroxide [**kar**-ba-mid]
Murine Ear
Classification:
Otic

Carbidopa-Levodopa [**kar**-bi-doe-pa] [**lee**-voe-doe-pa]
Sinemet, Sinemet CR
Classification:
Antiparkinsonian

Cefazolin [sef-**a**-zoe-lin]
Ancef, Kefzol, Zolicef
Classification:
Anti-infective (cephalosporin)

Cefoxitin [se-**fox**-i-tin]
Mefoxin
Classification:
Anti-infective (second-generation cephalosporin)

Ceftriaxone [cef-try-**ax**-one]
Rocephin
Classification:
Anti-infective (third-generation cephalosporin)

Chloramphenicol [klor-am-**fen**-i-kole]
AK-Chlor, Chlorofair, Chloromycetin, Chloroptic, Econochlor, {Fenicol}, {Novochlorocap}, Ocu-Chlor, Ophthochlor, {Pentamycetin}, {Sopamycetin}, Spectro-Chlor
Classification:
Anti-infective

Chlordiazepoxide hydrochloride [klor-dye-az-e-**pox**-ide]
Librium
Classification:
Antianxiety agent

Chlortetracycline [klor-te-tra-**sye**-kleen]
Aureomycin Ointment 3%, Aureomycin Ophthalmic 1%
Classification:
Anti-infective (tetracycline)

Cholestyramine [koe-less-**tear**-a-meen]
Cholybar, Questran, Questran Light
Classification:
Lipid-lowering agent

Cimetidine [sye-**met**-i-deen]
{Apo-Cimetidine}, {Novocimetine}, {Peptol}, Tagamet
Classification:
Antiulcer (histamine H_2 antagonist)

Clofibrate [kloe-**fye**-brate]
Atromid-S, Claripex, Novofibrate
Classification:
Cholesterol-lowering agent

Clotrimazole [kloe-**try**-my-zole]
{Canesten}, Gyne-Lotrimin, Lotrimin, Mycelex-7, Mycelex-G, Mycelex-OTC
Classification:
Anti-infective

Colchicine [**kol**-chi-seen]
Classification:
Antigout agent

Colestipol [koe-less-**tip**-ole]
Colestid
Classification:
Lipid-lowering agent

Cromolyn sodium [**kro**-my-lon]
Crolom, Gastrocrom, Intal Spray Aerosol, Nasalcrom
Classification:
Miscellaneous respiratory agent

Cyanocobalamin [sye-an-oh-koe-**bal**-a-min]
Anacobin, Bedoz, Berubigen, Betalin 12, Cobex,
Crystamine, Crysti-12, Cyanabin, Cyanoject,
Kayborite, Redisol, Rubesol, Rubion, Rubramin
PC, Sytobex, Vitamin B$_{12}$
Classification:
Vitamin B$_{12}$

Cyclobenzaprine [sye-kloe-**ben**-za-preen]
Cycloflex, Flexeril
Classification:
Skeletal muscle relaxant (centrally acting)

Cyclosporine [**sye**-kloe-spor-een]
Ciclosporin, Cyclosporin A, Sandimmune
Classification:
Immunosuppressant

Desoximetasone [des-ox-i-**met**-a-sone]
Topicort
Classifications:
Anti-inflammatory, topical glucocorticoid

Dexamethasone [dex-a-**meth**-a-sone]
Aeroseb-Dex, Decaderm, Decadron, Decaspray,
Deronil, Dexameth, Dexamethasone Intensol,
Dexasone, Dexone, Hexadrol, Maxidex,
Mymethasone
Classifications:
Anti-inflammatory, glucocorticoid, antiemetic,
corticosteroid, diagnostic

Dextroamphetamine [dex-troe-am-**fet**-a-meen]
Dexedrine, Ferndex, Oxydess II, Spancap #1
Classification:
CNS stimulant

Diazepam [dye-**az**-e-pam]
{Apo-Diazepam}, {Diazemuls}, {Novodipam},
T-Quil, Valium, Valrelease, Vazepam, {Vivol},
Zetran
Classifications:
Sedative/hypnotic (benzodiazepine), anticonvul-
sant (benzodiazepine), skeletal muscle relaxant
(centrally acting)

Diazoxide [dye-az-**ox**-ide]
Hyperstat, Proglycem
Classifications:
Antihypertensive (vasodilator), hyperglycemic

Digitoxin [di-ji-**tox**-in]
Crystodigin
Classifications:
Cardiac glycoside, inotropic agent, antiarrhythmic

Digoxin [di-**jox**-in]
Lanoxicaps, Lanoxin, {Novodigoxin}
Classifications:
Cardiac glycoside, inotropic agent, anti-
arrhythmic

Diltiazem [dil-**tye**-a-zeem]
{Apo-Diltiaz}, Cardizem, Cardizem SR, Cardizem
CD, Dilacor XR
Classifications:
Calcium channel blocker, antianginal, coronary
vasodilator

Diphenhydramine [dye-fen-**hye**-dra-meen]
{Allerdryl}, AllerMax, Belix, Bena-D, Benadryl,
Benahist, Ben-Allergin, Benaphen, Benoject,
Benylin, Bydramine, Dihydrex, Diphen,
Diphenacen, Diphenadryl, Dormarex 2, Genahist,
Gen-D-phen, Hydramine, Hydramyn, Hyrexin,
{Insomnal}, Maximum Strength Nytol, Nervine
Nighttime Sleep-Aid, Nidryl, Nordryl, Phendry,
Sleep-Eze 3, Sominex, Tusstat, Twilite, Valdrene,
Wehdryl
Classifications:
Antihistamine, antitussive

Diphenoxylate hydrochloride/atropine [dye-fen-
ox-i-late]
Diphenatol, Lofene, Logen, Lomanate, Lomotil,
Lonox, Lo-Trol, Normil
Classification:
Antidiarrheal

Disopyramide [dye-soe-**peer**-a-mide]
Norpace, Norpace CR, {Rythmodan},
{Raythmodan-LA}
Classification:
Antiarrhythmic (group I)

Disulfiram [dye-**sul**-fi-ram]
Antabuse
Classification:
Alcohol abuse deterrent

Divalproex Sodium [dye-val-**pro**-ex] [**soe**-dee-um]
Depakote, {Epival}
Classification:
Anticonvulsant

Docusate sodium [**dok**-yoo-sate]
Colace, Dioeze, Diocto, Diosul, Disonate, DOK,
DOS Softgels, DOSS, Doxinate, DSS, Laxinate
100, Modane Soft, Regulax SS, {Regulex}, Regutol,
Therevac, Therevac SB
Classification:
Laxative (stool softener)

Dopamine [**doe**-pa-meen]
Dopastat, Intropin, {Revimine}
Classifications:
Vasopressor, inotropic agent

Dornase alfa [**dor**-nas]
Pulmozyme
Classification:
Miscellaneous respiratory agent

Doxorubicin [dox-oh-**roo**-bi-sin]
Adriamycin PFS, Adriamycin RDF, Rubex
Classification:
Antineoplastic (anthracycline)

Edrophonium [ed-roe-**fone**-ee-yum]
Enon, Reversol, Tensilon
Classification:
Cholinergic (anticholinesterase)

Enalapril [e-**nal**-a-pril]
Vasotec

Classifications:
Antihypertensive, angiotensin-converting
enzyme (ACE) inhibitor

Epinephrine (parenteral) [ep-i-**nef**-rin]
Adrenalin, AsthmaHaler, Bronkaid, Dysne-Inhal,
Medihaler-Epi, Primatene
Classifications:
Bronchodilator (adrenergic), cardiac stimulant,
ophthalmic (antiglaucomal)

Erythromycin [er-ith-roe-**mye**-sin]
Base: {Apo-Erythro-EC}, E-Base, E-Mycin,
{Erybid}, Eryc, Eryc-Sprinkle, Ery-tab,
{Erythromid}, PCE Dispersatabs, Robimycin.
Estolate: Erythrozone, Ilosone, {Novorythro}.
Ethyl-Succinate: {Apo-Erythro-ES}, E.E.S,
EryPed, Erythro. **Lactobionate:** Erythrocin.
Stearate: Eramycin, Erythrocin, {Novorythro},
Erythrocot, My-E, Wintrocin, Wyamycin S.
Ophthalmic: Ilotycin. **Topical:** Akne-Mycin,
Erycette, Erygel, Erymax, ETS, Mythromycin,
Staticin, T-stat.
Classification:
Anti-infective (macrolide)

Ethinyl estradiol [**eth**-i-nil]
Estinyl
Classification:
Hormonal (estrogen)

Famciclovir [fam-**sys**-kloe-ver]
Famvir
Classification:
Antiviral

Famotidine [fa-**moe**-ti-deen]
Pepcid
Classifications:
Histamine H_2 receptor antagonist, antiulcer agent

Fentanyl (parenteral) [**fen**-ta-nil]
Sublimaze
Classification:
Opioid analgesic (agonist)

Fentanyl (transdermal) [**fen**-ta-nil]
Duragesic
Classification:
Opioid analgesic (agonist)

Ferrous sulfate [**fer**-us **sul**-fate]
{Apo-Ferrous Sulfate}, Feosol, Fer-In-Sol, Fer-Iron, {Fero-Grad}, Fero-Gradumet, Ferralyn, Ferra-TD, Mol-Iron, {Novoferrosulfa}, {PMS Ferrous Sulfate}, Slow Fe
Classifications:
Antianemic, iron supplement

Fluconazole [floo-**kon**-a-zole]
Diflucan
Classification:
Antifungal

Flucytosine [floo-**sye**-toe-seen]
Ancobon, {Ancotil}, 5-FC
Classification:
Antifungal

Fludarabine [floo-**dar**-a-been]
Fludara
Classification:
Antineoplastic (antimetabolite)

Flumazenil [flu-**maz**-e-nil]
Romazicon
Classification:
Antidote (benzodiazepine antagonist)

Fluorouracil [flure-oh-**yoor**-a-sil]
Adrucil, Efudex, Fluoroplex, 5-FU
Classification:
Antineoplastic (antimetabolite)

Fluoxetine [floo-**ox**-uh-teen]
Prozac
Classification:
Antidepressant

Folic acid [**foe**-lik **as**-id]
{Apo-Folic}, Folate, Folvite, {Novofolacid}, Vitamin B_9

Classifications:
Vitamin (water-soluble), antianemic

Furosemide [fur-**oh**-se-mide]
{Apo-Furosemide}, {Furoside}, Lasix, Myrosemide, {Novosemide}, {Uritol}
Classification:
Diuretic (loop)

Ganciclovir [gan-**sys**-kloe-vir]
Cytovene
Classification:
Antiviral

Gentamicin [jen-ta-**mye**-sin]
{Alcomicin}, {Cidomycin}, Garamycin, Genoptic, Gentafair, Gentak, Gentrasul, G-Mycon, Jenamicin, Ocu-Mycin, Spectro-Genta
Classification:
Anti-infective (aminoglycoside)

Glipizide [**glip**-i-zide]
Glucotrol
Classification:
Oral hypoglycemic agent (sulfonylureas)

Glucagon [**gloo**-ka-gon]
Classification:
Hormone (pancreatic)

Glyburide [**gli**-bu-ride]
Glynase, Glynase Pres Tab, Micronase
Classification:
Hormonal (antidiabetic)

Griseofulvin microsize [gris-ee-oh-**ful**-vin]
Grifulvin, Grisacton, Grisovin
Classification:
Local anti-infective

Haloperidol [ha-loe-**per**-i-dole]
{Apo-Haloperidol}, Haldol, Haldol Decanoate, {Haldo L.A.}, {Novoperidol}, {Peridol}
Classification:
Antipsychotic (butyrophenone)

Heparin sodium [hep-a-rin]
{Calcilean}, Calciparine, {Hepalean}, {Heparin Leo}, Liquaemin
Classification:
Anticoagulant

Hetastarch [het-a-starch]
Hespan
Classification:
Volume expander

Hydrochlorothiazide [hye-droe-klor-oh-**thye**-a-zide] {Apo-Hydro}, {Duiclor H}, Esidrex, Ezide, HCTZ, HydroDIURIL, Hydro-Par, {Natrimax}, {Neo-Codema}, Novo-Hydrazide, Oretic, {Urozide}
Classifications:
Diuretic (thiazide), antihypertensive

Ibuprofen [eye-byoo-**proe**-fen]
Aches-N-Pain, {Acitprofen}, Advil, {Amersol}, {Apo-Ibuprofen}, Children's Motrin, Excedrin IB, Genpril, Haltran, Ibuprin, Ibuprohm, Ibu-Tab, Medipren, Midol 200, Notrin, Motrin IB, {Novoprofen}, Nurpin, Pamprin-IB, Rufen, Saleto, Trendar
Classifications:
Nonsteroidal anti-inflammatory agent, nonopioid analgesic, antipyretic

Idoquinol [eye-oh-do-**kwin**-ole]
Diiodohydroxyquin, Diodoquin, Moebiquin, Sebaquin, Yodoxin
Classifications:
Anti-infective, antiprotozoal, amebicide

Indomethacin [in-doe-**meth**-a-sin]
Indocin, Indocin-SR
Classification:
Nonsteroidal anti-inflammatory

Insulin [in-su-lin]
Rapid-acting: Regular (Actrapid, Humulin R, Iletin I, Iletin II, Iletin II U-500 [concentrated], Novolin R, Velosulin); prompt zinc suspension (Semilente, Semilente Iletin, Semitard)

Intermediate-acting: isophane suspension (Humulin N, Iletin II, Insultard NPH, Lentard, Novolin N, NPH, NPH Purified); zinc suspension (Humulin L, Lente, Lente Iletin, Monotard, Novolin L)

Long-acting: extended zinc suspension (Humulin U, Ultralente, Ultralente Iletin, Ultratard)

Insulin Mixture: Regular plus NPH (Humulin 70/30, Mixtard 70/30, Novolin 70/30)
Classification:
Hormone (pancreatic)

Interferon Alpha-2b [in-ter-**feer**-on]
a-2-interferon, Intron A
Classifications:
Antineoplastic, antiviral, immunomodulator

Ipecac Syrup [ip-e-kak]
Classification:
Emetic

Iron Dextran [eye-ern **dex**-tran]
{Imferon}, InFeD
Classifications:
Antianemic, iron supplement

Ketorolac [kee-**toe**-role-ak]
Toradol
Classifications:
Nonopioid analgesic, nonsteroidal anti-inflammatory

Leucovorin [loo-koe-**vor**-in]
Citrovorum factor, 5-Formyl Tetrahydrofolate, Folinic Acid, Wellcovorin
Classifications:
Antidote (for methotrexate and folic acid antagonists), vitamin (folic acid analog)

Levamisole [lee-**vam**-i-sole]
Ergamisole
Classification:
Antineoplastic (immunomodulator)

Levodopa [**lee**-voe-doe-pa]
Dopar, Larodopa, L-Dopa
Classification:
Antiparkinsonian (dopamine agonist)

Levothyroxine [lee-voe-thye-**rox**-een]
{Eltroxin}, Levothroid, Levoxine, Synthroid, T_4
Classification:
Hormone (thyroid)

Lidocaine [**lye**-doe-kane]
Anestacon, Baylocaine, L-Caine, LidoPen,
Xylocaine, {Xylogard}
Classifications:
Antiarrhythmic (group IB), anesthetic (local)

Lindane [**lin**-dane]
Bio-well, Gamma benzene hexachloride, GBH,
G-well, Kwell, {Kwellada}, Kwildane, Scabene,
Thionex
Classification:
Antiparasitic

Mafenide acetate [**maf**-en-id]
Sulfamylon
Classification:
Local anti-infective

Mannitol [**man**-i-tol]
Osmitrol
Classification:
Diuretic (osmotic)

Mebendazole [me-**ben**-da-zole]
{Nemasole}, Vermox
Classification:
Antihelmintic

Meperidine Hydrochloride [me-**per**-I-deen]
[hy-droe-**klor**-ide]
Demerol, Pethadol, Pethidine
Classification:
Opioid analgesic (agonist)

Methocarbamol [meth-oh-**kar**-ba-mole]

Delaxin, Marbaxin, Robaxin, Robomol
Classification:
Skeletal muscle relaxant (centrally acting)

Methotrexate [meth-o-**trex**-ate]
Amethopterin, Folex, Folex PFS, Rheumatrex
Classifications:
Antineoplastic (antimetabolite),
immunosuppressant

Metolazone [me-**tole**-a-zone]
Mykrox, Zarozolyn
Classifications:
Diuretic (thiazide-like), antihypertensive

Metoprolol [me-**toe**-proe-lole]
{Apo-Metoprolol}, {Betaloc}, {Betaloc Durules},
Lopressor, {Lopressor SR}, {Novometoprol},
Toprop XL
Classifications:
Antihypertensive, antianginal, beta-adrenergic
blocker (selective)

Metronidazole [me-troe-**ni**-da-zole]
{Apo-Metronidazole}, Flagyl, Metizol, Metric 21,
MetroGel, Metro IV, Metryl, Metryl IV, {Neo-
Metric}, {Novonidazoel}, {PMS Metrodiazole},
Protostat, Satric, {Trikacide}
Classification:
Anti-infective

Morphine sulfate [**mor**-feen]
Astramorph PF, Duramorph, {Epimorph},
{Morphine H.P.}, {Morphitec}, {M.O.S.}, M.O.S.-
S.R.}, MS, MSO_4, MS Contin, MSIR, MSIR
Capsules, OMS Concentrate, Oramorph SR, RMS,
Roxanol, Roxanol SR {Statex}
Classification:
Opioid analgesic (agonist)

Nalbuphine [**nal**-byoo-feen]
Nubain
Classification:
Opioid analgesic (agonist/antagonist)

Naloxone [nal-**ox**-one]
Narcan
Classification:
Antidote (for opioids}

Naproxen sodium [na-**prox**-en]
Aleve, Anaprox, Anaprox DS, Naprelan
Classification:
Nonsteroidal anti-inflammatory

Neomycin [nee-oh-**mye**-sin]
Mycifradin, Myciguent
Classification:
Anti-infective (aminoglycoside)

Nifedipine [nye-**fed**-i-peen]
Adalat, Adalat CC, {Adalat P.A.}, {Apo-Nifed},
{Novo-Nifedin}, {NuNifed}, Procardia, Procardia
XL
Classifications:
Calcium channel blocker, antianginal, coronary
vasodilator, antihypertensive

Nitroglycerin [nye-troe-**gli**-ser-in]
Nitroglycerin extended-release capsules:
Nitrobid, Nitrocap T.D., Nitrocine, Nitroglyn,
Nitrolin; **Nitroglycerin extended-release tablets:**
Klavikordal, Niong, Nitronet, Nitrong; **Nitro-
glycerin extended-release buccal tablets:**
Nitrogard, {Nitrogard SR}; **Nitroglycerin intra-
venous:** Nitro-bid, Tridil; **Nitroglycerin lingual
spray:** Nitrolingual; **Nitroglycerin ointment:**
Nitro-bid, Nitrol, Nitrong; **Nitroglycerin sublin-
gual:** Nitrostat; **Nitroglycerin transdermal:**
Deponit, Minitran, Nitrodisc, Nitro-Dur, Nitro-
Dur II, NTS, Transderm-Nitro
Classifications:
Vasodilator (nitrate), antianginal, coronary
vasodilator

Nitroprusside [nye-troe-**pruss**-ide]
Nitropress
Classification:
Antihypertensive (vasodilator)

Nizatidine [ni-**za**-ti-deen]

Axid
Classifications:
Histamine H_2 antagonist, antiulcer

Norepinephrine [**nor**-ep-i-nef-rin]
Levarterenol, Levophed
Classification:
Vasopressor

Nortriptyline Hydrochloride [nor-**trip**-ti-leen]
[hy-droe-**klor**-ide]
Aventyl, Pamelor
Classification:
Antidepressant (tricyclic)

Nystatin [nye-**stat**-in]
Mycostatin, {Nadostine}, {Nyaderm}, Nystex
Classification:
Antifungal

Oxamniquine [ox-**am**-ni-kwin]
Vansil
Classification:
Anthelmintic

Oxytocin [ox-i-**toe**-sin]
Pitocin, Syntocinon
Classification:
Hormone (oxytocic)

Paclitaxel [pa-kli-**tax**-el]
Taxol
Classification:
Antineoplastic (antimicrotubule agent)

Pancrelipase [pan-kree-**li**-pase]
Catozym, Cotazym-S, Cotazym-65 B, Cotazym
E.C.S. 8, Cotazym E.C.S. 20, Enzymase-16,
Ilozyme, Ku-Zume HP, Pancrease, Pancrease
MT 4, Pancrease MT 10, Pancoate, Pancrease
MT 16, Protilase, Ultrase MT 12, Ultrase MT 20,
Ultrase MT 24, Viokase, Zymase
Classification:
Pancreatic

Paroxetine [par-**ox**-e-teen]
Paxil

Penicillin G Procaine [pen-i-**sill**-in] [jee] [**proe**-cane]
{Ayercillin}, Crysticillin A.S., Pfizerpen-AS, Wycillin
Classification:
Anti-infective (penicillin)

Pentaerythritol Tetranitrate [pen-ta-er-**ith**-ri-tole tet-ra-**nye**-trate]
Duotrate, Naptrate, Pentol, Pentritol, Pentylan, Peritrate, P.E.T.N.
Classifications:
Vasodilator, antianginal, nitrate

Pentamidine [pen-**tam**-i-deen]
Nebupent, Pentam, {Pentacarinat}, {Pneumopent}
Classification:
Anti-infective (antiprotozoal)

Phenytoin [**fen**-i-toyn]
Dyphenylhydantoin, DPH, Dilantin, Diphenylan
Classifications:
Anticonvulsant (hydantoin), antiarrhythmic (group IB)

Pilocarpine [pye-loe-**kar**-peen]
Adsorbocarpine, Akarpine, Isopto Carpine, Ocu-Carpine, Pilagan, Pilocar, Piloptic, Pilostat, Pilopto-Carpine, Ocusert-Pilo
Classification:
Ophthalmic cholinergic agent (direct-acting)

Piperazine Adipate [**pi**-per-a-zeen][**add**-i-pate]
{Entacyl}
Classification:
Anthelmintic

Potassium Chloride [poe-**tass**-ee-um]
Apo-K, Cena-K, Gen-K, K-10, {Kalium Durules}, Kaochlor, Kaochlor S-F, Kaon Cl, Kato, Kay Ciel, KCl, K-Dur, {K-Long}, K- Lor, Klor-10%, Klor-Con, Klorvess, Klotrix, K-Lyte/Cl Powder, K- Norm, K+Care, K+10, K-Lease, {K-Long], K-Tab, Micro-K, LS, {Novolente-K}, Potachlor, Potasalan, Rum-K, Slow-K, Ten-K
Classification:
Electrolyte (potassium supplement)

Prazosin [pra-**zoe**-in]
Minipress
Classification:
Antihypertensive (peripherally acting anti-adrenergic)

Prednisolone [pred-**niss**-oh-lone]
Articulose, Delta-Cortef, Hydeltra-T.B.A., Hyudeltrasol, Key-Pred, Nor-Pred T.B.A., Pediapred, Predaject, Predalone, Predalone T.B.A., Predate, Predocor, Predicort, Prednisol, Prelone
Classification:
Glucocorticoid (intermediate-acting)

Prednisone [**pred**-ni-sone]
{Apo-Prednisone}, Deltasone, Liquid Pred, Meticorten, Orasone, Panasol, Prednicen-M, Sterapred, {Winpred}
Classification:
Glucocorticoid (intermediate-acting)

Probenecid [proe-**ben**-e-sid]
Benemid, {Benuryl}, Probalan
Classification:
Antigout agent (uricosuric)

Procainamide [pro-**kane**-ah-mide]
Procan SR, Promine, Pronestyl, Pronestyl-SR
Classification:
Antiarrhythmic (group IA)

Prochlorperazine [proe-klor-**pair**-a-zeen]
Chlorpazine, Compa-Z, Compazine, Contranzine, {Provazin}, {Stemetil}, Ultrazine
Classifications:
Antiemetic (phenothiazine), antipsychotic

Promethazine [proe-**meth**-a-zeen]
Anergan, {Histanil}, Mallergan, Pentazine, Phenameth, Phenazine, Phencen-50, Phenergan, Phenergan Fortis, Phenergan Plain, Phenoject-50, {PMS Promethazine}, Pro-50, Prometh-25, Prometh-50, Prorex, Prothazine Plain, Remsed, V-Gan
Classifications:
Antihistamine (phenothiazine), antiemetic, sedative/hypnotic

Propranolol [proe-**pran**-oh-lole]
{Apo-Propranolol}, {Detensol}, Inderal, Inderal-LA, {Novopranol}
Classifications:
Antihypertensive, antianginal, beta-adrenergic blocker (nonselective), antiarrhythmic

Protamine Sulfate [**proe**-ta-meen]
Classification:
Antidote (antiheparin agent)

Pseudoephedrine [soo-doe-e-**fed**-rin]
Afrin, Drixoral
Classification:
Adrenergic (sympathomimetic)

Pyridostigmine bromide [peer-id-oh-**stig**-meen]
Mestinon, Mestinon Timespan, Regonol
Classification:
Cholinergic (anticholinesterase)

Quinidine gluconate [**kwin**-i-deen]
Duraquin, Quinaglute, Quinlan
Classification:
Antiarrhythmic

Ramipril [**ram**-i-pril]
Altace
Classification:
Antihypertensive (angiotensin-converting enzyme (ACE) inhibitor)

Ranitidine [ra-**nye**-te-deen]
{Apo-Ranitidine}, Zantac, {Zantac-C}
Classifications:
Histamine H_2 antagonist, antiulcer

Rh₀ (D) Immune Globulin [**arr**-aych-oh] {dee} [im-**yoon**] [**glob**-yoo-lin]
Standard dose: Gamulin Rh, HypRho-D, Rhesonativ, RhoGam; Microdose: HypRho-D Mini-Dose, MICRhoGam, Mini-Gamulin Rh
Classification:
Immune globulin

Ritodrine Hydrochloride [**ri**-toe-dreen] [hye-droe-**klor**-ide]
Yutopar
Classifications:
Beta-adrenergic agonist, tocolytic

Rubella virus vaccine [roo-**bel**-a]
Meruvax II
Classification:
Immunomodulator (vaccine)

Silver nitrate [**sil**-ver] [**nye**-trate]
Ophthalmic solution 1%
Classification:
Ophthalmic anti-infective

Silver Sulfadiazine [**sil**-ver] [sul-fa-**dye**-a-zeen]
{Flamazine}, Flint SSD, Silvadene, Thermazene
Classification:
Anti-infective (topical)

Sodium Bicarbonate [**soe**-dee-um] [bye-**kar**-boe-nate]
Baking Soda, Bellans, Citrocarbonate, Neut, Soda Mint
Classifications:
Electrolyte modifier (alkalinizing agent, antacid)

Sodium Polystyrene Sulfonate [**soe**-dee-um] [pa-lee-**stye**-reen] [sul-**fon**-ate]
Kayexalate, SPS
Classification:
Electrolyte modifier (cation exchange resin)

Spironolactone [speer-oh-no-**lak**-tone]
Aldactone, {Novospiroton}
Classification:
Diuretic (potassium-sparing)

Streptomycin [strep-toe-**mye**-sin]
Classifications:
Anti-infective (aminoglycoside), antitubercular

Sucralfate [soo-**kral**-fate]
Carafate, {Sulcrate}
Classification:
Antiulcer agent (protectant)

Sulconazole Nitrate [sul-**kon**-a-zole] [**nye**-trate]
Exelderm
Classification:
Antifungal (topical)

Sulfasalazine [sul-fa-**sal**-a-zen]
Azulfidine
Classification:
Miscellaneous uncategorized drug

Tamoxifen [ta-**mox**-i-fen]
Nolvadex, {Nolvades-D}, {Novo-Tamoxifen}, {Tamofen}, {Tamone}
Classification:
Antineoplastic (estrogen blocker)

Terbutaline [ter-**byoo**-ta-leen]
Brethaire, Brethine, Bricanyl
Classification:
Bronchodilator (beta-adrenergic agonist)

Terconazole [ter-**kon**-a-zole]
Terazol
Classification:
Antifungal (vaginal)

Tetracycline [te-tra-**sye**-kleen]
Achromycin, Alatet, {Apo-Tetra}, Nor-tet, {Novotetra}, {Nu-Tetra}, Panmycin, Robitet, Sumycin, Teline, Tetracap, Tetracyn, Tetralan, Topicycline
Classification:
Anti-infective (tetracycline)

Theophylline [thee-**off**-i-lin]
Accurbron, Aerolate, Aquaphyllin, Asmalix, Bronkodyl, Elixomin, Elixophyllin, Lanophyllin, Lixolin {Pulmophylline}, Slophyllin Syrup, Synophylate, Theoclear, Theolair, Theon, Theophyl, Theostat
Extended Release: Aerolate, Constant-T, Elixophyllin SR, LaBID, Quibron-T/SR, Respid, Slo-bid Gyrocaps, Slophyllin, Sustaire, T- Phyl, Theo-24, Theobid Duracap, Theobid Jr, Duracap, Theochron, Theoclear LA, Theoclear LA Cenules, Theo-Dur, Theo-Dur Sprinkle, Theolair-SR,

Theophyl-SR, Theospan-SR, Theo-Sav, Theo-Time, Theovent Long-Acting, Uniphyl
Classification:
Bronchodilator (phosphodiesterase inhibitor)

Thiabendazole [thye-a-**ben**-a-zole]
Mintezol
Classifications:
Anthelmintic, enzyme inhibitor

Tolbutamide [tole-**byoo**-ta-mide]
{Apo-Tolbutamide}, {Mobenol}, {Novobutamide}, Oramide, Orinase
Classification:
Oral hypoglycemic agent (sulfonylureas)

Torsemide [**tor**-see-mide]
Classification:
Loop diuretic

Tranylcypromine sulfate [tran-il-**si**-pro-men]
Parnate
Classification:
Antidepressant

Triazolam [trye-**az**-oh-lam]
{Apo-Triazo}, Halcion, {Novotriolam}, {Nu-Triazo}
Classification:
Sedative/hypnotic (benzodiazepine)

Trihexyphenidyl hydrochloride
[tyre-hex-ee-**fen**-i-dill]
Artane, Artane Sequels, Trihexane
Classification:
Antiparkinsonian

Trimethoprim [trye-**meth**-oh-prim]
Proloprim, Trimpex
Classification:
Anti-infective

Triprolidine hydrochloride [trye-**proe**-li-deen]
Actidil, Alleract, Myidl
Classification:
Antihistamine

Tuberculin purified protein derivative (PPD)
[too-**bur**-que-lin]
Aplisol, PPD-Stabilized Solution
Classification:
Diagnostic

Vasopressin [vas-o-**pres**-in]
Pitressin
Classification:
Hormonal (pituitary)

Vecuronium [ve-**kure**-oh-nee-yum]
Norcuron
Classification:
Neuromuscular blocking agent (nondepolarizing)

Verapamil [ver-**ap**-a-mil]
Calan, Calan SR, Isoptin, Isoptin SR, Verelan
Classifications:
Calcium channel blocker, antianginal, antihypertensive, antiarrhythmic, coronary vasodilator

Vincristine [vin-**kriss**-teen]
Oncovin, Vincasar PFS
Classification:
Antineoplastic agent (vinca alkaloid)

Vitamin A (beta carotene) [**vye**-ta-min A]
Aquasol A, Del-Vi-A
Classification:
Vitamin (fat-soluble)

Vitamin B (dexpanthenol) [dex-**pan**-the-nole]
Llopan, Panthoderm
Classifications:
Cholinergic (direct-acting); vitamin B complex

Vitamin B$_6$ (pyridoxine) [peer-i-**dox**-een]
Beesix, {Hexa-Betalin}, Nestrex, Rodex, Vitabee 6,
Vitamin B$_6$
Classification:
Vitamin (water-soluble)

Vitamin C (ascorbic acid) [as-**kor**-bic-] [**as**-id]
Vitamin C, {Apo-C}, Ascorbicap, Cecon, Cemill,
Cetane, Cevalin, Ce-Vi-Sol, Flavorcee
Classification:
Vitamin (water-soluble)

Vitamin D (dihydrotachysterol) [dye-hye-droe-
tak-**iss**-ter-ole]
DNT, DHT Intensol, Hytakerol
Classifications:
Vitamin D, serum calcium regulator

Vitamin K$_1$ (phytonadione) [fye-toe-na-**dye**-one]
AquaMEPHYTON, Konakion, Mephyton
Classification:
Vitamin (fat-soluble)

Warfarin sodium [**war**-far-in]
Coumadin, Sofarin, {Warfilone}
Classification:
Anticoagulant

FDA Pregnancy Risk Categories

The developing fetus of a pregnant woman is at potential risk for birth defects and death when exposed to medications. The U.S. Food and Drug Administration (FDA) has authorized five categories (Categories A, B, C, D, and X) that indicate some medications' potential for producing birth defects or fetal death. The identifying letters signal the level of risk to the fetus. The risks follow a continuum from safe to unsafe. Medications in Category A are generally viewed as safe for pregnant women, whereas medications in Category X are generally deemed unsafe and are contraindicated.

Category	Description
A	Controlled studies in pregnant women have not demonstrated a risk to the fetus. The potential for fetal harm appears remote.
B	Somewhat more of a risk to the fetus than Category A. Animal studies show no risk to a fetus. However, studies have not been completed in women—or, animal studies do indicate a risk to the fetus, but studies in women do not indicate a risk.
C	Greater risk than Category B. Animal studies do show a risk of fetal harm. However, no studies have been completed in women—or no studies have been completed in women or animals.
D	Proven risk of harm to the fetus. Studies in pregnant women provide proof of fetal damage. This medication should be used only if the risk of the untreated condition for the woman is greater than the risk of the medication for the fetus. A statement of fetal risk will appear in the WARNING section of medication labeling.
X	Proven risk of harm to the fetus. Studies in pregnant women and animals indicate definite risk of fetal abnormalities. Fetal risks outweigh all possible benefits. A statement of risk appears in the CONTRAINDICATIONS section of medication labeling.

Table of Measurement Equivalents

Health-care providers prescribing, dispensing, and/or administering medications should abide by the protocols of the facility where they work. When dosage calculations are required, they should be checked by a pharmacist before administering.

The following charts express approximate liquid and dry weights and their equivalents and conversions, with metric measures as the standard and apothecary and household (British imperial) measures afterward.

LIQUID MEASUREMENTS

Metric	Approximate Apothecary Equivalents	Approximate Household Equivalents
1000 ml	32 fluid ounces (1 quart)	1 quart
500 ml	16 fluid ounces (1 pint)	1 pint
250 ml	8 fluid ounces	1 cup
30 ml	1 fluid ounce	2 tablespoons
15 ml	4 fluid drams	1 tablespoon
4 or 5 ml	1 fluid dram	1 teaspoon
1 ml	15 or 16 minims	1/4 teaspoon
0.06 ml	1 minim	1 drop

[1 milliliter (ml) is the approximate equivalent of 1 cubic centimeter (cc).]

APPROXIMATE SOLID EQUIVALENTS

Avoirdupois	Apothecary
1 grain (gr)	1 grain (gr)
15.4 gr	15 gr
1 ounce	480 gr
1 pound (lb)	1.33 lb
2.2 lb	2.7 lb

WEIGHTS

Metric	Apothecary
30 gm	1 ounce
15 gm	4 drams
4 gm	60 grains (1 dram)
1 gm	15 or 16 grains
300 mg	5 grains
60 mg	1 grain
30 mg	1/2 grain
10 mg	1/6 grain
6 mg	1/10 grain
1 mg	1/60 grain
0.6 mg	1/100 grain
0.5 mg	1/120 grain
0.4 mg	1/150 grain
0.3 mg	1/200 grain
0.2 mg	1/300 grain
0.1 mg	1/600 grain

Metric Conversions

1 kg	=	1000 gm
1 gm	=	1000 mg
1 mg	=	0.001 gm
1 mcg	=	0.001 mg

1 gram (gm)	=	1000 milligrams (mg)
1000 grams	=	1 kilogram (kg)
.001 milligram	=	1 microgram (mcg)
1 meter	=	100 centimeters (cm)
1 meter	=	1000 millimeters (mm)

Conversion Equivalents

Metric	Metric Equivalents	Apothecary
1 gram (g)	1000 milligrams	15 grains
0.6 gram	600 milligrams	10 grains
0.5 gram	500 milligrams	7.5 grains
0.3 gram	300 milligrams	5 grains
0.06 gram	60 milligrams	1 grain

VOLUME

Metric	Apothecary	Household
1 milliliter	15 minims (M)	15 drops (gtt)
5 milliliters	1 fluid dram (ℨ)	1 teaspoon (tsp)
15 milliliters	4 fluid drams	1 tablespoon (T)
30 milliliters	1 ounce (oz)	2 tablespoons
500 milliliters	1 pint (pt)	1 pint (pt)
1000 milliliters	1 quart (qt)	1 quart (qt)

Conversion Equivalents

Metric	Metric Equivalents	Apothecary
1 liter (l)	1000 milliliters (ml)	1 quart (qt)
1 deciliter (dl)	100 milliliters (ml)	3.2 fluid ounces (fl oz)
1 milliliter (ml)	1 cubic centimeter (cc)	15 minims (M)

APOTHECARIES' METRIC

15 grains	=	1000 mg	1/6 grain	=	10 mg
10 grains	=	600 mg	1/10 grain	=	6 mg
5 grains	=	300 mg	1/15 grain	=	4 mg
1 1/2 grains	=	100 mg	1/20 grain	=	3 mg
1 grain	=	60 mg	1/30 grain	=	2 mg
3/4 grain	=	45 mg	1/60 grain	=	1 mg
2/3 grain	=	40 mg	1/100 grain	=	0.6 mg
1/2 grain	=	30 mg	1/200 grain	=	0.3 mg
3/8 grain	=	25 mg	1/250 grain	=	0.25 mg
1/3 grain	=	20 mg	1/300 grain	=	0.2 mg
1/4 grain	=	15 mg	1/600 grain	=	0.1 mg
1/5 grain	=	12 mg	1/1000 grain	=	0.06 mg

HOUSEHOLD METRIC

20 drops	=	1 ml
1 teaspoon	=	5 ml
1 tablespoon	=	15 ml

WEIGHT CONVERSIONS

1 oz	=	30 gm
1 lb	=	453.6 gm
2.2 lb	=	1 kg

LENGTH

1 cm	=	0.39 inch
1 inch	=	2.54 cm

CENTIGRADE/ FAHRENHEIT CONVERSIONS

C	=	$(F - 32) \times 5/9$
F	=	$(C \times 9/5) + 32$

Practice Exam disk for
The Chicago Review Press *Pharmacology Made Easy for NCLEX-PN*

1. To use this practice exam disk, you must have a PC with windows.
2. Insert the disk into Drive A.
3. Click on "Start" at the bottom of your screen.
4. Click on "Run."
5. When you are prompted to type in a program name, type **a:pronto** and then click "OK."

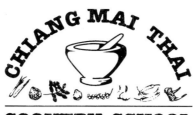

CHIANG MAI THAI

COOKERY SCHOOL

47/2 Moon Muang Road, Opp. Tha Phae Gate,
Chiang Mai 50200
Tel: (66-53) 206388 Fax: (66-53) 206387
Home: (66-53) 399036
Web-site : http:\\www.thaicookeryschool.com
e-mail: nabnian@loxinfo.co.th

Sompon and Elizabeth Nabnian
Established 1993

A Passion for Thai Cooking

Published in 2000 by Sompon and Elizabeth Nabnian

© Sompon and Elizabeth Nabnian 2000

ISBN 974-85886-4-5

Publisher   : Sompon and Elizabeth Nabnian
Cookery Editor : Sompon and Elizabeth Nabnian
Designer   : Sompon Nabnian
Photography   : Patinya Kongpitchayanon

Printed in Bangkok by Horatanachai Printing Ltd.,Part.

ACKNOWLEDGMENTS
The publisher would like to thank the following:
Gloy Pu-Sa aad and Sirisuda Phanthong

NOTES
For all recipes, quantities are given in both metric and imperial measures and, where appropriate, measures are also given in standard cups and spoons.

Standard spoon and cup measurements are level
1 tsp = 5 ml, 1 tbsp = 15 ml, 1 cup = 250ml/8fl oz

1

**To Benjamin, Emily and Charles
with all our love**

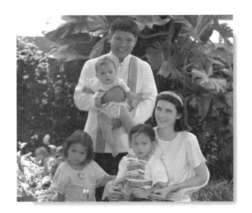

CONTENTS

INTRODUCTION

I have been dreaming of writing a Thai cook book ever since I opened the *Chiang Mai Thai Cookery School* in 1993. I have been teaching my students how to cook Thai food every day and I have always wanted to be able to give my students more knowledge and recipes. I have made the recipes simple and easy to follow so that everyone who loves Thai food as much as I do will be able to cook Thai food at home.

I first went to England in 1990 and was so excited to see all the Thai ingredients that were available in the Chinese shops. As I go back to visit my parents-in-law every year, I just cannot believe how widely available all the ingredients are, even in the supermarkets. You can get fresh chillies , ginza , lemongrass , kaffir lime leaves and the world famous Thai rice and fish sauce as well as many curry pastes.

Every year I notice that more and more people are travelling to Thailand to learn more about Thai food. Many people who have done my courses can not wait to return home and successfully cook some of the dishes they learnt. Learning to cook Thai food is a highlight of their trip and being able to reproduce the food at home in their own country will make their trip to Thailand even more memorable.

I have been selecting the dishes to include in my book for many years and the recipes have been cooked many times so that I am sure that you will be able to successfully cook all the dishes. Thai cooking is easy but it is important to prepare all the ingredients before beginning to cook as the cooking time is very short.

Thai food has so many different flavours such as hot, spicy, sweet, sour, salty and bitter and two or more flavours are often mixed together in one dish so that the flavours in Thai food are quite different to those of any other cuisine. Thai food uses a mixture of fresh and dried ingredients which makes its flavors unique.

I hope that you will enjoy using my cook book *" A PASSION FOR THAI COOKING "* and I hope that it will introduce you to lots of new dishes. I have always believed that the taste of the food is influenced by the mood of the cook so "keep smiling" (not difficult in the Land of Smiles!) .

Sompon Nabnian

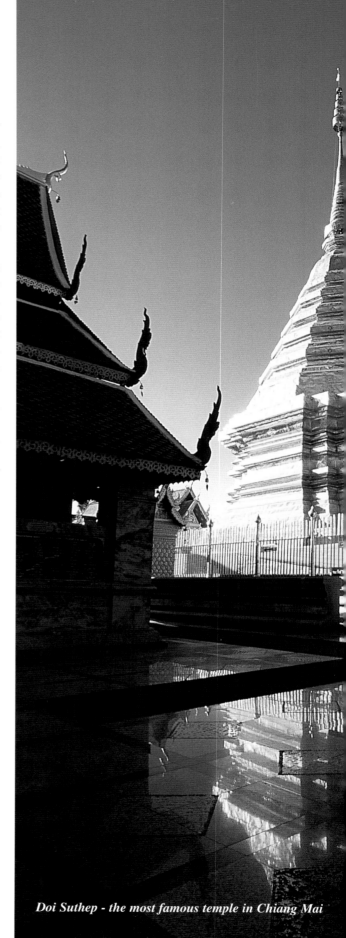

Doi Suthep - the most famous temple in Chiang Mai

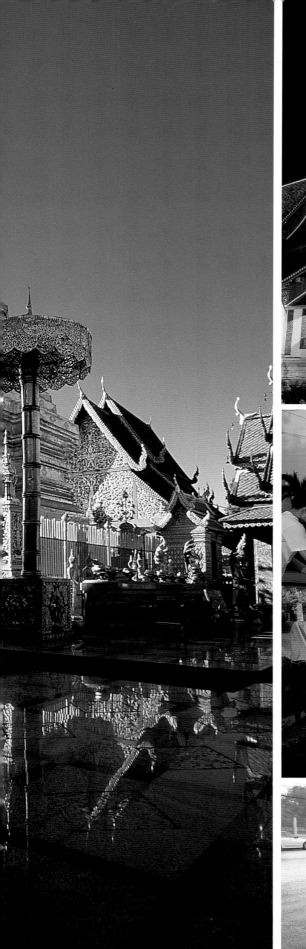

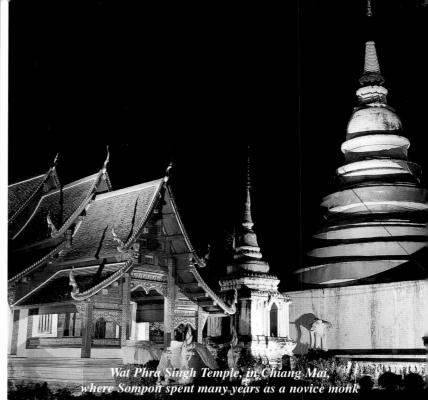

*Wat Phra Singh Temple, in Chiang Mai,
where Sompon spent many years as a novice monk*

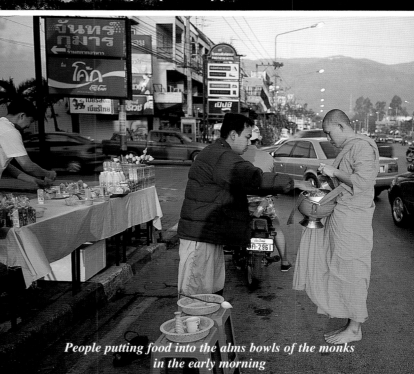

*People putting food into the alms bowls of the monks
in the early morning*

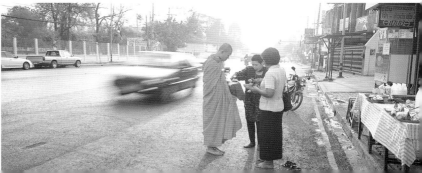

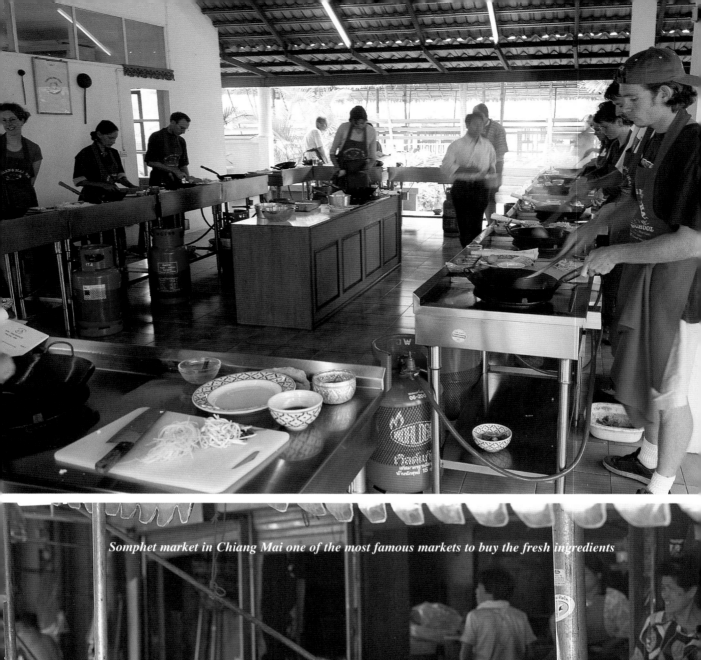

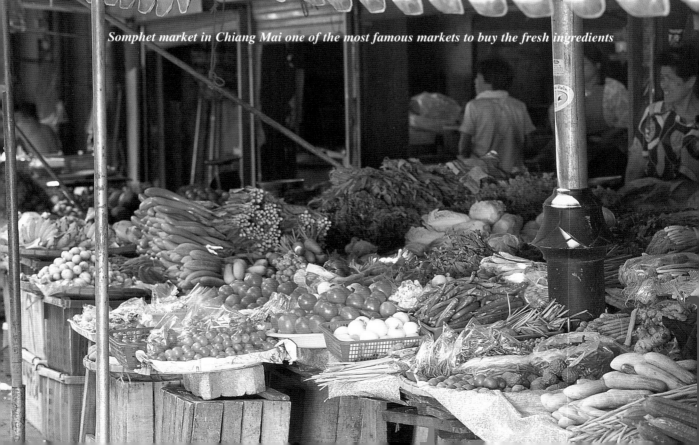

Somphet market in Chiang Mai one of the most famous markets to buy the fresh ingredients

COOKING AND EATING THAI FOOD

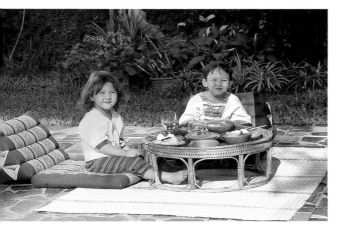

Food is an integral part of Thai life and you will find Thai people eating at all times of the day. You can eat out 24 hours a day as food stalls are open all night long. Thais tend to eat a little and often and will have many snacks in a day such as a plate of fried rice or papaya salad. Apart from the snacks they will on the whole eat 3 meals a day but the food served at each meal is fairly similar and it is definitely always rice or noodles.

Cooking is a sociable pastime in Thai society and often the whole family will congregate in the kitchen to help with the cooking although in the countryside it is often the women who are left cooking while the men folk sit and drink! Recipe books are never in evidence and most of the cooking is done by recipes handed down through generations. I have never seen any Thai people using measuring scales and measuring spoons as Thai cooking is done by taste or people just have a feel for how much of any one ingredient to put in. Consequently the measurements in this book are all approximate and you do not need to worry if you put in a little bit too much or too little. Once you have cooked a dish you will need to taste it and see if it needs more fish sauce, lime juice, palm sugar, chilli etc.

Thai people normally sit on the floor to eat. Sometimes they will have a little table to put the food on or sometimes they will just put the dishes of food straight on to the floor. If you ever eat with Thai people sitting on the floor then you should try not to point your feet at anybody as this is considered to be impolite. Thais are very forgiving and easy-going and they do not really mind how you eat. As a rule if there is a serving spoon in the dish of food then you should use this spoon to put some of the food onto your plate and then put the spoon back. Thais share their food and this is a way of not passing germs on but in many families they make do without serving spoons in which case you just use your normal spoon.

Thai people use a spoon and fork to eat rice with and will only use chop sticks to eat noodles so they are different from the Chinese who use chop sticks for rice too. The fork is just used to help to get the food onto the spoon in the same way that westerners would eat a dessert. In the north and north-east of Thailand everybody eats sticky rice which is eaten using your hand. It is important to roll the rice into a small ball so that when you dip the rice into a soup or curry you will not leave any of the rice behind in the soup and lose face! The ball of sticky rice that you make should be enough for one mouthful, not more so that there is no double dipping! As everybody eats from communal bowls you need to try not to touch the food too much and only touch the piece of meat or vegetable that you are going to eat. It may take a bit of practice but it is worth it. My children love sticky rice as it gives them an excuse to eat with their hands.

A Thai meal will consist of a variety of dishes such as a curry, a soup, a stir-fry and a dipping sauce or salad. There is normally a balance of spicy and mild dishes with at least one mild dish to counter the spicy dishes. When you eat Thai food you eat one dish at a time and it is not normal to spoon 2 or 3 different foods onto your rice at the same time. If you do that the sauces will all mix together and the food will not taste as good.

Thai cooking is not difficult once you are familiar with the main ingredients and I can guarantee that you will amaze yourself with the delicious food that you can cook. The Thai way of life is laid back and this translates into their cooking too so don't worry too much, relax, keep a smile on your face and enjoy!

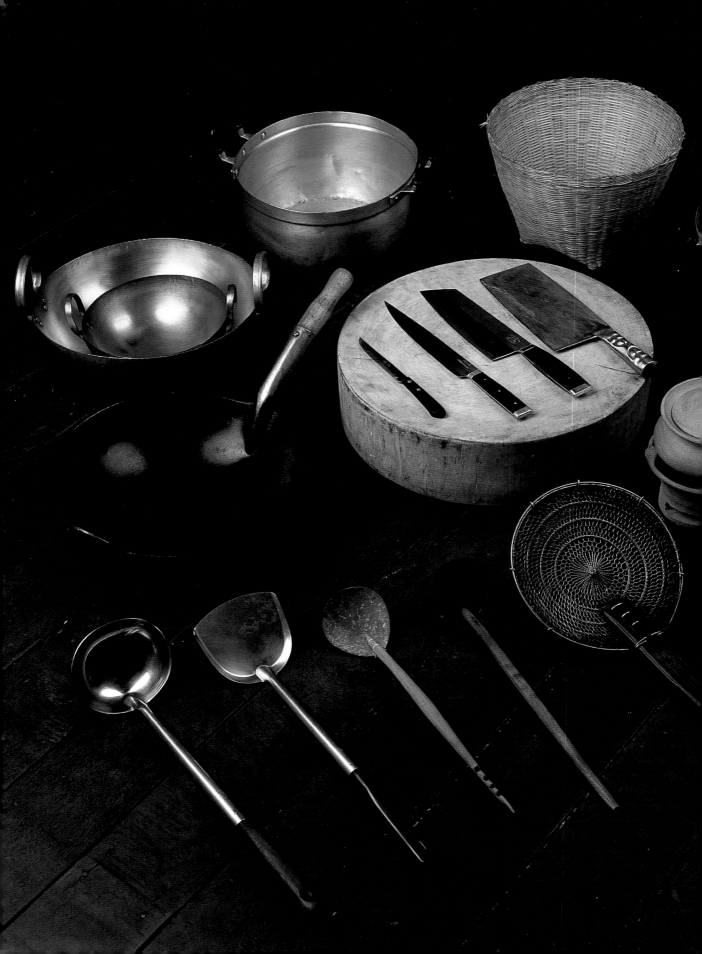

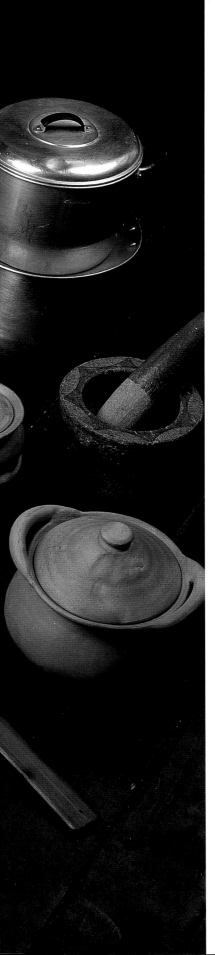

THAI COOKING UTENSILS

Thai cooking is very easy and it is not really necessary to have any special equipment in order to cook Thai food. Any pots and pans that you have at home will do but I would like to introduce you to some of the utensils that are commonly used in Thailand.

Thai cooking involves making curry pastes and all the ingredients need to be combined together so that they form a paste. A large, heavy granite pestle and mortar is used for this. Thai families will always have one in their kitchen and they can also be used for grinding dried spices. If you do not have one, you can use an electric blender to make the pastes and a coffee grinder to grind the dried spices. Wooden pestle and mortars are used for making salads, most notably, papaya salad.

Chopping boards are big and heavy and are made of tamarind wood. We use big chefs knives and cleavers to do our cutting and chopping but any knife will do.

The most important and most used cooking utensil is probably the wok. If you are thinking of investing in some cooking equipment especially for cooking Thai food, I would suggest purchasing a wok. They are very versatile and can be used for all sorts of cooking. They distribute the heat evenly and are excellent for stir-fries. When I was a trekking guide the only piece of cooking equipment that I took with me was my wok. If you do not have one then you can use a frying pan instead but you may find that bits go flying everywhere!

Woks can be made of iron, aluminium or brass. Personally I like to use an iron wok and most restaurants in Thailand will use these too. However, they have to be burnt in a flame until they are red hot and the outside is black before they are used. Once they have been burnt they need to be seasoned by putting a little oil into the wok and heating it gently for a couple of minutes. Aluminium and brass woks also need to be seasoned with a little oil as above. If you have a non-stick wok, it can be used straight away. Brass woks look absolutely beautiful and I love to use them. They are excellent for making soups, curries and sweet desserts and they can also be used as a serving dish. Aluminium or stainless steel pans can be used for making curries and soups too.

A steamer or double boiler is used to steam sticky rice, fish and vegetables. A bamboo basket is used to drain the water out of the sticky rice after it has been soaked.

Big, clay pots can be used to make soups and curries. Before they are used the first time they need to be soaked in water so that they do not crack. The smaller versions are used as serving dishes and often have stands that enable them to be lit so that the dish can be kept warm. They are too small to use to cook with.

Spoons made from coconut shells are often used for stirring as they do not scratch. A wire draining spoon with a wooden handle is used to remove food from the wok after it has been deep-fried.

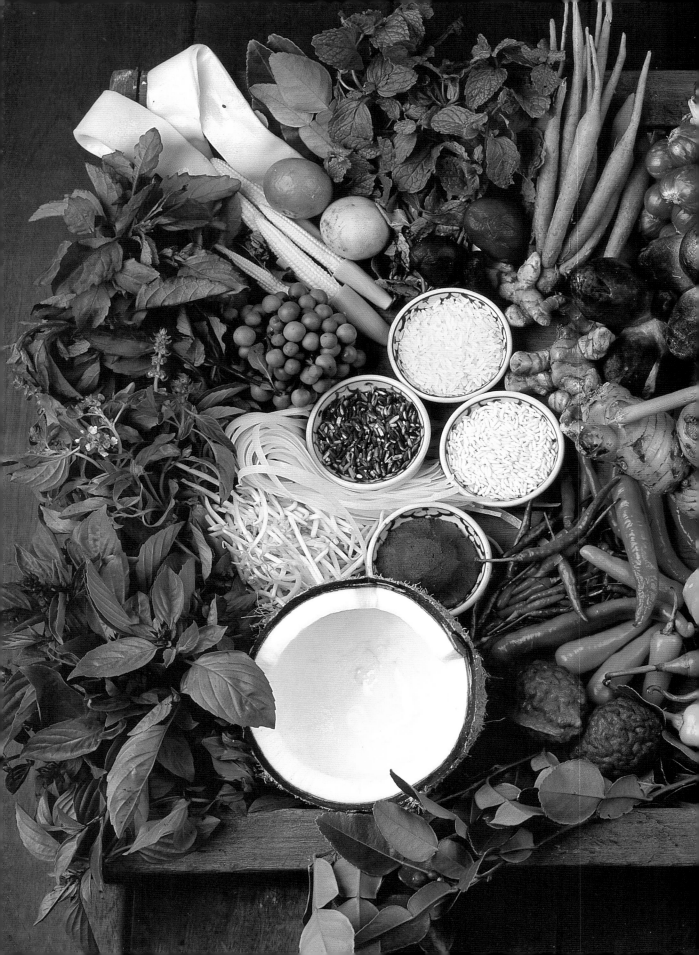

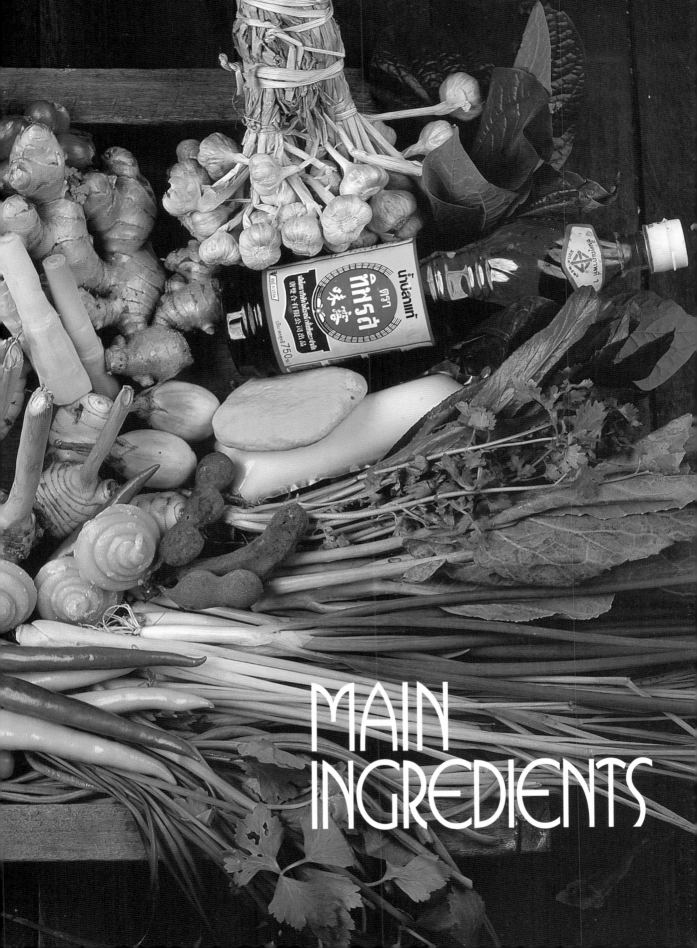

MAIN
INGREDIENTS

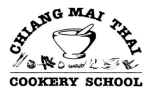

MAIN INGREDIENTS

BASIL
(BAI KAPROW) ใบกะเพรา

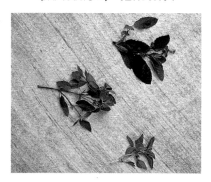

There are 3 different types of basil. The first is called holy or purple basil (bai kaprow) and it has a purple stem and purple leaves. It has a hot flavour and is used in stir-fries. It is added at the last minute.

The second is called lemon basil (bai manglak) and is has a light green stem and light green leaves. It has a lemony flavour and is used in soups, salads and curries especially those containing seafood. It is added at the end.

The third is called sweet basil (bai horapa) and it has a purple stem and dark green leaves. It has an aniseed flavour and can be used in all types of dishes including curries, stir-fries and curry pastes. It is often used as a garnish. This is the type of basil most commonly found abroad.

Basil is stored by wrapping it in tissue paper and then by putting it into a plastic bag. It can be stored in the refrigerator for about one week. It can also be frozen.

Sweet basil can be used as a substitute for the other kinds. Dried basil and mint can also be used as substitutes if none of the fresh forms are available.

BAMBOO SHOOTS
(NOH MAAI) หน่อไม้

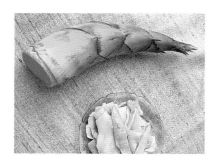

Bamboo shoots are the young shoots of the bamboo plants and are edible. They are a creamy or bright yellow colour when they are fresh. They are used in soups and curries or can be pickled. Sometimes they are boiled in the water for a few hours and eaten with a dipping sauce.

Tinned bamboo shoots can be used as a substitute for the fresh

ones but try to get the whole ones as they seem to be better quality than the ready-sliced tinned ones.

BEAN SPROUTS
(TUA NGORK) ถั่วงอก

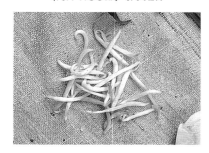

Bean sprouts are the fresh sprouts of the mung bean or soya bean. They are used in stir-fry and noodle soup dishes and spring rolls. They are added at the end to keep them crunchy.

They should be stored in water and kept in the refrigerator where they will last for a few days. The water should be changed daily.

CHILLI
(PRIK) พริก

There are a number of different types of chillies used in Thai cooking. Young chillies are green in colour and are spicier than the red ones which are ripe.

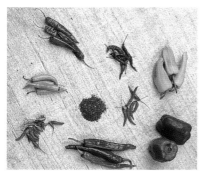

However the small chillies are much more spicy than the big chillies whatever the colour.

The small chillies or birds eye chillies (prik khii noo) are the spiciest and are often used for their colour when making pastes. They are also used in spicy soups and salads. They are used in their fresh form.

The medium or jalapeno chillies (prik chee faa) are used for their colour when making pastes and may be used instead of the small ones if you do not want the paste to be too spicy.

The big chillies (prik num) are not spicy and are used in stir-fries or as a garnish. Dried chillies are obtained by drying the big, red chillies in the sun for 4-5 days. Dried chillies usually have their seeds removed so that they are not so spicy.

The big chillies (prik num) are not spicy and are used in stir-fries or as a garnish. Dried chillies are obtained by drying the big, red chillies in the sun for 4-5 days. Dried chillies usually have their seeds removed so that they are not so spicy. They need to be soaked in cold water for at least 10 minutes (or in hot water for 5 minutes) to soften them before they are used. They are usually used for making pastes.

The big, red dried chillies are used to make chilli powder. They need to be dried in the sun for 2 hours or roasted in a wok until the outside is a dark, crisp colour. The stem is then removed and the chillies can be pounded or blended into a powder.

Chillies can be made less spicy by removing the seeds. If they are being added to a soup they can be left whole, as opposed to slicing them, to make the soup less spicy but care must be taken not to eat the entire chilli. The fewer chillies used the less spicy the dish will be.

Fresh chillies can be stored in the refrigerator for a couple of weeks or can be frozen in plastic containers.

Chilli powder and green and red peppers can be used as substitutes.

CHINESE CELERY
(KHUNCHAI) ขึ้นฉ่าย

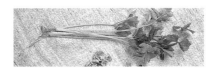

Chinese celery looks similar to coriander but has bigger leaves. However it has a flavour similar to celery.

The stalks and leaves of normal celery may be used as a substitute.

COCONUT MILK
(GATI) กะทิ

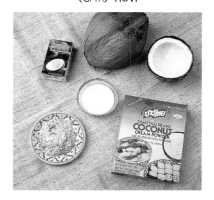

In Thailand it is possible to get fresh coconut milk but it also comes in tins, as a dried powder and in a creamed form. It is used in soups, curries and desserts. Fresh coconut milk is made from the coconut flesh. The flesh is grated or chopped by putting it into an electric blender.

To make 750mls (3 cups, 24 fl oz) of coconut milk you need 500g (1 lb 2 oz) of grated coconut. Then add 500mls (2 cups, 16 fl oz) of warm water to the grated coconut. This then needs to be squeezed by hand for about 10 minutes or longer to obtain the milk. It is then put through muslin or a strainer. It needs to be squeezed hard to make sure that the thick coconut milk (also called coconut cream) is obtained. It is then left for 10 minutes and the thick coconut milk and thin coconut milk will separate out.

Tinned coconut milk needs to be shaken before using. To separate the thick and thin coconut milk the tin can be frozen for 10 minutes.

Powdered and creamed coconut milk need to have water added to them and then they are used as normal. Instructions will be given on the packet.

Soya bean milk or milk can be used as alternatives if you do not want to use coconut milk as coconut milk is very high in cholesterol.

CORIANDER
(PHAK CHEE) ผักชี

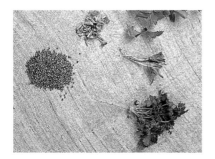

This is also known as cilantro or Chinese parsley. The root, stem and seeds are used for making curry pastes. The root has a stronger flavour and aroma than the leaves and the stem can be used as a substitute for the root. The leaves are a dark green colour and are used as a garnish. If the leaves are a pale green or yellow colour then the coriander is not fresh. The seeds need to be roasted in a wok over a low heat until they go a brown colour. They can then be crushed and made into a powdered form. They are then ready to be used in curry pastes.

Coriander is stored by wrapping it in tissue paper and then by putting it into a plastic bag. It can be stored in the refrigerator for 1 week. It can also be frozen.

The dried coriander seeds can be used as a substitute for the root. Dried coriander and parsley can be used as a substitute. One tablespoon of dried coriander is the equivalent of 2 tablespoons of fresh coriander. However coriander is widely available abroad.

EGG PLANT
(MAKUA PROH) มะเขือเปราะ

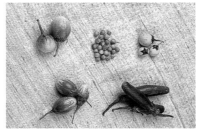

Egg plants come in many sizes. They can be white, green or purple. They vary in size. The very big, purple ones are also called aubergines.

Big egg plants are a green and white colour and are the same size as tomatoes. The stalk is cut off the top and then the egg plant is cut into bite-sized pieces. Big egg plants are used in all types of dishes.

The small or pea egg plants are green. They are crunchy on the outside and have a bitter taste. They are used in soups, stir-fries, curries and dipping sauces.

The small or pea egg plants are green. They are crunchy on the outside and have a bitter taste. They are used in soups, stir-fries, curries and dipping sauces.

Once the egg plants have been cut they will go brown very quickly. If egg plants are to be prepared in advance they should be stored in water with salt, lemon juice, lime juice or vinegar to prevent them going brown. This also removes the bitter flavour. The other option is to prepare them just before they are to be used.

They can be stored in the refrigerator for 1 week and they can also be frozen.

Big, purple aubergines, bamboo shoots or peas can be used as substitutes.

FISH SAUCE
(NAM PLAA) น้ำปลา

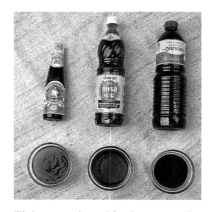

Fish sauce is a thin, brown, salty liquid which is made from fermented or pickled fish. It is used instead of salt in nearly every dish. The darker the colour of the fish sauce, the higher the quality. High quality fish sauces are also more expensive than the low quality ones. The high quality fish sauces have a strong, fishy taste as more fish and less salt is used to make them. They can be stored at room temperature.

Soy sauce or salt can be used as a substitute.

GARLIC
(KRATIEM) กระเทียม

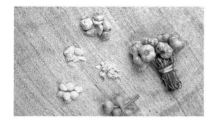

In Thailand there are several different varieties of garlic. One variety has very small cloves and a slightly pink skin. When used in cooking Thai people do not remove the skin. It is often used in stir-fries. Another variety is round in shape but has no cloves and it has a stronger taste than some other types. It is often pickled. Other varieties are bigger and are similar to garlic that can be found abroad.

GINZA
(KHA) ข่า

This is also known as galangal, Siamese ginger, kha or laos powder (Indonesia). It is a pale, yellow root similar to ginger but it has a very distinctive taste. The

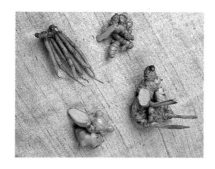

outside skin is removed before using it. It is used for making curry pastes and it is also used in soups. If it is being used in the curry pastes then it needs to be well chopped as it is quite hard to pound. If it is in slices in a soup it is not eaten.

It will keep for 2-3 weeks in the refrigerator and it can be cut into thin slices and frozen.

Dried sliced ginza needs to be soaked in water first. One teaspoon of dried ginza powder is the equivalent of 5 slices of fresh ginza.

Ginger can also be used as a substitute.

KAFFIR LIME
(MAGROOD) มะกรูด

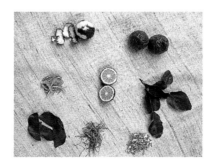

A kaffir lime is a dark, green, knobbly lime. The skin is used

for making curry pastes. The juice is sometimes used in soups and the leaves are used in curries and soups. The kaffir lime leaves should be torn into pieces, discarding the stem and are often added at the end of cooking for their aroma.

The leaves can be stored in the refrigerator for 2 weeks and they can be frozen.

Dried kaffir lime leaves need to be soaked in water before using.

Lemon leaves or finely grated lemon or lime rind can be used as a substitute. A kaffir lime leaf is the equivalent of ½ teaspoon of lemon rind.

LEMONGRASS
(TAKRAI) ตะไคร้

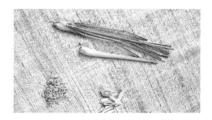

Lemongrass or citronella is a straw-like grass which has a distinctive, lemony flavour. The outer layer is discarded along with the straw-like top. Only the bottom one third is used. It can be sliced or chopped. It is used in soups and curry pastes and is also used to make drink or tea. If it is in big slices it is not eaten.

Lemongrass can be stored in the refrigerator for 2-3 weeks and it can also be frozen.

Dried sliced lemongrass should be soaked in water before using. One tablespoon of dried lemongrass powder is the equivalent of 2 stalks of fresh lemongrass.

Lemon peel can be used as a substitute.

MUSHROOMS
(HED) เห็ด

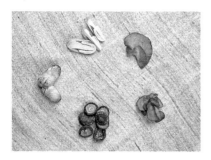

Tinned straw mushrooms, button mushrooms and oyster mushrooms can be used as substitutes. Straw mushrooms are often used in Thai cooking and are used in stir-fries, soups and curries.

Chinese mushrooms are used in stir-fries. Dried Chinese mushrooms should be soaked in water for 10 minutes before using.

NOODLES
(KWITHIAW) ก๋วยเตี๋ยว

There are many different sorts of noodles and many different sizes. They come in fresh and dried forms and are made from rice, wheat or mung beans. If it is possible it is best to use fresh

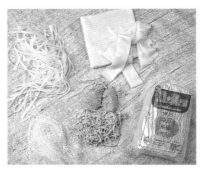

noodles. Yellow or egg noodles are yellow because egg yolk is added and they are used for noodle soup. Noodles are used in stir-fries, soups and salads.

If you use dried noodles then they need to be soaked in water for 15-20 minutes before using. They are then ready to be stir-fried. If they are to be used for noodle soup, they need to be put into the hot soup for about 2 minutes. Fresh noodles do not need to be soaked and can be put straight into the soup.

If they are needed quickly then the dried noodles can be put into boiling water for 3-5 minutes and once they are soft they are transferred into cold water and then they are ready to be used.

Bean vermicelli or glass noodles are made from mung beans. They need to be soaked in water for 5 minutes before using. If they are going to be used for a salad then they need to be put into boiling water after they have been soaked and then transferred into cold water.

Rice vermicelli which are to be deep-fried for a crispy noodle dish do not need to be soaked. They can just be fried in hot oil.

PALM SUGAR
(NAM TAAN PEEP) น้ำตาลปีบ

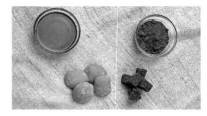

Sugar from the palm tree is a light brown, raw sugar which comes in two different forms. One form is hard and comes in lumps. The other form is softer and is more like a paste. It comes from the trunk of the coconut tree. The juice from the sap is collected and boiled in water until all the water has evaporated. It is used in curries and desserts.

Brown sugar, maple syrup or honey can be used as a substitute.

SHALLOTS
(HOM DAENG) หอมแดง

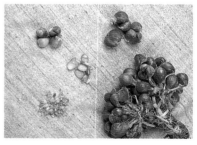

Shallots or purple onions are small onions which have a purple skin. The outside skin is removed and they are used in the same way as normal onions.

Normal onions, chives, spring or scallion onions can be used as substitutes.

SHRIMP PASTE
(KAPI) กะปิ

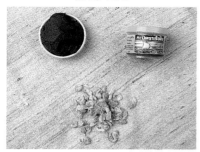

Shrimp paste is made from fermented dried shrimps and it is a dark coloured paste with a strong smell. It is used for making curry pastes, dipping sauces and it is also used in soups. Only a small amount is used.

It can be stored at room temperature for up to 1 year.

A tin of anchovies can be mixed with 2 tablespoons of water and used as a substitute. Anchovy or soya bean paste can also be used.

TAMARIND
(MAKHAM) มะขาม

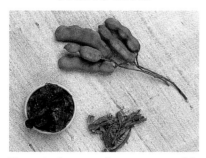

Tamarind comes from a tree and it looks like brown long beans. It is peeled and inside is the flesh which has seeds in it.

There are two varieties. One is sweet and one is sour. The sweet one is eaten as a fruit and the sour one is made into a juice and used in cooking.

To make tamarind juice, hot water is poured on to the sour tamarind and then the tamarind is squeezed so as to extract the juice.

It can be stored for 2 or 3 weeks in the refrigerator.

Tamarind paste may be diluted with water and used as a substitute. Lime or lemon juice can also be used as substitutes.

TOFU
(TAO HOO) เต้าหู้

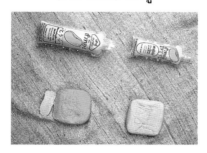

Tofu is also know as soya bean curd as it is made from soya beans. There are 2 different types of tofu. The first is called soft tofu and it can have either a bean or an egg flavour. It is used for soups. The second is called firm tofu and is used as a meat substitute. It can be either white or yellow (food colouring is added) and it is used for stir-fries.

Once a packet of tofu has been opened the tofu should be stored in a bowl of water and kept in the refrigerator. The water should be changed daily and it will keep for about 5 days. It can also be put into a plastic bag and frozen.

TUMERIC
(KHAMIN) ขมิ้น

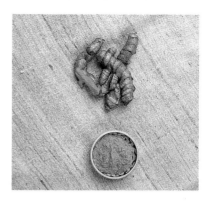

Tumeric is a small root and it is a bright orange colour. It looks similar to ginger. Before it is used the outside skin needs to be removed. It is used for its colour when making pastes and it is also used in fish dishes to take away the smell of the fish.

It can be stored in the refrigerator for 2-3 weeks and it can also be frozen.

Tumeric powder can be used as a substitute.

RICE

Rice comes in many different forms.
There is long and short grain rice
and it can be white, brown,
red or black in colour.

PLAIN RICE
(KHAO PLAO) ข้าวปล่าว

Plain rice is most popular in central and southern Thailand. To cook it, for every single measure of rice you put two measures of water into a pan and bring the water to a boil. Boil the water until the rice is soft on the outside but still hard in the centre for about 10-15 minutes. The time will vary depending on how much rice is being cooked. Put the lid on the pan, turn the heat right down and let the rice cook until the water has evaporated for about 5-10 minutes. If the rice on the top is cooked, then all the rice in the pan will be cooked as well.

Once all the water has evaporated care must be taken not to burn the rice at the bottom of the pan.

STICKY OR GLUTINOUS RICE
(KHAO NEOW) ข้าวเหนียว

Sticky rice is a different grain of rice from plain rice and it is eaten mainly in the north and north-east of Thailand. It is eaten using your hands. The sticky rice needs to be soaked in water for at least 3 hours or overnight before it is cooked.

Drain the water out of the sticky rice and put the sticky rice into the top part of a steamer. If the steamer has big holes in it, then put a muslin cloth in the steamer first, to stop the rice falling through the holes. Then bring the water in the bottom part of the steamer to the boil. Once the water is boiling, it will start to cook the rice. When you can see steam coming through the sticky rice then put the lid on the steamer for 5 minutes. Check the rice and if it is not hard in the middle it is cooked. If the middle of the rice is still hard then you need to replace the lid another few minutes.

Once it is cooked turn the heat off and put the sticky rice onto a tray or plate. Use a spoon to move the rice around to get rid of all the hot steam. If you do not do this, the sticky rice will go soggy.
The sticky rice is then ready to be eaten. It can also be kept to eat later in the day.

ROASTED GROUND STICKY RICE

Roasted, ground sticky rice used to be used in curries and stir-fries to make the sauce thicker instead of tapioca flour or corn flour. It is still used in some dishes today to give the sauce a thicker texture.

To make roasted, ground sticky rice, put some grains of sticky rice (uncooked) into a wok over a low heat and roast until they become a brown colour. Then put the roasted sticky rice into a mortar and pound well with a pestle until it becomes a powder.

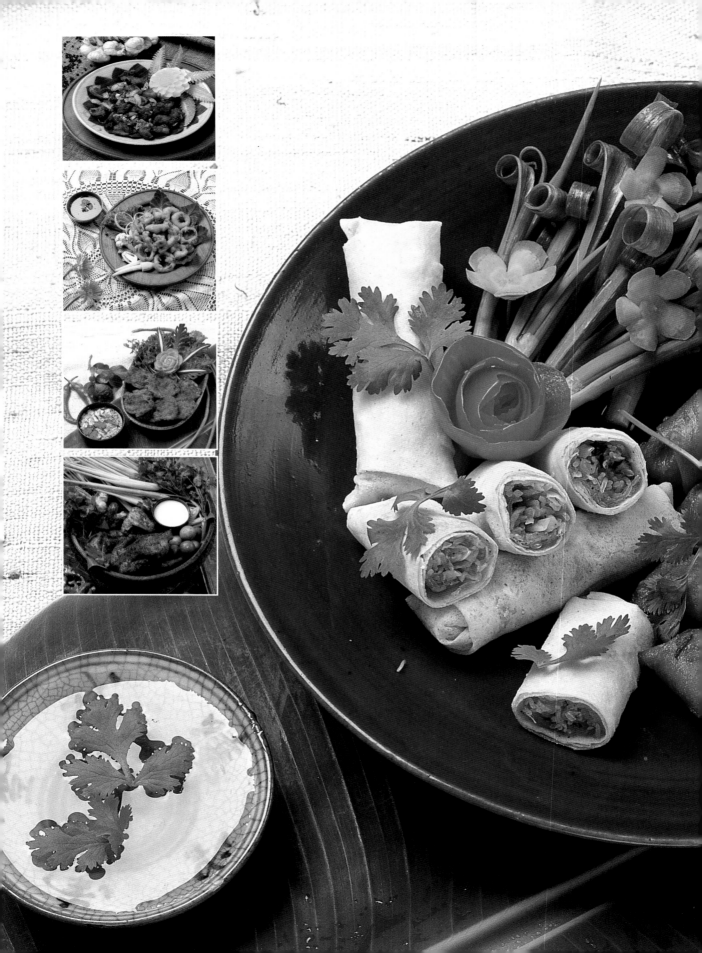

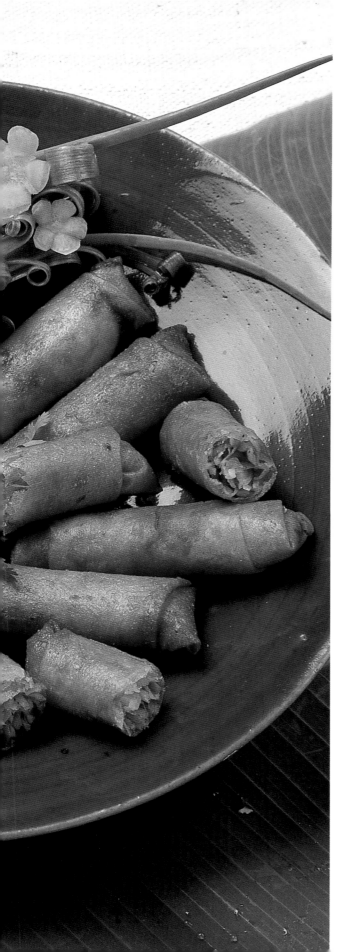

APPETIZERS

Thai people do not usually have appetizers. They tend to order a variety of dishes and the dishes are all served at the same time or as they are ready. However many restaurants realize that there are some dishes that foreigners order expecting that they will come as a starter so they will try to make sure that these dishes are ready first. The dishes contained in this section are a selection of dishes that I think can be served very successfully as appetizers. They can also be eaten as snacks.

FRIED SPARERIBS WITH GARLIC

SEE KRONG TORD GRATIUM - ซี่โครงทอดกระเทียม

This dish makes a really good starter and if you like garlic you will love this.

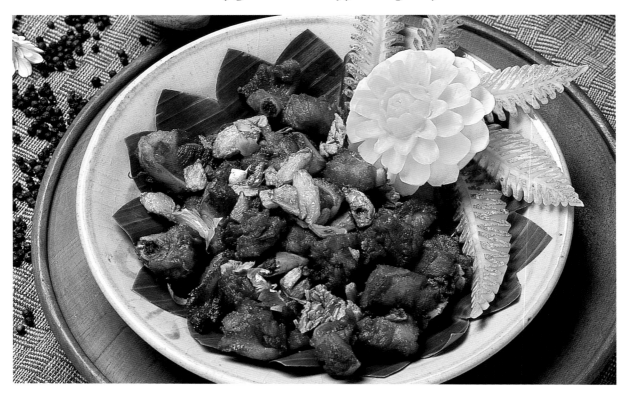

INGREDIENTS
Serves 4

500g (4 cups, 1lb 2 oz) pork spareribs - cut into 2cm (1 inch) pieces
Enough oil to deep fry
750mls (3 cups, 24 fl oz) chicken stock or water
125mls (1/2 cup, 4 fl oz) oil
50g (1/2 cup, 2oz) garlic with skin on - chopped

Sauce

50g (1/2 cup, 2oz) garlic - chopped
50g (1/4 cup, 2oz) coriander root and stem - roughly chopped
1 teaspoon white peppercorns - crushed
30mls (2 tablespoons) oyster sauce
15mls (1 tablespoon) light soy sauce
15mls (1 tablespoon) soy sauce
1/4 teaspoon sweet soy sauce

METHOD

Mix the spareribs together with all the sauce ingredients and then put them into a pan along with the chicken stock and simmer for 20 minutes. Drain out the stock and set the spareribs aside.

Put 125mls (1/2 cup, 4 fl oz) oil into a wok and when it is hot add the unpeeled garlic and cook on a high heat until the garlic starts to turn brown. Turn down the heat and keep stirring until the garlic is crispy (about 2-3 minutes). Drain out the oil and put the garlic on some kitchen paper.

Put the oil for deep frying into a wok and when it is hot fry the spareribs until they are golden brown (4-5 minutes) and then drain.

To serve, put the spareribs on a plate and sprinkle the garlic over the top.

CHICKEN IN PANDANUS LEAVES
GAI HOR BAI TOEY - ไก่ห่อใบเตย

If you cannot get pandanus leaves or do not want to fry the chicken, then this dish is also excellent when the marinated chicken is baked in the oven covered (for about 30 minutes until cooked). If this dish is served in pandanus leaves then remove them before eating the chicken - they are not edible!

INGREDIENTS
Serves 4

200g (1 cup, 7 oz) chicken breast - cut into 20 equal pieces
20 pandanus leaves
20g (4 tablespoons) roasted sesame seeds
1 teaspoon ground, black pepper
250mls (1 cup, 8 fl oz) oil

Sauce

15mls (1 tablespoon) light soy sauce
1 tablespoon tapioca flour
15mls (1 tablespoon) sesame oil

METHOD

Put the chicken into a bowl, add the sauce ingredients and mix well together. Leave to marinate for at least 10 minutes. Then add the sesame seeds and black pepper and mix well together.

Wrap each piece of chicken in a pandanus leaf and cut off the ends if they are too long. The chicken can be stored in the refrigerator like this until you are ready to fry it.

When you want to fry it, put the oil into a wok and turn on a medium heat. When the oil is hot put in the chicken pieces and fry for about 5 minutes until the chicken is cooked. Drain on some kitchen paper and serve immediately with some sweet chilli dipping sauce *(see p.48)*.

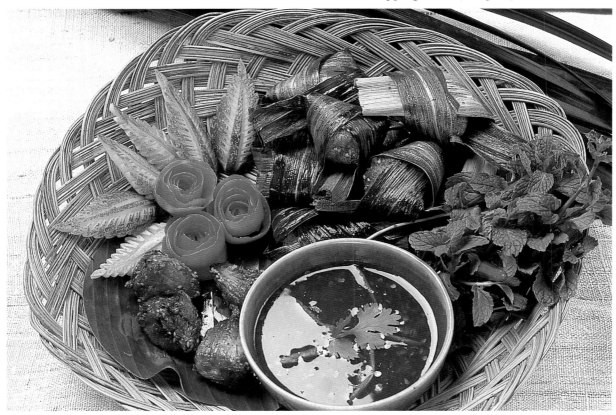

VEGETABLES FRIED IN BATTER
TEMPURA PHAK - ผักชุบแป้งทอด

You can use any selection of vegetables you like. Prawns and squid rings are very popular too.

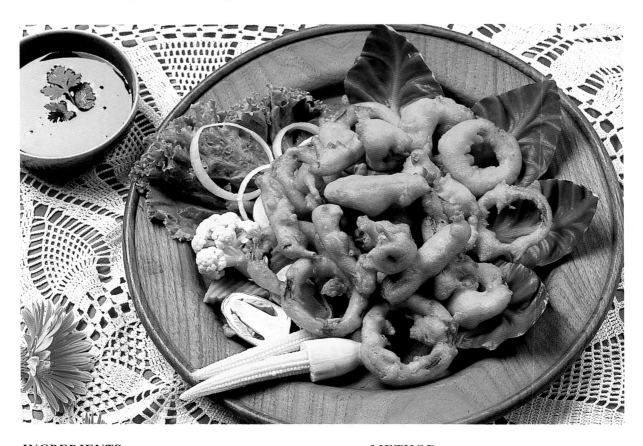

INGREDIENTS
Serves 4

150g (11/2 cups, 5oz) tempura flour or self-raising batter
1 egg - beaten
180mls (3/4 cup, 6 fl oz) water
1/4 teaspoon baking powder

Enough oil to deep-fry
8 baby corn
1 onion - turned on its side and cut into 6 slices
50g (1/2 cup, 2 oz) long beans - cut into 2cm (1 inch) pieces
50g (1/2 cup, 2oz) carrot - cut lengthways into strips

METHOD

Put the tempura flour, egg and water into a bowl and mix thoroughly. Add the baking powder and mix again.

Put all the vegetables into the batter and make sure they are all well covered.

Put the oil into a wok and when it is hot add the vegetables and keep stirring until they are golden brown. Once cooked put them on some draining paper and then serve with some plum dipping sauce *(see p.48)*.

SPRING ROLLS
PAW PIA TORD - ปอเปี๊ยะทอด

Although Chinese in origin, spring rolls are now widely available in Thailand. They can also be made by adding minced pork or tofu. The spring rolls can be frozen before and after frying. They will need heating up after they have defrosted if they have already been fried.

INGREDIENTS
Makes 8

60mls (4 tablespoons) oil
60g (1 cup, 2oz) carrot - finely shredded
60g (1 cup, 2oz) cabbage - finely shredded
60g (1 cup, 2oz) bean sprouts
60g (1 cup, 2oz) glass noodles - soaked in cold water for at least 5 minutes

Sauce
¼ teaspoon ground, black pepper
1 tablespoon sugar
15mls (1 tablespoon) light soy sauce
15mls (1 tablespoon) oyster sauce

8 spring roll wrappers
1 egg - beaten
Enough oil for deep frying

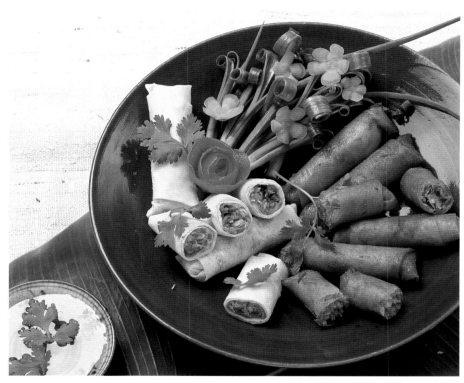

METHOD

Put the oil into a wok and on a low heat add the carrot and cabbage. Stir-fry together and add the bean sprouts and glass noodles. Stir-fry the mixture for about 3-5 minutes and then add the sauce ingredients. Stir-fry to combine and then put the mixture onto a plate.

Divide the mixture into 8 portions. Put the mixture into the middle of the spring roll wrapper and fold one side over the mixture and pull back slightly and then fold in the edges and roll tightly. When the wrapper is rolled up use the beaten egg to seal the edge. Do this for all 8 portions. The spring rolls can be prepared in advance and kept in the refrigerator until you are ready to fry them.

When you are ready to fry the spring rolls, put the oil into a wok and heat on a medium heat. When the oil is hot put in the spring rolls and keep turning them until they start to turn golden brown. Take them out of the oil and put them onto some kitchen paper to drain. Cut each spring roll into 3 pieces and put onto a serving dish. Serve immediately with some plum dipping sauce *(see p.48)*.

THAI STYLE FISH CAKES

TORD MAN PLAA - ทอดมันปลา

Thai style fish cakes are one of the most famous starters. Once they have been deep-fried and left to cool they can be frozen so you can make this dish in big batches. Let them unfreeze when you want to use them and put them in a warm oven to heat through. They are very good for parties. They can also be made using chicken, pork, prawns or crab.

INGREDIENTS   *Makes 40*

500mls (2 cups, 16 fl oz) oil

Fish cakes
500g (2½ cups, 1lb 2oz) any white fish fillets - minced
130g (5 tablespoons) red curry paste *(see p.105)*
60mls (4 tablespoons) fish sauce
1 egg - beaten
80g (8 tablespoons) tapioca flour
10g (2 teaspoons) baking powder
20g (1 tablespoon) palm sugar
10 kaffir lime leaves - thinly sliced discarding the stem
8 long beans - thinly sliced

Sauce
90mls (6 tablespoons) water
60g (6 tablespoons) sugar
15mls (1 tablespoon) vinegar
5g (1 teaspoon) chilli powder
30g (2 tablespoons) roasted peanuts - chopped
10g (1/2 cup, 1/2 oz) coriander - chopped
30g (2 tablespoons) cucumber - thinly sliced

METHOD

To make the dipping sauce, put the water, sugar and vinegar into a pan and dissolve the sugar over a low heat. Once the sugar has dissolved bring the water to the boil and boil for 5 minutes. Turn off the heat and add the chilli powder, peanuts and cucumber. Leave to cool and serve garnished with the coriander.

Mix all the ingredients for the fish cakes together in a bowl until they are thoroughly combined.

Make the fish cake mixture into small, flat cakes about 5cm (2½ inches) in diameter. Put the oil into a wok and when it is hot add the fish cakes. Fry them until they start to turn golden brown (about 2-3 minutes). Then take them out and put them on kitchen paper to drain. It is best to fry the above quantity in about 5-6 batches.

Serve the fish cakes while they are still hot with the dipping sauce.

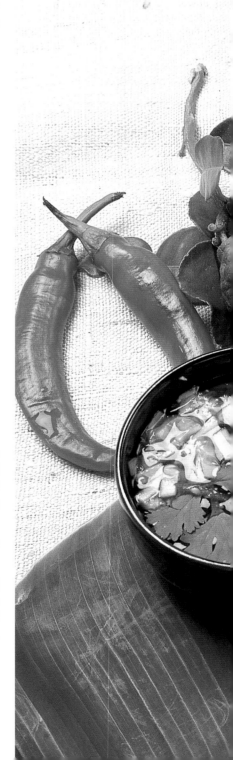

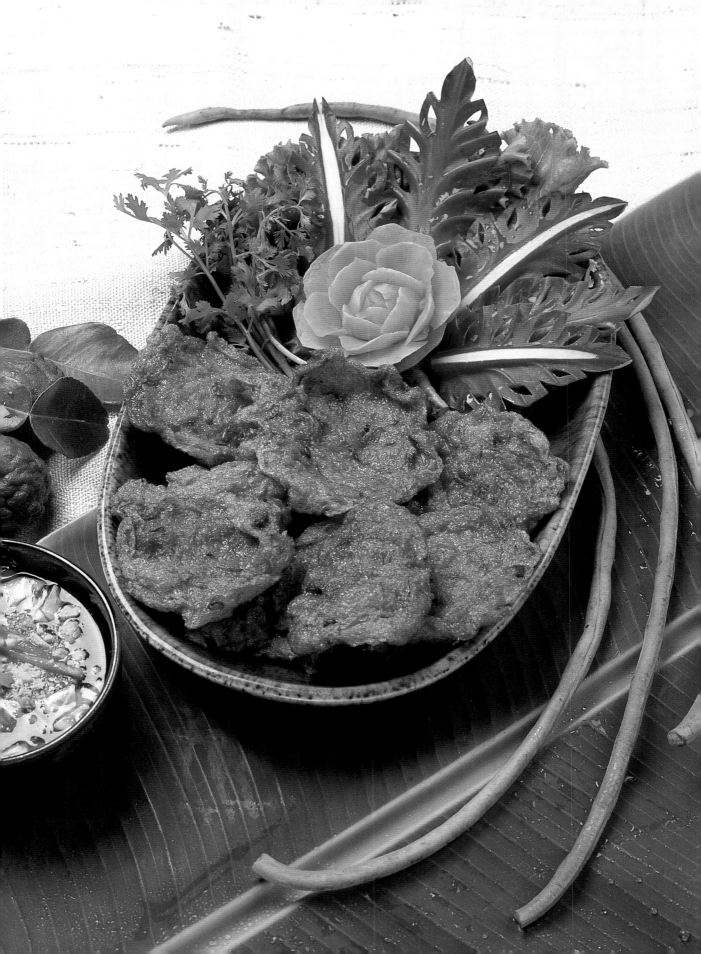

BEEF SATAY
SATAY NEUA - สะเต๊ะเนื้อ

Satay is a dish that is found in many Asian countries including Malaysia and Indonesia as well as Thailand. You can use peanut butter instead of ground, roasted peanuts if you like. Satay is also made using chicken or pork.

INGREDIENTS
Serves 4

500g (21/2 cups, 1 lb 2 oz) beef - cut into thin slices

Marinade
90mls (6 tablespoons) thick coconut milk
30mls (2 tablespoons) fish sauce
30mls (2 tablespoons) condensed, sweetened milk
15mls (1 tablespoon) oil
20g (2 tablespoons) sugar
30g (2 tablespoons) curry powder

Sauce
500mls (2 cups, 16 fl oz) thick coconut milk
30g (1 tablespoon) red curry paste *(see p.105)*
30mls (2 tablespoons) fish sauce
30g (3 tablespoons) sugar
125g (1/2 cup, 4 oz) finely ground, roasted peanuts

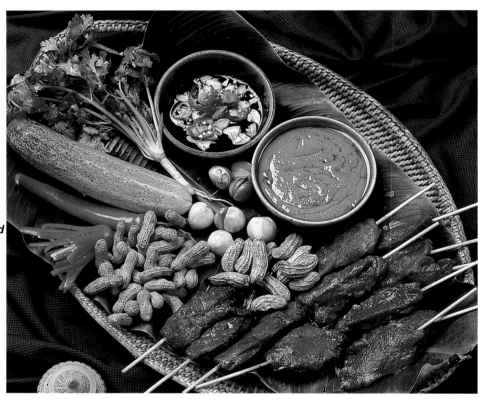

METHOD

Mix all the ingredients for the marinade together and then cover the beef with the marinade. Leave for at least 30 minutes.

To make the sauce, put the coconut milk into a wok and bring to the boil. Add the red curry paste and stir to combine. Add the fish sauce, sugar and peanuts and simmer for 10-15 minutes until the sauce is thick. Stir continuously.

The beef can be either barbecued, grilled or shallow fried. To barbecue or grill put the meat on to skewers (if you are using wooden skewers you will need to soak them in water first to stop them burning) and cook for 3 minutes each side until the meat is cooked. Spoon the marinade over the beef as it is cooking. To shallow fry put 45mls (3 tablespoons) oil into a wok and add the meat and the marinade and stir-fry until cooked.

Serve with the peanut dipping sauce.

GRILLED CHICKEN WITH LEMONGRASS
GAI YANG TAKRAI - ไก่ย่างตะไคร้

This dish is excellent for barbecues and is really simple to make. The lemongrass flavour really comes through and the longer it can be left to marinate the better. It can also be made using chicken breast, pork chops or spareribs.

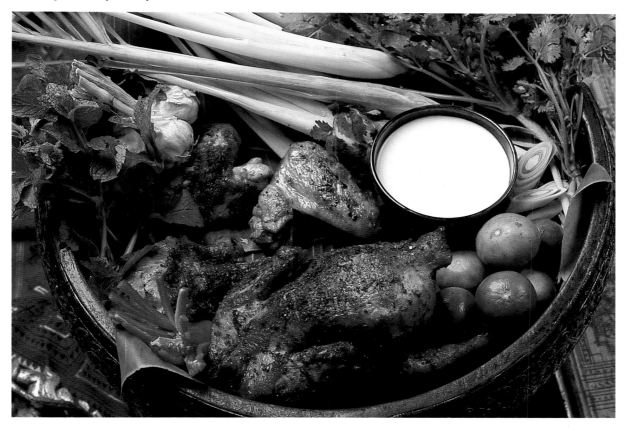

INGREDIENTS
Serves 4

8 chicken legs

Marinade
10 cloves of garlic - chopped
3 stalks of lemongrass - lower 1/3 only, finely chopped
2 spring onions - finely chopped
30mls (2 tablespoons) fish sauce
30mls (2 tablespoons) lime juice
30mls (2 tablespoons) white wine
75mls (5 tablespoons) coconut milk
15mls (1 tablespoon) sesame oil
1/2 teaspoon ground, black pepper

METHOD

Mix all the ingredients for the marinade together and then cover the chicken legs with the marinade. Leave for 30 minutes or overnight.

Grill or barbecue the chicken legs until they are completely cooked. Spoon the marinade over the chicken legs while they are cooking. Serve this dish hot or cold.

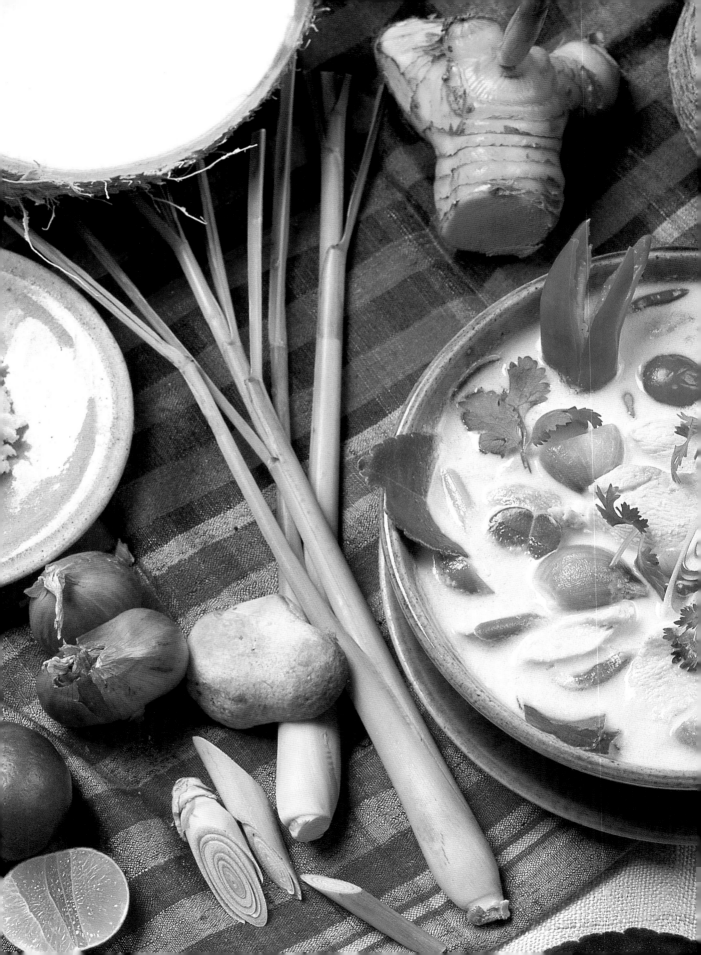

SOUPS

Thai soups are becoming very popular abroad as most of them are easy to make and healthy to eat. Thai soups are made with either water or coconut milk as the base. Some soups are spicy such as Hot and Sour Prawn Soup which combines many Thai flavours. Other soups are not spicy, such as Clear Soup with Minced Pork, and are a good choice when the other dishes being eaten are spicy. Another popular soup is Chicken in Coconut Milk Soup which is a thick, creamy soup. Soups are eaten as part of a main meal and will be one of several dishes at any meal. However, at home you may want to serve the soup as a starter as many people are not used to eating soup along with rice.

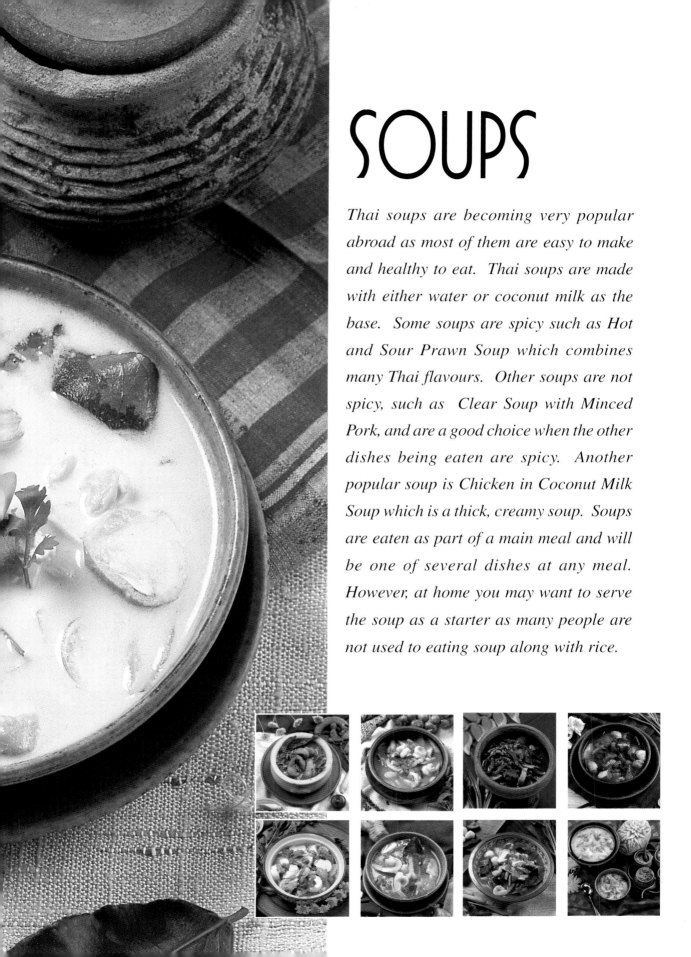

SPICY MIXED VEGETABLE SOUP WITH PRAWNS
GAENG LIANG GOONG - แกงเลียงกุ้ง

This is a simple and healthy dish to make. The sauce is a mix of water and vegetables which makes it taste completely different from all the coconut milk curries.

INGREDIENTS
Serves 4

120g (1 cup, 4 oz) prawns - washed, peeled and deveined
500mls (2 cups, 16 fl oz) chicken stock or water
100g (1 cup, 31/2 oz) pumpkin - cut into bite-sized pieces
6 baby corn - each cut into 3
50g (1/2 cup, 2 oz) straw mushrooms - cut in 1/2
2 courgettes - sliced
30mls (2 tablespoons) fish sauce
30g (1 cup, 1 oz) lemon basil

Paste

20g (2 tablespoons) coriander root - chopped
15g (3 tablespoons) shallots - chopped
15g (3 tablespoons) garlic - chopped
1 big, red chilli - chopped
10g (1/2 oz) or 3 stalks of young, green peppercorns
10g (3 tablespoons) ground, dried shrimps
1 teaspoon white peppercorns - crushed
250mls (1 cup, 8 fl oz) water

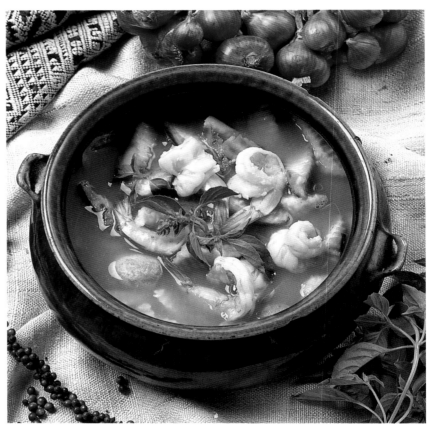

METHOD

Put all the ingredients for the paste into a blender and blend until smooth. Once it is smooth put the paste into a pan along with the chicken stock and bring to the boil. Add the pumpkin and babycorn and cook for 2 minutes. Then add the mushrooms and courgettes and cook for a further 2 minutes.

Add the lemon basil and fish sauce followed by the prawns and cook for 2 minutes. Serve.

THAI HOT AND SOUR PRAWN SOUP
TOM YAM GOONG - ต้มยำกุ้ง

This soup combines all the exotic flavours of Thailand bringing together ingredients such as lemongrass, chillies, ginza and coriander. You can make it as spicy as you like. You can also try adding some chilli jam in for a different version of this soup.

INGREDIENTS
Serves 4

300g (2 cups, 10 oz) prawns - washed, peeled and deveined. Keep the peelings

750mls (3 cups, 24 fl oz) water or chicken stock

6 cloves of garlic - crushed

6 shallots - sliced

2 stalks of lemongrass - lower 1/3 only, slice into 2cm (1 inch) pieces.

10 thin slices of ginza - skin removed

200g (2 cups, 7 oz) straw mushrooms - cut in half

2 tomatoes - each one cut into 8 pieces

20 small, green chillies - cut in 1/2 lengthways

45mls (3 tablespoons) fish sauce

5 kaffir lime leaves - torn into pieces discarding the stem

30mls (2 tablespoons) lime juice

10g (1/2 cup, 1/2 oz) coriander - chopped

METHOD

Put the heads and peelings of the prawns in a pan with the water and bring to the boil. Remove the prawn peelings from the pan and bring the stock back to the boil. Add the garlic, shallots, lemongrass and ginza and bring to the boil. Then add the mushrooms and tomatoes and bring back to the boil . Add the chillies and fish sauce followed by the kaffir lime leaves. Cook gently for 2 minutes, then add the prawns and cook for about 1 minute. Turn off the heat and stir in the lime juice. Serve garnished with the coriander.

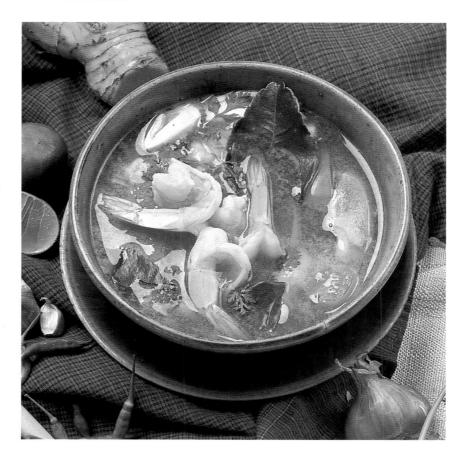

SOUR SOUP WITH FISH
TOM SOM PLAA - ต้มส้มปลา

This soup is quite similar to hot and sour prawn soup but tamarind juice is used instead of lime juice making it more sour and it is not usually as spicy.

INGREDIENTS
Serves 4

300g (2 cups, 10 oz) fish fillets - cut into 2 cm (1 inch) pieces
Enough oil to deep-fry the fish
750mls (3 cups, 24 fl oz) chicken or fish stock
40g (4 tablespoons, 1 1/2 oz) ginza - skin removed and sliced
4 kaffir lime leaves - stem removed
2 stalks of lemongrass - lower 1/3 only, sliced
4 shallots - smashed
5 cherry tomatoes - cut in 1/2
60g (3/4 cup, 2 oz) straw mushrooms - cut in 1/2
30-45mls (2-3 tablespoons) tamarind juice *(see p.17)*
2 big, red dried chillies - roasted and chopped
20g (1 cup, 1oz) young tamarind leaves
10g (1/2 cup, 1/2 oz) coriander - chopped

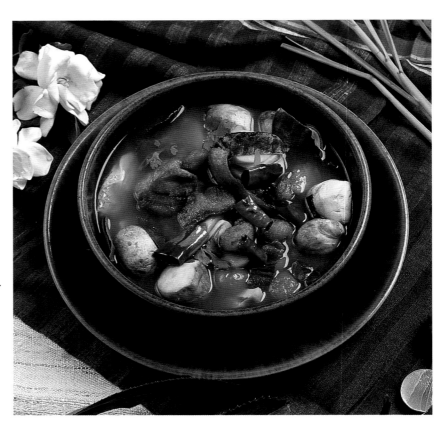

METHOD

Put the oil into a wok and when it is hot deep-fry the fish until it is golden brown (about 2-3 minutes). Remove the fish from the oil and drain.

Put the stock into a pan and bring to the boil. On a high heat add the ginza, kaffir lime leaves, lemongrass, shallots, cherry tomatoes, mushrooms and fried fish and boil for about 3 minutes. Then add the fish sauce and tamarind juice and boil for another 2 minutes. Add the dried, roasted chillies and young tamarind leaves and turn the heat off.

Serve garnished with the chopped coriander leaves.

SPICY SEAFOOD SOUP
PO TAEK - โป๊ะแตก

This is a wonderful dish for people who like seafood. All the different seafood is mixed together in one dish and it is usually served still bubbling hot. I would highly recommend this dish.

INGREDIENTS
Serves 4

750mls (3 cups, 24 fl oz)
chicken stock or water
1 crab (including shell) - cut
into chunks
100g (3/4 cup, 31/2 oz)
squid - cut into pieces
50g (1/2 cup, 2 oz) mussels
100g (3/4 cup, 31/2 oz)
prawns
50g (1/4cup, 2 oz) fish fillet -
cut into pieces
10 slices of ginza
1 stalk of lemongrass -
lower 1/3 only, sliced
5 shallots - smashed
20-30 small green and red
chillies - smashed
4 kaffir lime leaves - torn into
pieces discarding the stem.
50g (1/2cup, 2 oz) straw
mushrooms - cut in 1/2
1 tomato - cut lengthways
into 8 pieces
45mls (3 tablespoons) fish
sauce
20g (1/2 cup, 1oz) eryngo
leaves - roughly chopped
30g (1 cup, 1oz) holy basil
45mls (3 tablespoons) lime
juice

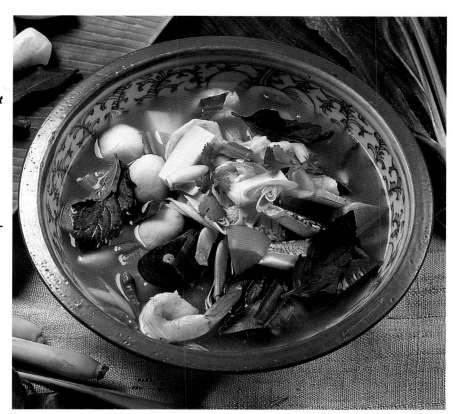

METHOD

Put the stock into a pan and bring to the boil. Then add the ginza, lemongrass, shallots, chillies, kaffir lime leaves, mushrooms and tomato and simmer for 5 minutes. Then add the crab followed by the squid and mussels and simmer for 2 minutes. Add the prawns and then the fish fillet and simmer for a further 2 minutes.

Add the fish sauce, eryngo leaves and holly basil and bring back to the boil. Turn the heat off, add the lime juice and serve.

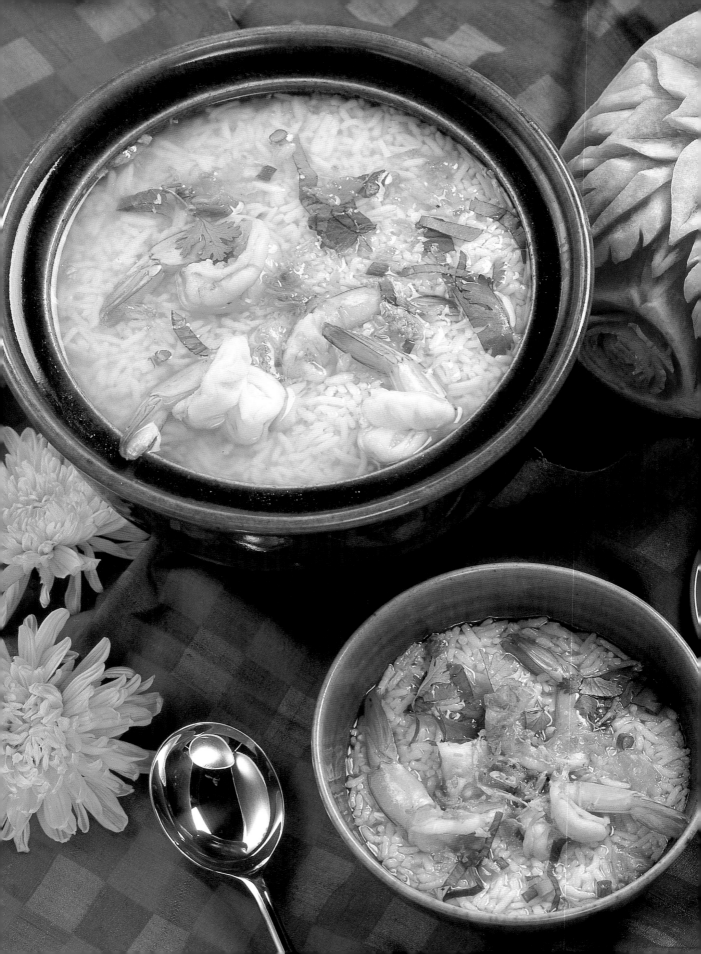

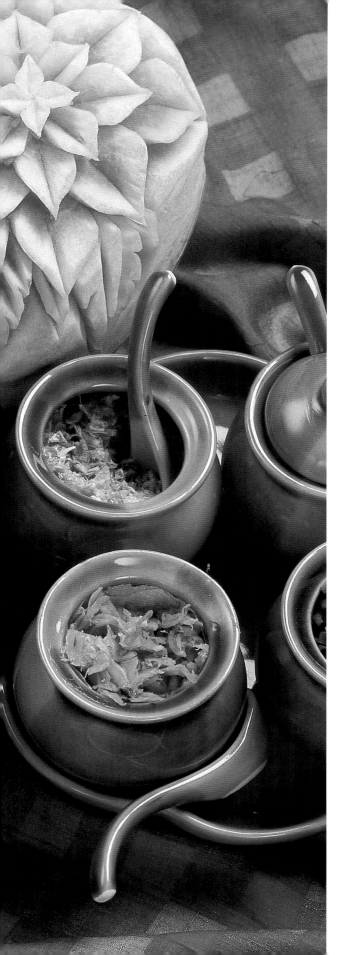

RICE SOUP WITH PRAWNS
KHAO TOM GOONG - ข้าวต้มกุ้ง

This dish is a very simple, plain dish and is often eaten by Thai people for breakfast. People who are ill and need plain food will also eat this dish although the smell of the garlic may be a bit off-putting if you are not used to it. It can also be made with chicken, fish or squid. You can also break an egg into it while it is still hot.

INGREDIENTS
Serves 4

150g (1 cup, 5 oz) prawns - peeled and deveined
750mls (3 cups, 24 fl oz) chicken stock, fish stock or water
500g (2 cups, 1 lb 2 oz) precooked rice
Pinch of salt
45mls (3 tablespoons) light soy sauce
1 teaspoon ground pepper
5g (1 teaspoon) pickled radish root - chopped
5g (1 teaspoon) crispy, fried garlic - chopped

METHOD

Put the stock into a pan and bring to the boil. Then add the precooked rice and boil for 2 minutes. Add the salt, light soy sauce, pepper and prawns and simmer for 1 minute. Turn off the heat and garnish with the pickled radish root and crispy fried garlic.

Serve immediately.

CLEAR SOUP WITH MINCED PORK
TOM JUED - ต้มจืด

This is one of the few Thai soups that are not spicy. It is good to eat as an accompaniment to spicy salads and curries to counter balance the spiciness.

INGREDIENTS
Serves 4

150g (3/4 cup, 5oz) minced pork

20g (2 tablespoons) coriander root - finely chopped

5 cloves of garlic - chopped

750mls (3 cups, 24 fl oz) chicken stock or water

120g (2 cups, 4 oz) Chinese cabbage

120g (1 cup, 4 oz) soft tofu - cut into 8 pieces

50g (1 cup, 2 oz) glass noodles - cut into 8cm (3 inch) pieces

45mls (3 tablespoons) light soy sauce

½ teaspoon ground, black pepper

10g (1/2 cup, 1/2 oz) Chinese celery - chopped

2 spring onions - chopped

METHOD

Mix the pork, coriander root and garlic together and then chop together so that it is well combined. Separate the mixture into about 15 meatballs.

Put the stock into a pan and bring to the boil. Add the meat balls and cook for 2 minutes. Then add the Chinese leaves and tofu and simmer for another 2 minutes. Add the glass noodles followed by the light soy sauce and ground, black pepper. Turn off the heat and garnish with the Chinese celery and spring onions.

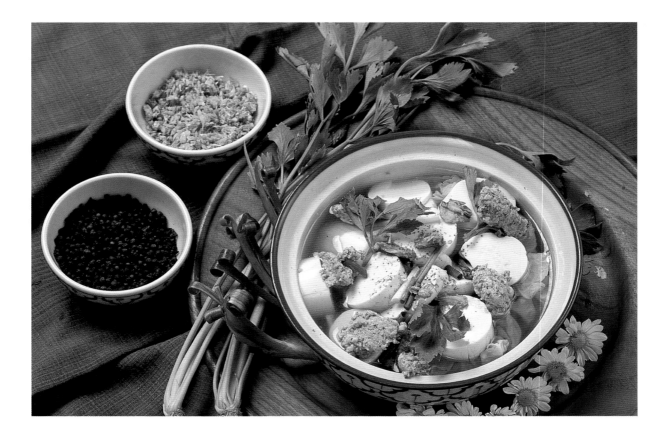

TAMARIND FLAVOURED SOUP WITH FISH
GAENG SOM PLAA CHON - แกงส้มปลาช่อน

This soup is made using a paste which gives the soup lots of flavour.

INGREDIENTS
Serves 4

300g (2 cups, 10oz) fish fillets - thinly sliced
750mls (3 cups, 24 fl oz) chicken stock or water
40g (2 tablespoons) palm sugar
60mls (4 tablespoons) fish sauce
100g (1 cup, 31/2 oz) carrot - sliced
2 long beans - chopped in 2cm (1 inch) pieces
60g (1/2 cup, 2 oz) white radish root - sliced
180mls (3/4 cup, 6 fl oz) tamarind juice (see p.17)
50g (2 cups, 2 oz) water mimosa

Paste

3 shallots - chopped
10g (2 tablespoons) garlic - chopped
10g (1 teaspoon) shrimp paste
6 big, red dried chillies - seeds removed and soaked in water for at least 10 minutes and then finely chopped
40g (1/2 cup, 11/2 oz) lesser ginger - chopped
20g (6 tablespoons) ground, dried shrimps
250mls (1 cup, 8 fl oz) water

METHOD

Put all the ingredients for the paste into a blender and blend until smooth. Put the paste into a pan along with the stock and bring to the boil. When it is boiling, add the palm sugar and stir gently. Add the fish sauce, followed by the carrot, long beans and white radish root and simmer for 5 minutes. Add the tamarind juice and stir. Then add the fish and cook for 5 minutes.

Put the water mimosa into a serving bowl and pour the soup over the top. Serve.

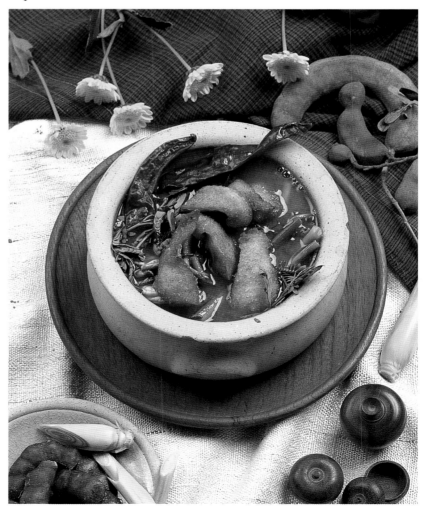

CHICKEN IN COCONUT MILK SOUP
TOM KHA GAI - ต้มข่าไก่

This soup is one of the most well known soups in Thailand. It has a creamy consistency and has a lovely lemony flavour to it. It is not as spicy as the hot and sour prawn soup but you can add extra chillies if you want. If you do not want to make the soup so rich and creamy then you can use equal quantities of thick and thin coconut milk.

INGREDIENTS
Serves 4

300g (11/2 cups, 10 oz) chicken breast - sliced
500mls (2 cups, 16 fl oz) thick coconut milk
250mls (1 cup, 8 fl oz) thin coconut milk
5 thin slices of ginza - cut in half
2 stalks of lemongrass - lower 1/3 only, sliced into 2 cm (1 inch) pieces
4 shallots - sliced
10 -15 small chillies - cut in 1/2 lengthways
200g (2 1/4 cups, 7 oz) straw mushrooms - cut in half
45mls (3 tablespoons) fish sauce
3 kaffir lime leaves - torn into pieces discarding the stem
30mls (2 tablespoons) lime juice
10g (1/2 cup, 1/2 oz) coriander leaves - chopped
2 spring onions - sliced - optional

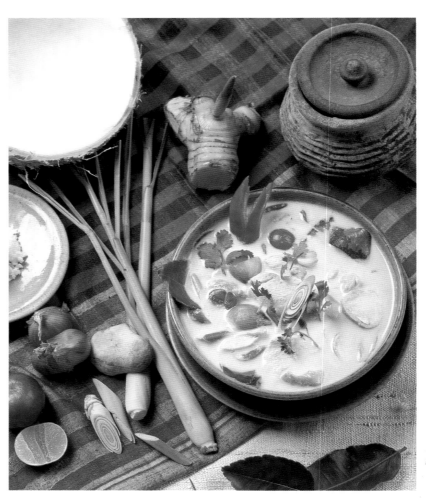

METHOD

Put the thick and thin coconut milk into a wok on a high heat. Add the ginza, lemongrass, shallots, chillies and mushrooms and bring to the boil. Simmer for about 3-5 minutes and add the chicken and stir. Then add the fish sauce and kaffir lime leaves and bring back to the boil. Add half the coriander leaves and turn off the heat. Stir in the lime juice. Serve garnished with the remaining coriander leaves and spring onions.

SPICY CHICKEN SOUP NORTHERN STYLE

YAM JIN GAI - ยำจิ้นไก่

This is one of my favourite dishes and I love it to be really spicy. I would recommend eating it with sticky rice.

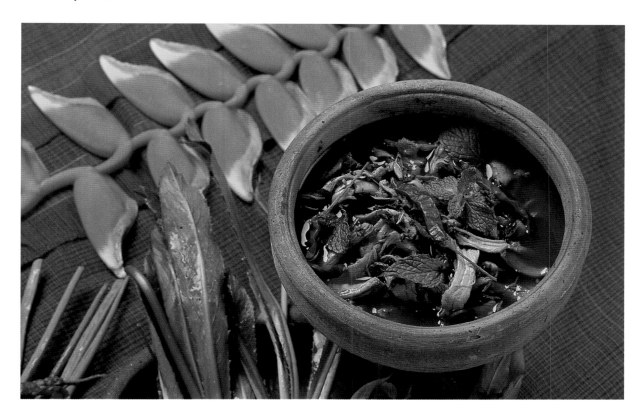

INGREDIENTS

Serves 4

300g (21/2 cups, 10oz) pre-cooked chicken breast - thinly sliced
750mls (3 cups, 24 fl oz) chicken stock or water
3 shallots - thinly sliced
2 tablespoons Northern chilli powder - a mixture of coriander seeds, cumin seeds, prickly ash, long green peppers, and dried red chillies. They all need to be roasted and ground.
30mls (2 tablespoons) fish sauce
15mls (1 tablespoon) soy sauce
20g (1/ 1/2 cup, 1oz) mint leaves - chopped
20g (½ cup, 1oz) Vietnamese mint leaves - chopped
2 spring onions - chopped
10g (1/2 cup, 1/2 oz) coriander - roughly chopped

METHOD

Put the stock into a pan and when it is boiling add the chicken, shallots, Northern chilli powder, fish sauce and soy sauce and simmer for 1 minute. Add the mint and Vietnamese mint and simmer for 1 more minute. Serve garnished with the spring onions and coriander.

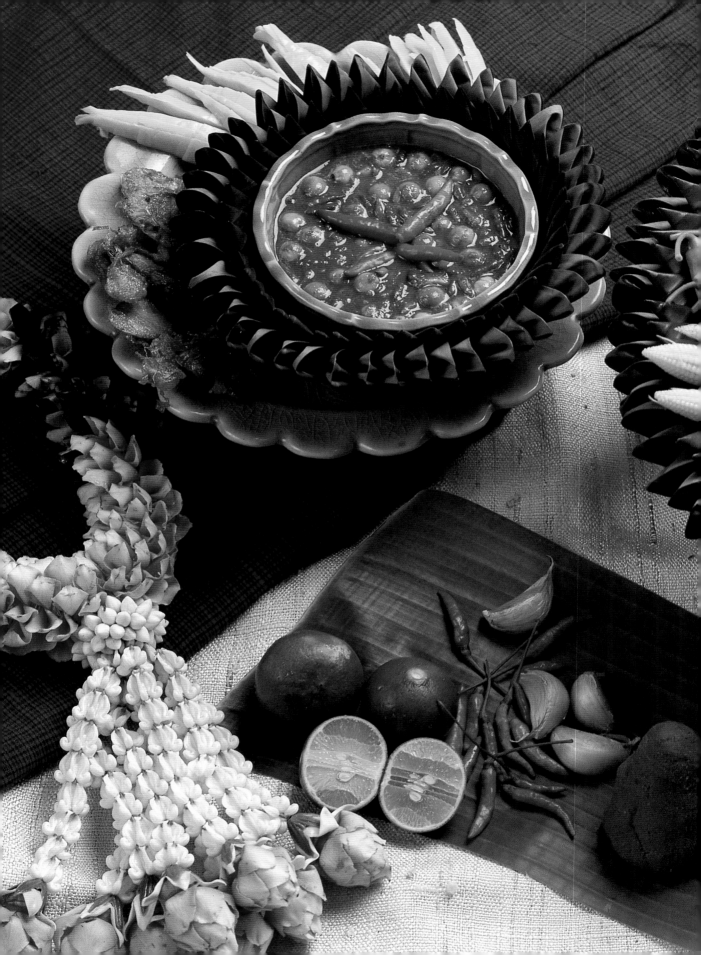

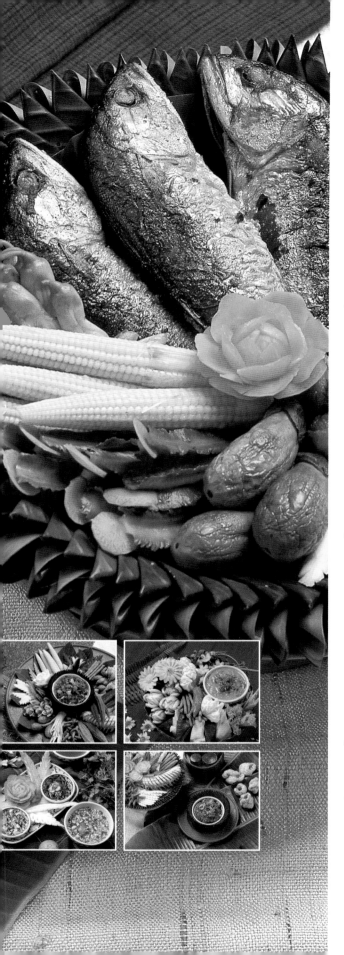

DIPPING SAUCES

Dipping sauces are normally eaten as part of a meal along with a few other dishes. They are nearly always spicy and are often eaten along with sticky rice and a selection of fresh, boiled or steamed vegetables. It is up to you what selection of vegetables you would like to use. If you are not used to them you will definitely need to eat them along with rice. They are served in fairly small portions as you only eat a little bit at a time. In many poor villages in the countryside they will eat these dipping sauces virtually every day as they use very small amounts of meat so they are cheap to make. There are over 100 different sorts of dipping sauces but I have chosen a few of my favourites for you in this section.

This section also includes some dipping sauces that are served as accompaniments to other dishes.

43

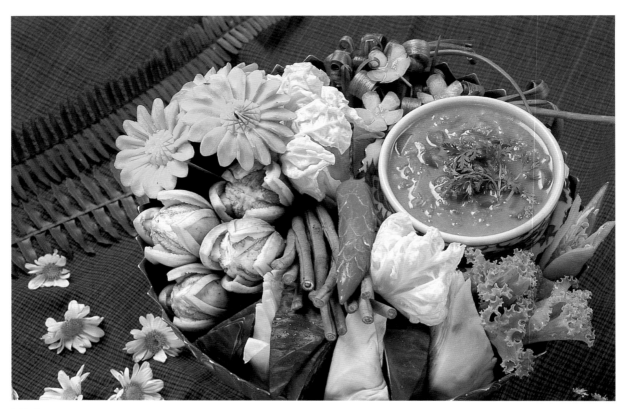

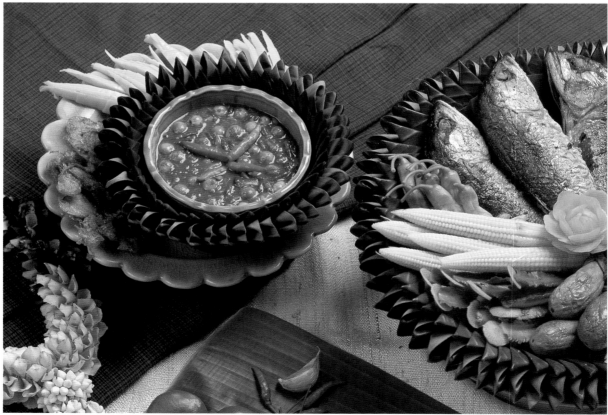

SOYA BEAN DIPPING SAUCE
LON TAO JEOW - หลนเต้าเจี้ยว

This dish is easy to make and is different from most dipping sauces because it has coconut milk in it.

INGREDIENTS
Serves 4

500mls (2 cups, 16 fl oz) thick coconut milk
90mls (6 tablespoons) soya bean paste
70g (3/4 cup, 21/ oz) minced pork
3 stalks of lemongrass - lower 1/3 only, sliced
4 shallots - sliced
1 big, red chilli - sliced
40g (2 tablespoons) palm sugar
10g (1 tablespoon) sugar

A selection of fresh, steamed or boiled vegetables such as long beans, egg plants, cabbage and cucumber.

METHOD

Put the thick coconut milk into a pan and bring to the boil. Add the soya bean paste and cook for about 1 minute. Then add the pork, lemongrass, shallots and chilli and cook for about 2 minutes. Add the palm sugar and sugar and stir until the sugar has melted. Turn off the heat and serve with a selection of vegetables.

SHRIMP PASTE DIPPING SAUCE
NAM PRIK KAPI - น้ำพริกกะปิ

Many foreigners are put off this dish due to the strong smell of the shrimp paste but this is no deterrent to Thai people. They think that this dipping sauce is wonderful especially when eaten along with fresh vegetables and fried mackerel. This is one of my favourite dipping sauces and I would recommend trying it rather than judging it by its name!

INGREDIENTS
Serves 4

30g (1 tablespoon) shrimp paste
7 cloves of garlic
20 small green and red chillies
5g (2 tablespoons) dried shrimps - very finely chopped
30g (1/2 cup, 1 oz) small, green egg plants
10g (2 teaspoons) palm sugar
45mls (3 tablespoons) fish sauce
45mls (3 tablespoons) lime juice

A selection of fresh, steamed or boiled vegetables such as cabbage, babycorn, cauliflower and long beans.
Mackerel fish - deep fried

METHOD

Put the shrimp paste, garlic, chillies and half the dried shrimps into a mortar and roughly pound with a pestle. Add the small, green egg plants and palm sugar and pound again. Then add the remaining dried shrimps, fish sauce and lime juice and stir to mix together. Serve with a selection of vegetables.

YOUNG CHILLI DIPPING SAUCE
NAM PRIK NUM - น้ำพริกหนุ่ม

This is a northern dipping sauce and whenever Thai people come up to the north it is one of the dishes that they like to eat.

INGREDIENTS
Serves 4

15 big, green chillies - roasted and then peeled

60g (1/2 cup, 2oz) garlic - roasted and then peeled

9 shallots - roasted and then peeled

1/4 teaspoon shrimp paste

1/2 teaspoon salt

15mls (1 tablespoon) fish sauce

A selection of fresh, steamed or boiled vegetables such as eggplants, cucumber, carrot, cabbage, long beans, pumpkin, bamboo shoot, etc.

METHOD

Put the big, green chillies into a mortar and pound gently with a pestle until they are broken up. Then add the garlic and pound. Add the shallots and pound again. Add the shrimp paste and salt and pound to combine all the ingredients together. Add the fish sauce and mix in.

Serve with a selection of vegetables.

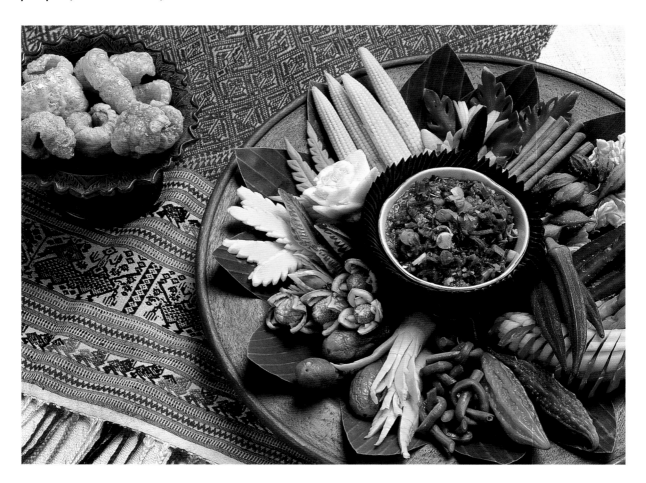

MINCED PORK NORTHERN STYLE

NAM PRIK ONG - น้ำพริกอ่อง

This dipping sauce is made using dried chillies and is a dish that is used on ceremonial occasions in the north. It reminds me of my childhood and all the temple ceremonies that I used to attend. It is eaten along with sticky rice. In the country side it is made with eggs added so that the dish will feed more people. If you want a change from rice then it also makes an amazing sauce for spaghetti but you will need to add more water (this quantity is enough for 2 people).

INGREDIENTS

Serves 4

100g (3/4 cup, 5 oz) pork - finely minced

30mls (2 tablespoons) oil

3 shallots - chopped

2 cloves of garlic - chopped

8 cherry tomatoes - cut in half

2 eggs - beaten - optional

45mls (3 tablespoons) water

15mls (1 tablespoon) fish sauce

2 spring onions - chopped

10g (1/2 cup, 1/2 oz) coriander - chopped

A selection of fresh, steamed or boiled vegetables such as carrots, cucumber, beans, egg plants, cauliflower, broccoli etc.

Paste

Dried

1/2 teaspoon salt

13 big, red, dried chillies - seeds removed and soaked in water for at least 10 minutes and finely chopped

Fresh

10g (1 tablespoon) coriander root - chopped

3 shallots - chopped

2 cloves of garlic - crushed

5g (1/2 teaspoon) shrimp paste

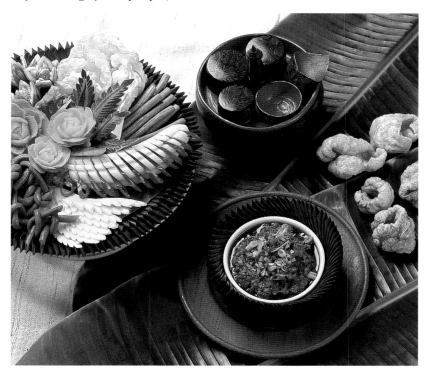

METHOD

Put all the ingredients for the paste together into a mortar and pound using a pestle until a smooth paste is formed. Add the cherry tomatoes and pound well to combine. Add the beaten eggs and mix thoroughly. Spoon the paste out into a bowl. Put the water into the empty mortar to rinse it out and spoon the water into another bowl.

Put the oil into a wok and over a low heat fry the shallots and garlic until they are brown and crispy. Remove them from the pan and put them onto a piece of kitchen paper to drain. Fry the pork for about 3 minutes until it is cooked. Then add the paste and fry for another 3 minutes. Add the fish sauce and water and cook for about 1 minute.

Turn off the heat and serve garnished with the crispy shallots and garlic, spring onions and coriander. Serve with a selection of vegetables and sticky rice.

FISH SAUCE WITH CHILLIES
NAM PLAA PRIK - น้ำปลาพริก

This sauce is served along with most Thai dishes and is added individually in the same way that salt and pepper are used in the west. It can be stored at room temperature.

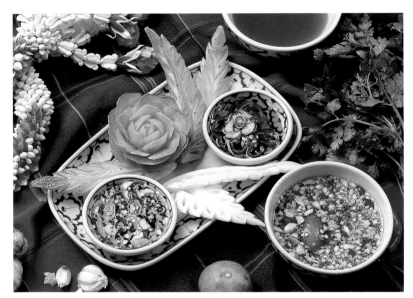

INGREDIENTS

250mls (1 cup, 8 fl oz) fish sauce
130g (1 cup, 41/2 oz) medium
chillies - thinly sliced
25g (1/4 cup, 1 oz) garlic - chopped
45mls (3 tablespoons) lime juice

METHOD

Mix all the ingredients together.

PLUM SAUCE
NAM JIM BUOY - น้ำจิ้มบ๊วย

INGREDIENTS
350g (21/2 cups, 12 oz) sweet pickled plums - remove stones
250mls (1 cup, 8 fl oz) juice from the sweet pickled plums
700g (31/2 cups, 1 lb 6 oz) sugar
180mls (3/4 cup, 6 fl oz) vinegar
125mls (1/3/4 cup, 4 fl oz) water

METHOD

Put all the ingredients into a pan and simmer on a low heat for about 20 minutes, until the sauce is thick. Stir occasionally.

Once cooked this can be stored in a bottle for about 1 month.

SWEET CHILLI DIPPING SAUCE
NAM JIM GAI - น้ำจิ้มไก่

INGREDIENTS
100g (3/4 cup, 31/2 oz) coriander root - finely chopped
250g (5 cups, 81/2 oz) pickled garlic - chopped
7 big, red chillies - finely chopped
700g (31/2 cups, 1 lb 6oz) sugar
150g (2 cups, 5 oz) white radish - cut into thin strips
375mls (11/2 cups, 12 fl oz) vinegar
1/4 teaspoon salt

METHOD

Put all the ingredients into a pan and simmer on a low heat for about 20 minutes, until the sauce is thick. Stir occasionally.

Once cooked this can be stored in a bottle for about 1 month.

CHILLI JAM
NAM PRIK POW - น้ำพริกเผา

Chilli jam is added to many Thai dishes and some people like to eat it with sticky rice.

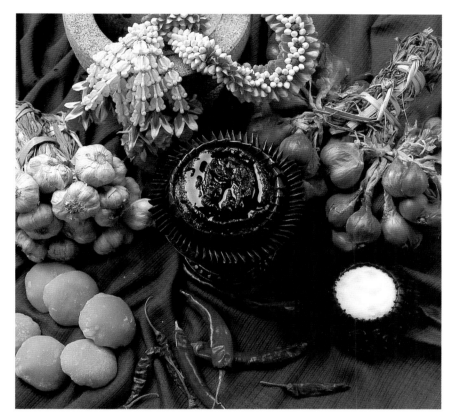

INGREDIENTS

100g (1 cup, 31/2 oz) garlic - peeled and roasted
100g (3/4 cups, 31/2 oz) shallots - peeled and roasted
15 big, red dried chillies - roasted and then chopped
250mls (1 cup, 8 fl oz) oil
40g (2 tablespoons) melted palm sugar
10g (1 tablespoon) sugar
1/4 teaspoon salt

METHOD

Put the big, red, dried chillies into a mortar and pound with a pestle until they become a powder. Add the garlic and the shallots and pound until smooth.

Put the oil into a wok and when it is hot add the chilli paste. Cook it on low heat for about 5 minutes, stirring occasionally. Then add the melted palm sugar and salt and stir to combine. Once the sugar has melted turn off the heat.

The chilli jam should be stored in a jar with a lid and will last for about 3 months outside the refrigerator or for 6 months in the refrigerator.

SUGAR SYRUP
NAM CHEUM - น้ำเชื่อม

This is used is Thai desserts and is also added to fruit shakes.

INGREDIENTS
90mls (6 tablespoons) water
80g (6 tablespoons) sugar

METHOD

To make the sugar syrup put the water and the sugar into a pan and dissolve the sugar over a low heat. Once the sugar has dissolved bring the water to the boil and simmer for about 5 minutes or until the syrup is thick.

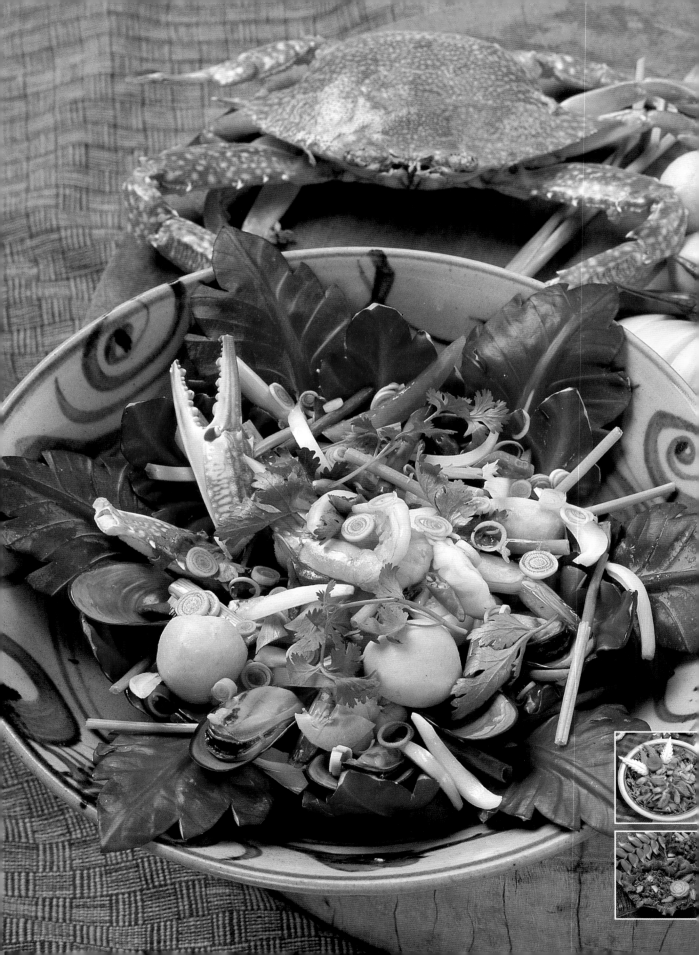

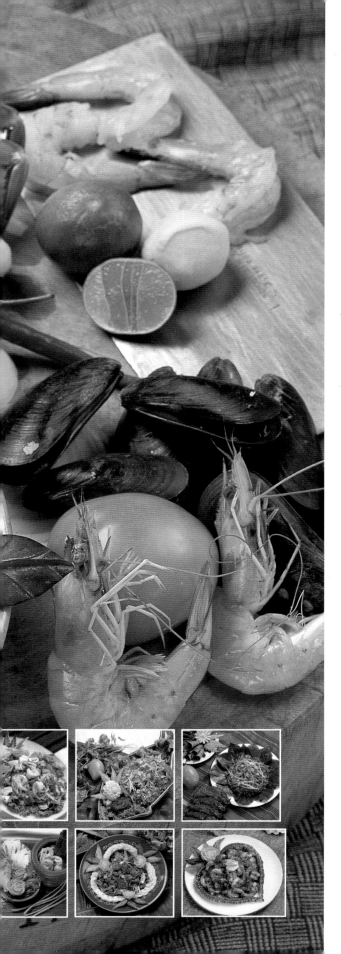

SALADS

Spicy salads are very popular with Thai people and are usually eaten as snacks. They are also eaten as an accompaniment to whisky if people are drinking as opposed to having crisps or peanuts. They are always spicy and Thai people like to have a sense of satisfaction after having eaten a spicy salad. If the salad is not spicy enough then they feel let down!

Salads are very simple to make and taste wonderful. Everybody likes their salads to have a different emphasis and it is up to you which flavours you want to emphasize. Thai people nearly always like them to be very spicy and sour and then it is up to the individual if they want it to be sweet or salty. Personally I do not like the salads to be sweet so I do not add very much palm sugar. If you are not sure how you like them then experiment by adding more or less chillies, lime juice, sugar and fish sauce. Remember though if you are cooking for people who are not used to eating spicy food that you need to go easy on the chillies or they will not be able to taste the rest of the meal. If you are not sure how spicy you want the salad to be then you can always add the chillies bit by bit.

Thai people also believe that eating a spicy salad will help clear your head if you have a cold. It does not get rid of the cold but it will make you feel a bit better. At least if you are eating something spicy it will take your mind off your cold for a while! Also Thai people like to eat spicy food as it is a good way of cooling down in the hot weather!

If you want to make a salad then you can do the preparation in advance and prepare all the ingredients but do not mix them together until the last minute as you want the salads to taste as fresh as possible.

51

CATFISH SALAD
YAM PLAA DUK FOO - ยำปลาดุกฟู

I love this salad as it is slightly different from the others are the fried fish gives it an unusual texture. I would highly recommend having a go at making this dish.

INGREDIENTS
Serves 4

300g (2 cups, 10 oz) catfish fillet
Enough oil to deep-fry
5g (3 tablespoons) dried bread crumbs
1/4 teaspoon baking powder
75mls (5 tablespoons) melted palm sugar
90mls (6 tablespoons) fish sauce
75mls (5 tablespoons) lime juice
10 small green chillies - thinly sliced
4 shallots - thinly sliced
70g (1 cup, 21/2 oz) sour, green mango - peeled and grated or thinly sliced
50g (3 tablespoons, 2oz) peanuts - roasted
1 big, red chilli - sliced
10g (1/2 cup, 1/2 oz) coriander

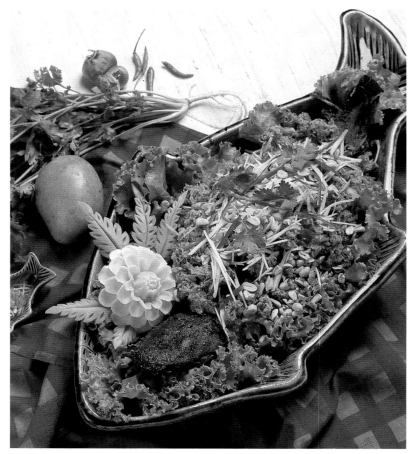

METHOD

Put the oil into a wok and heat it until it has smoke coming out. Deep-fry the fish fillets until they are golden brown and then drain and leave to cool.

When the fish is cool put it into a mortar and roughly pound with a pestle or chop to break it up. Add the bread crumbs and baking powder and mix together.
Reheat the oil and when it is very hot, carefully add the fish mixture. Deep-fry for 2-3 minutes. Then drain and put on a serving dish.

Put the melted palm sugar, fish sauce and lime juice into a bowl and mix together. Add the chillies, shallots and sour, green mango and mix together again.

Pour the mixture over the fish and sprinkle the peanuts on top.
Serve immediately garnished with the red chilli and coriander.

GREEN MANGO SALAD
TAM MAMUANG - ตำมะม่วง

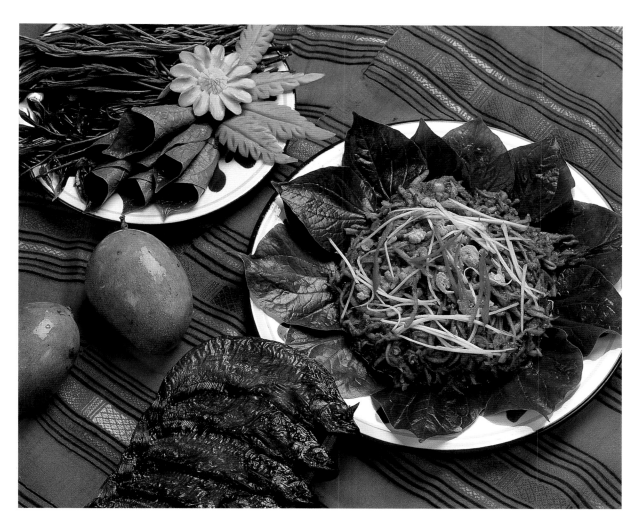

INGREDIENTS
Serves 4

250g (31/2 cups, 81/2 oz) sour green mango - peeled and grated

6 shallots

5g (1 teaspoon) shrimp paste

10g (3 tablespoons) ground dried shrimps - reserve 1 tablespoon for garnish

10g (4 tablespoons) ground, dried fish

5g (2 tablespoons) roasted chilli powder

30mls (2 tablespoons) fish sauce

30mls (2 tablespoons) lime juice

15mls (1 tablespoons) melted palm sugar

15g (3 tablespoons) dried shrimps

METHOD

Put the shallots into a mortar and pound with a pestle until completely smashed. Add the shrimp paste and pound again. Add the sour green mango and roughly pound. Add the remaining ingredients and roughly pound to combine.

Serve immediately with the remaining ground, dried shrimps sprinkled on top.

BEEF SALAD
YAM NEUA - ยำเนื้อ

This is a delicious salad but you need to make sure that the beef that you use is tender and sliced thinly.

INGREDIENTS
Serves 4

250g (11/4 cups, 81/2 oz) of medium rare roasted or grilled beef - thinly sliced
75mls (5 tablespoons) fish sauce
90mls (6 tablespoons) lime juice
25 small green and red chillies - finely chopped
5mls (1 teaspoon) melted palm sugar
5 shallots - thinly sliced
80g (3/4 cup, 3 oz) cucumber - cut in 1/2 lengthways and thinly sliced
1 tomato - cut in 1/2 and thinly sliced lengthways
20g (1/2cup, 1oz) Chinese celery - roughly chopped
5 spring onions - cut into 2cm (1 inch) pieces

METHOD

Put the fish sauce, lime juice, chillies and melted palm sugar into a bowl and mix together. Add the beef and stir well so that the beef is well covered in the sauce. Add the shallots and mix together. Then add the cucumber and the tomato and mix again. Finally add the Chinese celery and spring onions.

Mix together and serve immediately.

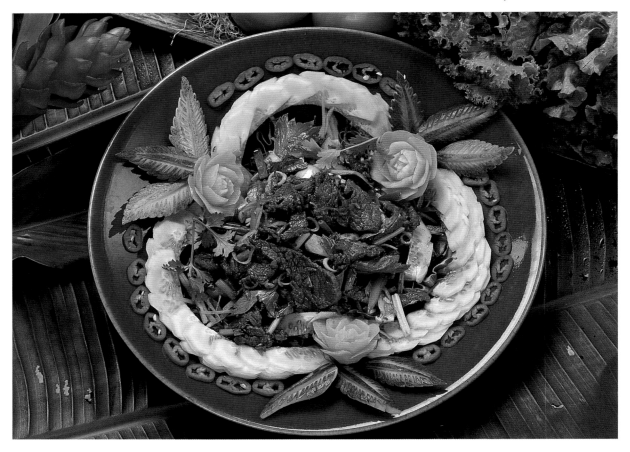

SEAFOOD SALAD
YAM TALAY - ยำทะเล

You can use any selection of seafood that you like. All the seafood needs to be cooked before it is added to the salad.

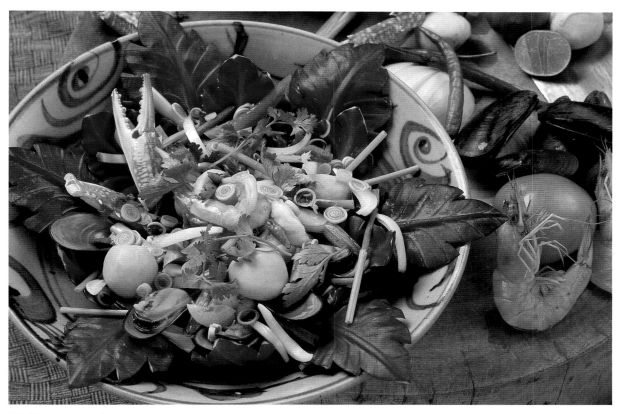

INGREDIENTS
Serves 4

150g (1 cup, 5 oz) crab meat

150g (1 cup, 5 oz) squid - cut into pieces

50g (1/2 cup, 2 oz) mussels

50g (1/2 cup, 2 oz) fish fillet - cut into pieces

100g (3/4 cup, 31/2 oz) prawns - washed, peeled and deveined

60mls (4 tablespoons) fish sauce

75mls (5 tablespoons) lime juice

20 small green and red chillies - finely chopped

5mls (1 teaspoon) melted palm sugar

3 stalks of lemongrass - lower 1/3 only, thinly sliced

1/2 medium onion - thinly sliced

1 tomato - cut in 1/2 and thinly sliced lengthways

20g (1/2 cup, 1oz) Chinese celery - roughly chopped

4 spring onions - cut into 2 cm (1 inch) pieces

METHOD

Put some water into a pan and bring to the boil. Cook the crab meat, squid, mussels, fish and prawns separately. Once cooked, mix the seafood together and set aside.

Put the fish sauce, lime juice, chillies and melted palm sugar into a bowl and mix together. Add the seafood and stir well so that the seafood is well covered in the sauce. Add the lemongrass and mix together. Then add the onion and mix again. Finally add the tomato, Chinese celery and spring onions.

Mix together and serve immediately.

SPICY PRAWN SALAD NORTH-EASTERN STYLE
PLAAH GOONG - พล่ากุ้ง

This salad is different from a normal spicy prawn salad as it has chilli jam in it which is what gives it its unique flavour.

INGREDIENTS
Serves 4

300g (2 cups, 10 oz) prawns - washed, peeled, deveined and boiled in water until cooked (about 1 minute)
45mls (3 tablespoons) fish sauce
90mls (6 tablespoons) lime juice
40g (4 tablespoons) chilli jam *(see p.49)*
40g (1/2 cup, 11/2 oz) lemongrass - lower 1/3 only, thinly sliced
6 shallots - thinly sliced
15-20 small chillies - finely chopped
10g (1/2 cup, 1/2 oz) coriander leaves - chopped
20g (1/2 cup, 1 oz) mint leaves - chopped
4 spring onions - chopped
8 kaffir lime leaves - stem removed and shredded

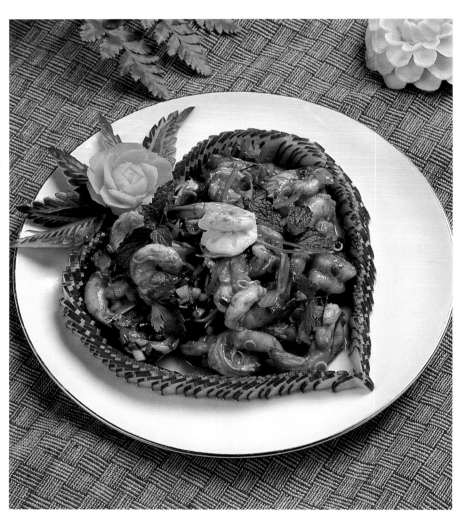

METHOD

Put the fish sauce, lime juice and chilli jam into a bowl and mix together well. Then add the prawns and mix together. If it is too thick add a bit of water or stock. In a separate bowl mix the lemongrass, shallots, small chillies, coriander leaves, mint leaves and spring onions together. Add the prawn mixture to the other ingredients and mix together. Put onto a plate and garnish with the kaffir lime leaves.

Serve immediately.

SPICY GLASS NOODLE SALAD
YAM WUN SEN - ยำวุ้นเส้น

This salad is a bit unusual because it is made using glass noodles. It is vital that you do not mix this salad in advance as the noodles will soak up all the sauce and become very stodgy. You can also add cooked prawns or dried shrimps to this salad to make it a bit different. In Thailand it is often served with fungus or ear mushrooms in it.

INGREDIENTS
Serves 4

100g (1 cup, 31/2 oz) glass noodles - soak in water for 10 minutes and then cut into 15 cm (6 inch) lengths
100g (1/2 cup, 31/2 oz) pork - finely minced and boiled in water or coconut milk until it is cooked. Reserve 60mls (4 tablespoons) of the water/coconut milk.
5 cloves of garlic or pickled garlic - crushed
3 shallots - sliced
10-20 small, red chillies - thinly sliced
30g (1/2 cup, 1 oz) Chinese celery - chopped
45mls (3 tablespoons) fish sauce
30mls (2 tablespoons) lime juice
1 tomato - cut in 1/2 lengthways and then thinly sliced
10g (1/2 cup, 1/2 oz) coriander leaves

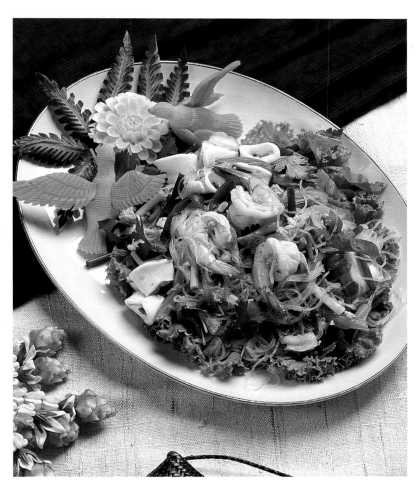

METHOD

Put the glass noodles into some boiling water and leave for about 1 minute and then drain. Transfer the glass noodles into a bowl of cold water and leave for 1 minute.

Strain the glass noodles and put them into a bowl along with the pork, water, garlic, onion, chillies, Chinese celery, fish sauce, lime juice and tomato. Mix thoroughly and check the seasoning.

Serve garnished with the prawns and coriander leaves.

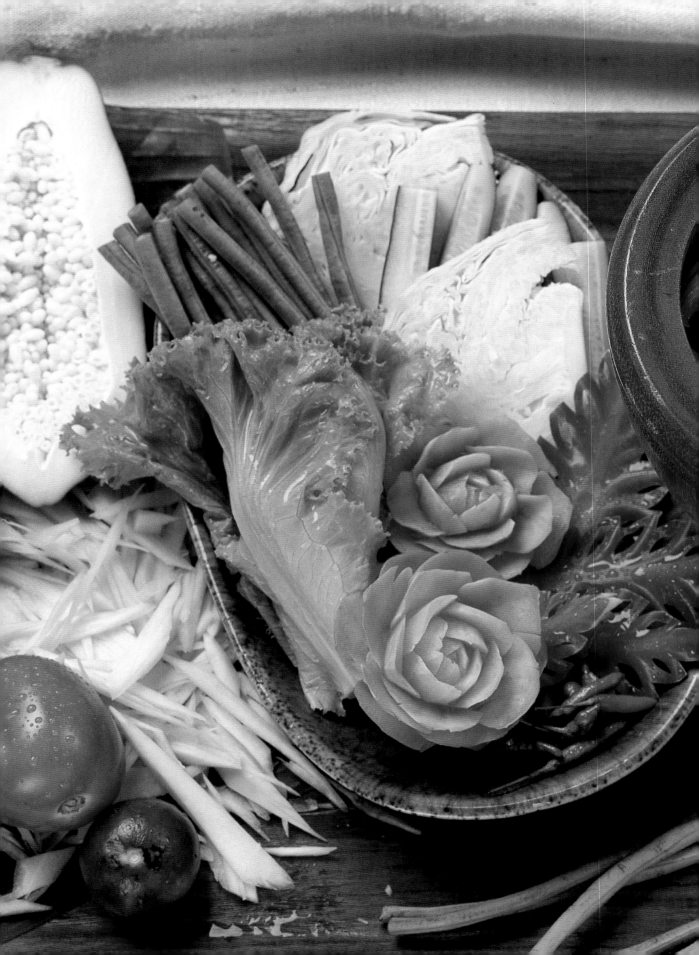

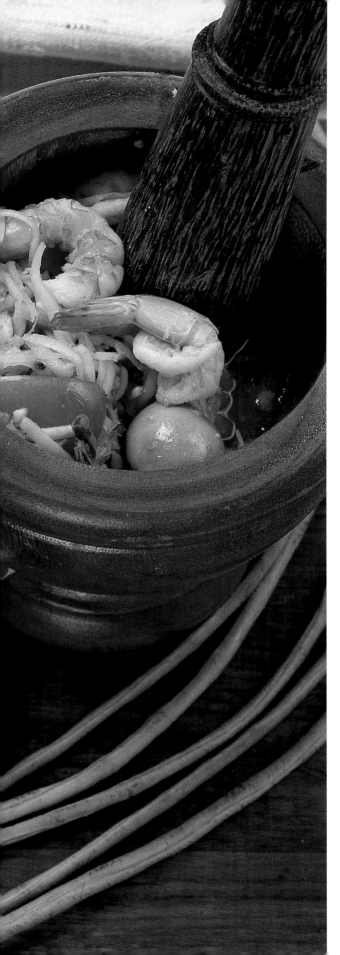

PAPAYA SALAD
SOM TAM - ส้มตำ

This salad is very popular with both Thais and foreigners. Unripe, green papaya is becoming more widely available abroad now so there is every chance that you will be able to reproduce this at home. Thais like to eat it with sticky rice and barbecued chicken.

INGREDIENTS
Serves 2

200g (3 cups, 7oz) green papaya - peeled and grated into thin strips (cucumber, carrot or melon can be substituted)
3 cloves of garlic
10 small, green chillies
2 long beans - cut into 2cm (1 inch) pieces
5g (2 tablespoons) dried shrimps
30mls (2 tablespoons) fish sauce
30mls (2 tablespoons) lime juice
10g (1 teaspoon) palm sugar
15mls (1 tablespoon) anchovy sauce - optional
1 tomato - cut in half and sliced
30g (2 tablespoons) peanuts - roasted

METHOD

Put the garlic, chillies and long beans into a mortar and pound roughly. Add the papaya and pound again to bruise the ingredients. Then add the dried shrimps, fish sauce, lime juice and palm sugar and stir together using the pestle and a spoon until the palm sugar has melted. Add the anchovy sauce and tomatoes and pound to combine. Then add the peanuts and mix together. Serve with sticky rice.

SAUSAGE SALAD
YAM SAI GROK - ยำไส้กรอก

This sausage salad can be made using any sort of sausages that you like. It is really good if you make it using a mixture of sausages such as salami, brokwurst, English sausages.

INGREDIENTS

Serves 4

300g (3 3/4 cups, 10 oz) hot dog sausages - thinly sliced

10 small, green chillies - thinly sliced

10 small, red chillies - thinly sliced

3 shallots - thinly sliced

2 stalks of lemongrass - lower 1/3 only, thinly sliced

3 cloves of garlic - chopped

30mls (2 tablespoons) lime juice

30mls (2 tablespoons) fish sauce

1 large tomato - cut in 1/2 lengthways and then thinly sliced

2 small cucumbers - cut in 1/2 lengthways and then thinly sliced

1/2 teaspoon salt

2 spring onions - thinly sliced

10g (1/2 cup, 1/2 oz) coriander - chopped

METHOD

Put all the ingredients except for the spring onions and coriander into a bowl and mix thoroughly. Check the seasoning.

Serve garnished with spring onions and coriander.

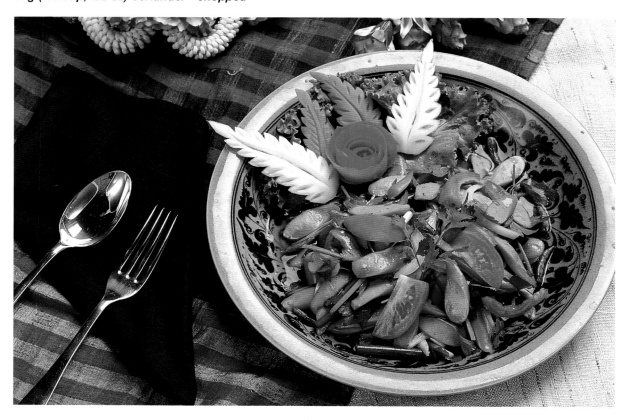

MINCED CHICKEN SALAD
LAAP GAI - ลาบไก่

This is a really fresh tasting salad and is slightly different from the other spicy salads as it has ground, roasted sticky rice in it. I love the fresh mint that is served with this dish.

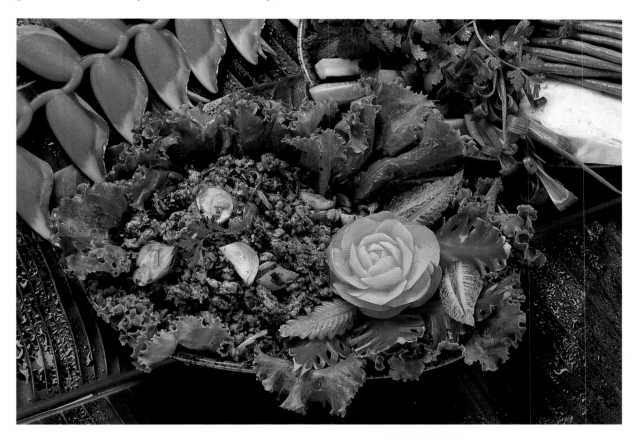

INGREDIENTS
Serves 4

300g (11/2 cups, 10 oz) chicken breast - minced

4 shallots - thinly sliced

2 slices of ginza - finely chopped

45mls (3 tablespoons) fish sauce

30mls (2 tablespoons) lime juice

15g (1 tablespoon) chilli powder

5g (1 tablespoon) coriander - chopped

1 spring onion - chopped

5g (1 tablespoon) mint leaves - chopped

30g (2 tablespoons) sticky rice - roasted and ground *(see p.19)*

Mint leaves - for garnish

A selection of fresh vegetables

METHOD

Put the chicken, shallots, ginza, fish sauce, lime juice and chilli powder into a bowl and mix thoroughly. Heat a wok and on a medium heat cook the chicken mixture for about 5 minutes until the chicken is cooked. Transfer the cooked chicken mixture into a bowl and add the coriander, spring onion, chopped mint leaves and ground, roasted sticky rice and mix well.

Serve garnished with some mint leaves and a selection of fresh vegetables such as long beans, cabbage, lettuce, spinach, cucumber, etc.

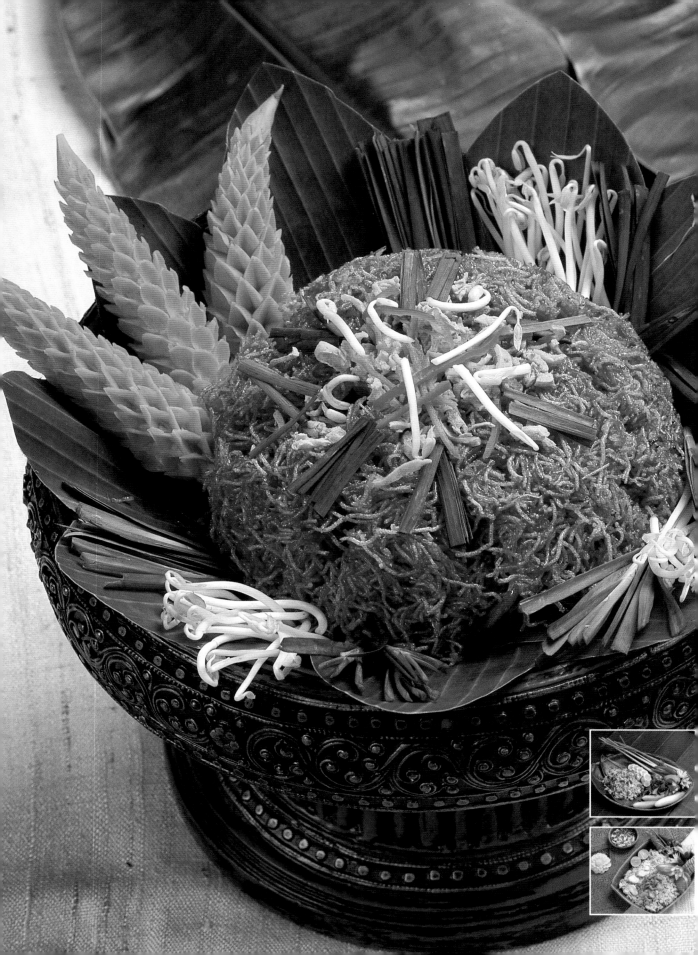

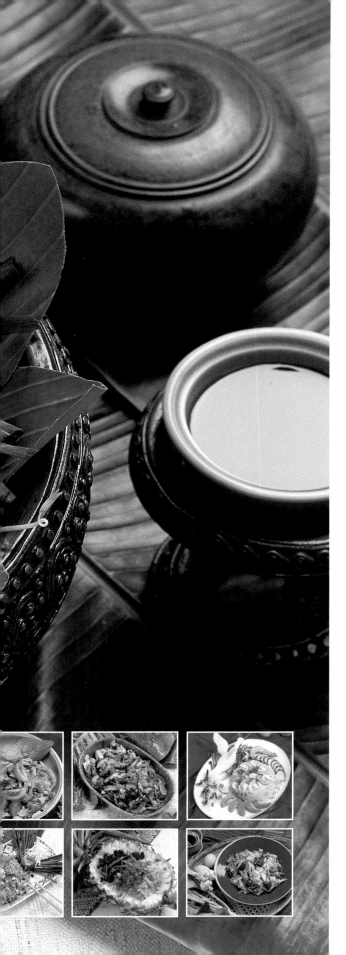

RICE AND NOODLES

Rice is used in many different ways in Thai cooking. It is often fried with meat and vegetables to make a quick and easy lunch dish. It is also used to make noodles which are very popular in Thailand. Noodles are also often stir-fried and there are many different sorts of noodles. The dishes included in this section are a selection of stir-fried rice and noodle dishes which I think you will find simple to cook and delicious to eat.

FRIED RICE WITH PRAWNS
KHAO PHAD GOONG - ข้าวผัดกุ้ง

This version of fried rice is a plain version and is what is often served in hotels.

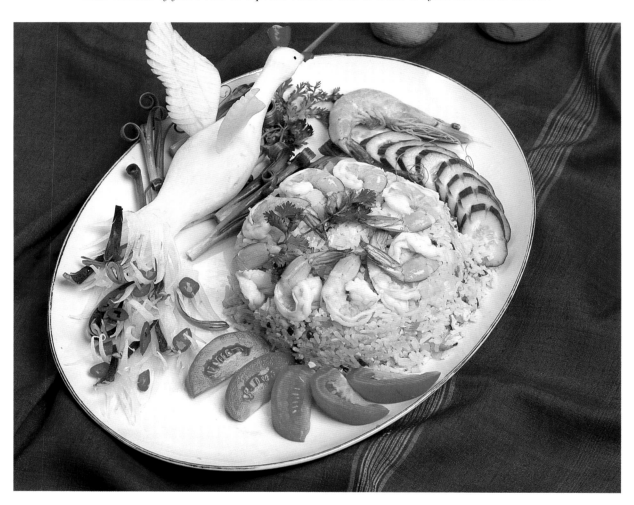

INGREDIENTS
Serves 4

700g (4 cups, 1lb 6oz) precooked rice
**250g (1/2 cups, 81/2 oz) prawns - peeled, deveined
and boiled in water for 1 minute**
120mls (1/2 cup, 4 fl oz) oil
4 eggs - beaten
5 spring onions - chopped
1/2 teaspoon salt
1/2 teaspoon ground pepper
1/2 teaspoon sugar
2 limes - cut into wedges

METHOD

Put the oil into a wok and on a high heat, add the egg and stir rapidly for 5 seconds. Then add the rice and stir-fry rapidly, turning the rice over as it is cooked, for about 2 minutes. Add the prawns, spring onions, salt, pepper and sugar and stir-fry again.

Serve garnished with the wedges of lime and some fish sauce and chillies *(see p.48)*.

FRIED RICE WITH CHICKEN
KHAO PHAD GAI - ข้าวผัดไก่

This version of fried rice is similar to the sort of fried rice that you would find on market stalls in Thailand. It is usually eaten as a quick snack or light lunch dish.

INGREDIENTS
Serves 4

700g (4 cups, 1lb 6oz) precooked rice
300g (11/2 cups, 10 oz) chicken - thinly sliced
15mls (1 tablespoon) soy sauce
120mls (1/2 cup, 4 fl oz) oil
1 onion - sliced
4 eggs - beaten
2 tomatoes - each cut into 8 pieces
200g (21/2 cups, 7 oz) Chinese leaves - roughly chopped
3 spring onions - chopped
2 limes - cut into wedges

Sauce
15mls (1 tablespoon) soy sauce
15mls (1 tablespoon) fish sauce
15mls (1 tablespoon) sweet soy sauce
1 teaspoon sugar
1/4 teaspoon pepper

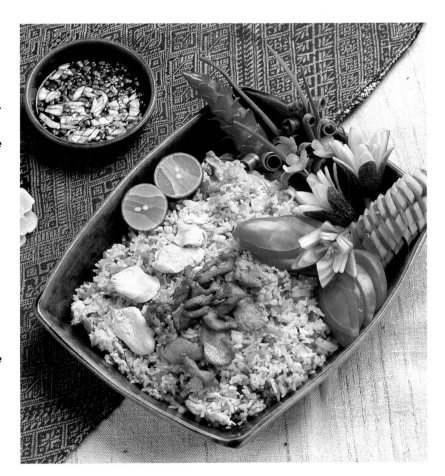

METHOD

Mix the chicken with 15mls (1 tablespoon) soy sauce.

Put the oil into a wok and when it is hot add the onion and fry for 1 minute. Add the chicken and when it starts to go brown (about 3 minutes) add the eggs and stir-fry rapidly to cook. Add the tomato and stir-fry to combine.

Add the rice and on a high heat and stir-fry rapidly, turning the rice over, for about 2 minutes. Turn the heat down and add the Chinese leaves and spring onion. Stir-fry together and add the sauce ingredients and stir to combine.

Serve garnished with the lime wedges and some fish sauce and chillies *(see p.48)*.

FRIED RICE WITH LEMONGRASS
KHAO PHAD TAKRAI - ข้าวผัดตะไคร้

I first had this dish in the clubhouse in the village where I live. It was cooked by the chef Oran and this is his recipe. I think it is a good way of making a plain dish like fried rice into something quite special.

INGREDIENTS
Serves 4

700g (4 cups, 1lb 6oz) precooked rice
4 stalks of lemongrass - lower 1/3 only, finely chopped and fried in oil until it is a light brown colour. Drain.
60mls (4 tablespoons) oil
2 eggs - beaten
50g (1/3 cup, 2 oz) prawns - cut into cubes
50g (3/4 cup, 2 oz) hot dog sausages - cut into cubes
50g (1/2 cup, 2 oz) Chinese sausages - cut into cubes
60mls (4 tablespoons) light soy sauce
5g (1 teaspoon) sugar
15g (1/2 cup, 1/2 oz) sweet basil leaves
1 lime - cut into quarters

Sauce
80g (1 cup, 3 oz) green mango - peeled and shredded
2 shallots - thinly sliced
2 small chillies - thinly sliced

METHOD

Put the oil into a wok and when it is hot add the eggs and stir-fry to cook. Add the prawns, hot dog sausages and Chinese sausages and stir-fry for 1 minute.

Add the rice on a high heat and stir-fry rapidly, turning the rice over, for about 2 minutes. Then add the lemongrass, light soy sauce and sugar and stir-fry to combine. Turn off the heat and serve garnished with the basil leaves and lime.

Mix all the ingredients for the sauce together and serve as an accompaniment to the fried rice.

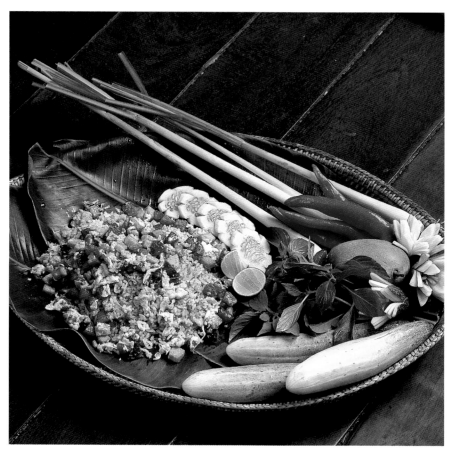

FRIED RICE IN PINEAPPLE
KHAO OP SAPPAROT - ข้าวอบสับปะรด

Despite its name this dish is not actually baked in the oven. It always looks impressive served in the pineapple and it has an unusual combination of ingredients.

INGREDIENTS
Serves 2

450g (3 cups, 1lb) precooked rice

1 big pineapple

60mls oil (4 tablespoons) oil

50g (1/2 cup, 2 oz) Chinese sausage - chopped into little pieces (keep a little to use as garnish)

10g (2 tablespoons) butter

1/2 teaspoon curry powder

1 small onion - cut into small chunks (keep a little to use as garnish)

3 spring onions - chopped (keep a little to use as garnish)

1 tomato - chopped (keep a little to use as garnish)

30g (1/2 cup, 1 oz) raisins (keep a little to use as garnish)

5g (1 teaspoon) sugar

30mls (2 tablespoons) soy sauce

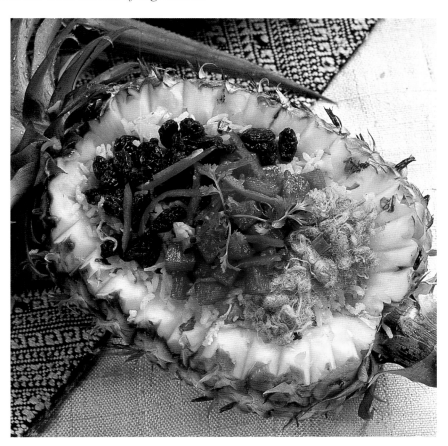

METHOD

Cut off one side of the pineapple and cut all the flesh out of the bigger half of the pineapple. Cut into bite-sized pieces and use 60g (½ cup, 2 oz). Keep the side of the pineapple to use as a lid.

Put the oil into a wok and fry the Chinese sausage until it is cooked (about 1 minute) and then remove the Chinese sausage from the oil and set aside. Add the butter to the same oil and when it is hot add the curry powder and mix together. Then add the precooked rice and stir-fry until the rice is well covered in oil. Add the Chinese sausage, pineapple, onion, spring onion, tomato, raisins and stir-fry for about 4 minutes. Then add the sugar and soy sauce and stir-fry to combine.

Put the rice into the pineapple and sprinkle on the remaining pineapple, Chinese sausage, onion, spring onion, tomato and raisins. Put the lid on the pineapple and serve.

FRIED BIG NOODLES WITH SWEET SOY SAUCE
PHAD SIEWE - ผัดซีอิ๊ว

This dish is quite dry but is excellent for people who like noodles as the full taste and texture of the noodles really comes through.

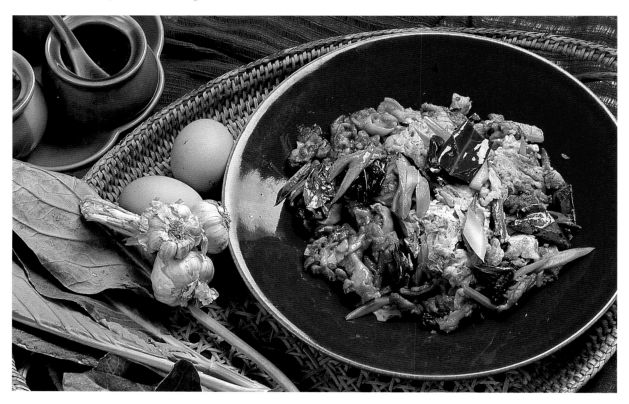

INGREDIENTS
Serves 4

400g (4 cups, 14 oz) fresh big noodles (or dried noodles, soaked in water for about 10-15 minutes before being used)
200g (1 cup, 7 oz) pork - thinly sliced
90mls (6 tablespoons) oil
6 cloves of garlic - crushed
250g (3 cups, 81/2 oz) Chinese leaves - roughly chopped (or cauliflower, carrot or mushroom)
4 eggs - beaten

Sauce
45mls (3 tablespoons) oyster sauce
5mls (1 teaspoon) sweet soy sauce
30mls (2 tablespoons) light soy sauce
10g (2 teaspoons) sugar
1 teaspoon ground, black pepper

METHOD

Put 60mls (4 tablespoons) oil into a wok and turn on a medium heat. When the oil is hot add garlic followed by the pork and stir-fry for 2 minutes. Add the noodles and stir-fry for another 2-3 minutes until they are brown and soft. Then add the Chinese leaves and stir-fry to combine. Then add the sauce ingredients and stir-fry to combine.

Move the stir-fry mixture to one side of the wok and add the remaining oil. Add the beaten egg and fry for 1 minute and then combine with the rest of the noodle mixture. Stir-fry to combine and serve.

FRIED DRUNKEN NOODLES WITH CHICKEN
PHAD KII MAW GAI - ผัดขี้เมาไก่

This dish combines many different ingredients together in an unusual way. It is a good dish to give you a kick and get you going again if you have a hangover but you would probably have to get somebody else to cook it for you!

INGREDIENTS
Serves 4

350g (3½ cups, 12 oz) big, flat noodles
300g (1½ cups, 10 oz) chicken - thinly sliced
180mls (¾ cup, 6 fl oz) oil
9 cloves of garlic - roughly chopped
4 shallots - roughly chopped
1 big, green chilli - sliced
1 big, red chilli - sliced
6 medium chillies - roughly chopped
60g (1 cup, 2 oz) lesser ginza - shredded
20g (¼ cup, 1 oz) fresh young green peppercorn
30g (½ cup, 1 oz) dried shrimps
1 tomato - cut into wedges
6 long beans - sliced
4 baby corn - each one sliced into 3
150g (2 cup, 5 oz) straw mushrooms - cut in quarters
100g (1 cup, 3½ oz) carrots - sliced
½ teaspoon sweet soy sauce
4 eggs - beaten
100g (½ cup, 3½ oz) peanuts - roasted and crushed
30g (1 cup, 1oz) holly basil

Sauce
60mls (4 tablespoons) oyster sauce
30mls (2 tablespoons) soy sauce,
60mls (4 tablespoons) fish sauce
½ teaspoon sugar

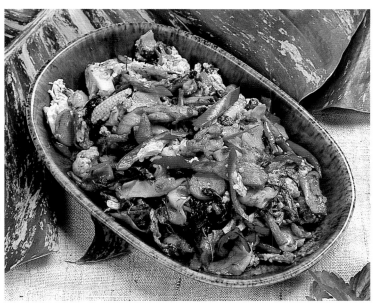

METHOD

Put 60mls (4 tablespoons) of oil into a wok and when it is hot, add the garlic, shallots, big red and green chillies and the medium chillies and fry on high heat for 1 minute. Add the chicken and stir-fry until the outsides turns to white (2-3 minutes). Add the lesser ginza, green peppercorns and dried shrimps and stir-fry for 2 minutes.

Turn the heat down and add the tomato, long beans, baby corn, mushrooms, and carrots cook for 3 minutes. Turn off the heat and set aside.

Put the remaining oil into a wok and when it is hot add the big noodles and the sweet soy sauce. Stir-fry over high heat for 1 minute, stirring continuously. Turn the heat down and add the eggs and stir to cook.

Then add the above vegetable mixture and over a high heat stir to mix everything together well. Add the sauce ingredients and stir-fry to combine. Finally add the peanuts and basil leaves and stir once again.

Turn off the heat and serve.

THAI FRIED NOODLES
PHAD THAI - ผัดไทย

Phad Thai is now very well known and is one of the dishes that foreigners love to eat when they come to Thailand. Everybody has a different version of this and this is mine. It can also be made using fresh prawns instead of dried shrimps.

INGREDIENTS
Serves 2

300g (10 oz) fresh rice noodles - (or dried noodles, soaked in water for about 10-15 minutes)
45mls (3 tablespoons) oil
5g (1 tablespoon) garlic - chopped
5g (1 tablespoon) dried shrimps
80g (1 cup, 3 oz) tofu - chopped into small pieces
90mls (6 tablespoons) chicken stock or water
2 eggs - beaten
45g (3 tablespoons) roasted peanuts - chopped
20g (1/4 cup,1oz) chives - cut into 2cm (1 inch) pieces
60g (1 cup, 2 oz) bean sprouts
2 limes - cut into wedges
Fresh vegetables (bean sprouts, cabbage and chives)

Sauce
30g (3 tablespoons) sugar
45mls (3 tablespoons) fish sauce
15mls (1 tablespoon) soy sauce
30mls (2 tablespoons) tamarind juice *(see p.17)*

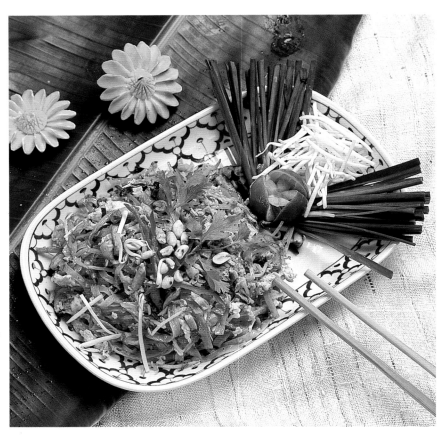

METHOD

Put the oil into a wok and fry the garlic, dried shrimps and tofu until the garlic turns golden brown and then add the rice noodles. Keep stirring over a high heat. Then add the chicken stock and stir-fry until the noodles are soft. Then turn the heat down and add the sauce ingredients and stir well to combine.

Add the eggs and stir-fry until the eggs are cooked and well combined with the noodles. Add the peanuts and chives. Stir-fry to combine and then add the bean sprouts and stir together. Turn off the heat and serve garnished with the lime wedges and fresh vegetables.

FRIED BIG NOODLES WITH THICK SAUCE AND PORK

RAAD NAH MUU - ราดหน้าหมู

This dish is usually eaten as a snack and can be made with any vegetables you like. It has a thick gravy-like sauce which makes it different from some of the other stir-fried noodle dishes.

INGREDIENTS
Serves 4

500g (5 cups, 1lb 2oz) flat
noodles
15mls (1 tablespoon) sweet
soy sauce
60mls (4 tablespoons) oil

250g (11/4 cups, 81/2 oz) pork -
thinly sliced
45mls (3 tablespoons) oil
3 cloves of garlic - chopped
100g (1 cup, 31/2 oz)
cauliflower - cut into bite
sized pieces (can also use
broccoli, carrots, peas,
mushrooms)
500mls(2 cups, 16 fl oz)
chicken stock or water
30g (2 tablespoons) tapioca
flour - dissolved in 45mls
(2 tablespoons) water

Sauce
30mls (2 tablespoons) fish
sauce
30mls (2 tablespoons) oyster
sauce
30mls (2 tablespoons) soya
bean paste
1/2 teaspoon pepper
10g (1 tablespoon) sugar

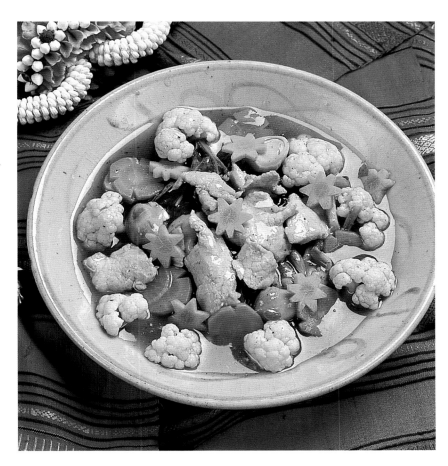

METHOD

Mix the noodles and sweet soy sauce together. Put the oil into a wok and fry the noodles on a medium heat for about 2-3 minutes. Set aside.

Put the oil for the sauce into a wok and fry the garlic on a high heat until it starts to turn golden brown. Add the pork and fry for about 3 minutes until the pork is cooked. Then add the cauliflower and keep stirring and add the stock. Add the sauce ingredients and stir-fry for 2 minutes. Add the tapioca flour and bring to the boil. Cook for about 1 minute until the sauce is thick.

Divide the noodles into 4 portions and pour the sauce over them and serve with chilli powder and chillies in vinegar.

FRIED GLASS NOODLES
PHAD WUN SEN - ผัดวุ้นเส้น

The glass noodles will stick together when you fry them so you need to keep stirring all the time while you are cooking them.

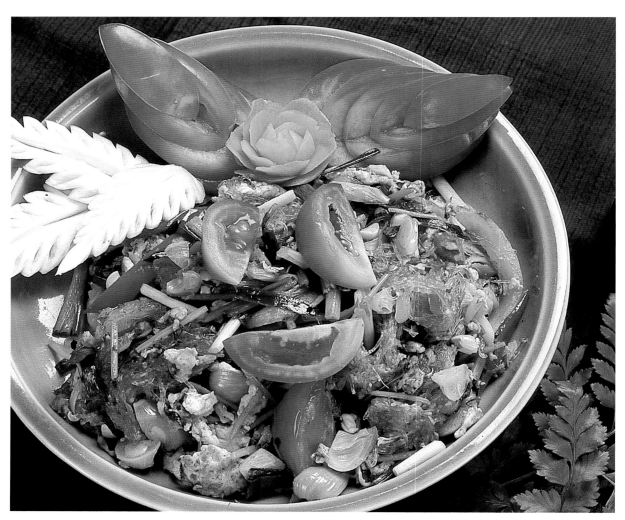

INGREDIENTS
Serves 2

160g (1½ cup, 5½ oz) glass noodles - soaked in water for at least 15 minutes
60mls (4 tablespoons) oil
3 eggs - beaten
1 onion - sliced
3 tomatoes - sliced
3 cloves of pickled garlic
½ teaspoon pepper powder

Sauce
30mls (2 tablespoons) fish sauce
45mls (3 tablespoons) oyster sauce
1 teaspoon sugar

METHOD

Put the oil into a wok and when it is hot, add the eggs and stir. Then add the glass noodles, onions, tomatoes and pickled garlic. Stir-fry to combine. Add the sauce ingredients and the pepper powder. Stir again to combine all the ingredients and then turn down the heat and serve.

CRISPY RICE VERMICELLI NOODLES
MEE GROB - หมี่กรอบ

This is a dish that I hear many foreigners talking about so here is a recipe for you to try at home.

INGREDIENTS
Serves 4

500mls (2 cups, 16 fl oz) oil
150g (11/2 cups, 5oz) rice vermicelli noodles

45mls (3 tablespoons) oil
60g (1/4 cup, 2 oz) pork - finely minced
60g (1/4 cup, 2 oz) chicken - finely minced
60g (1 cup, 2 oz) prawns - finely minced

2 eggs - beaten
5g (1 teaspoon) chilli powder
20g (1/4 cup, 1oz) chives - cut into 2cm (1 inch) pieces
20g (1/4 cup, 1oz) tofu - chopped into small pieces and fried until brown and crisp
5 cloves of garlic - chopped and fried until brown and crisp
3 shallots - chopped and fried until brown and crisp
1 big, red chilli - sliced
1 spring onion - chopped
10g (1/2 cup, 1/2 oz) coriander

Sauce
15mls (1 tablespoon) fish sauce
15mls (1 tablespoon) lime juice
15mls (1 tablespoon) vinegar
15mls (1 tablespoon) yellow bean sauce
20g (2 tablespoons) sugar

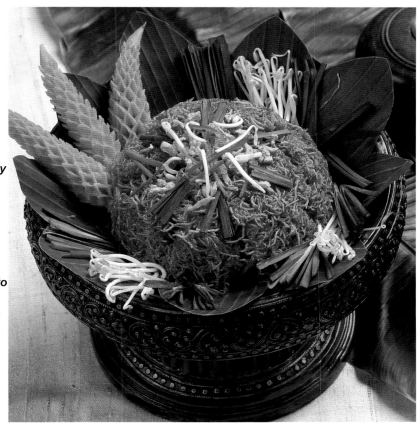

METHOD

Put the oil into a wok and when it is hot add the rice noodles in small quantities. Fry the noodles until they puff up and are crispy - this takes only a matter of seconds. Once the noodles are cooked, remove them from the oil and leave to drain.

Put the oil into a wok and add the pork, chicken and prawns and stir-fry for about 2 minutes. Then add the sauce ingredients. Stir-fry to combine. Then add the eggs and stir-fry for 1 minute until the eggs are cooked. Add the chilli powder, chives, tofu, garlic and shallots and stir -fry again to combine.

Once the sauce is cooked, add the crispy noodles to the sauce mixture and stir-fry quickly and gently to combine. Once they are combined put the noodles onto a plate and serve garnished with the big, red chilli, spring onion and coriander.

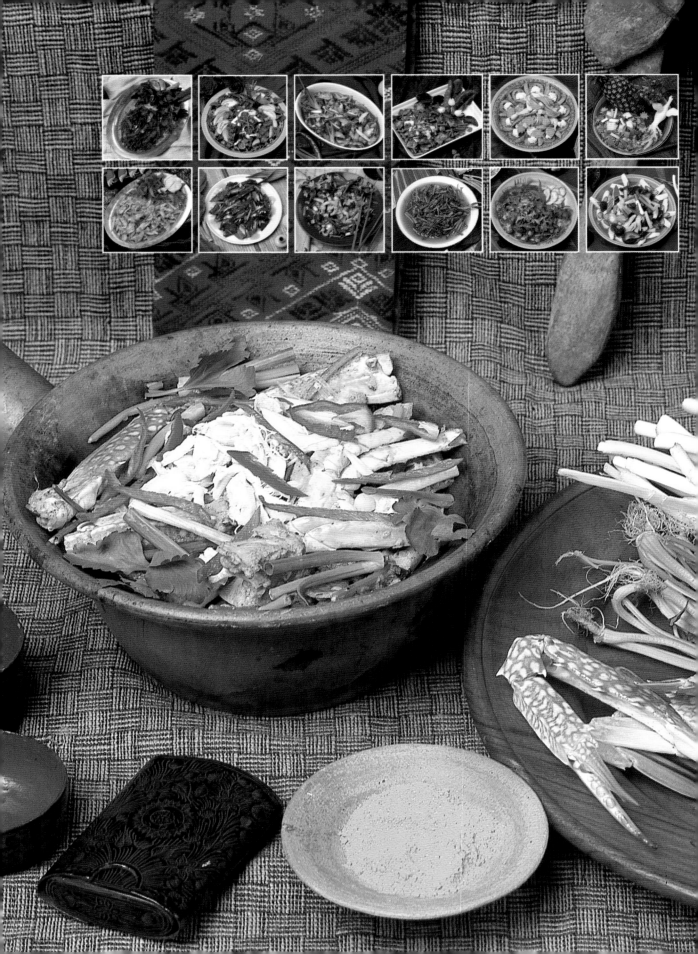

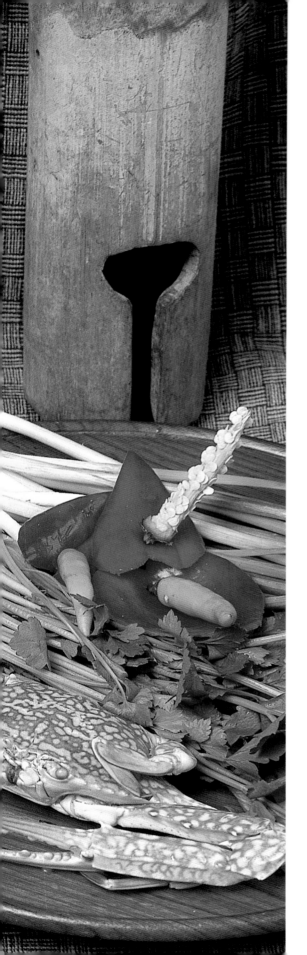

STIR FRIED DISHES

Stir-fried dishes are very popular in Thailand as they are quick, easy and cheap to make. Thai people will often have stir-fried dishes for lunch and many restaurants serve the dish on top of rice with a fried egg on top. If Thais are having a proper meal with several dishes then there will nearly always be a stir-fry included in the dishes. Stir-fries do not use very much meat so they are economical to make too.

In Thailand you will often see chefs cooking stir-fries over a very high heat often with the flames encircling the wok and lots of smoke spiraling up into the sky. They like to cook over a high heat as they do not want the oil to soak into the vegetables so they try to cook the dish quickly so that the vegetables are still crunchy. If you are not used to cooking then it is best to start with a low heat until you get used to it but once you get the idea then try to use a high heat so that the vegetables do not go soggy. If things start to burn turn the heat off quickly. If you find that the stir-fry is too dry and looks as if it may burn then you can add some chicken stock or water and you can also add the sauce ingredients which will help the temperature cool down a bit.

If you are cooking a stir-fry with vegetables in it then you need to add the vegetables that will take the longest to cook first and then add the ones that only need a little bit of cooking at the end.

It is important to prepare all the ingredients for a stir-fry before you start to cook so that you can add the ingredients quickly over a high heat. If you have to keep stopping to prepare vegetables then the ingredients will end up being soggy and full of oil. Once you have got used to cooking over a high heat you will find that stir-fried dishes are really very easy to cook and also very quick. If possible it is best to use a non-stick wok when cooking stir-fries.

CHICKEN WITH GREEN CURRY PASTE

PHAD KHEO WAN GAI - ผัดเขียวหวานไก่

This is a good dish if you want some food that is not too rich as it does not use very much coconut milk but still has a subtle flavour of coconut milk. It is also really nice eaten cold and makes an unusual dish for a cold buffet.

INGREDIENTS
Serves 4

300g (11/2 cups, 10 oz) chicken - thinly sliced
60mls (4 tablespoons) oil
100g (4 tablespoons) green curry paste *(see p.104)*
3 big egg plants - cut in quarters and then sliced
120g (11/4 cups, 4 oz) small egg plants
4 kaffir lime leaves - stem removed
60mls (4 tablespoons) chicken stock or water
1 big, red chilli - sliced
30g (1 cup, 1 oz) sweet basil leaves
120mls (1/2 cup, 4 fl oz) thick coconut milk - keep 30mls (2 tablespoons) for garnish

Sauce
20g (1 tablespoon) palm sugar
15mls (1 tablespoon) fish sauce
15mls (1 tablespoon) soy sauce
10g (1 tablespoon) sugar

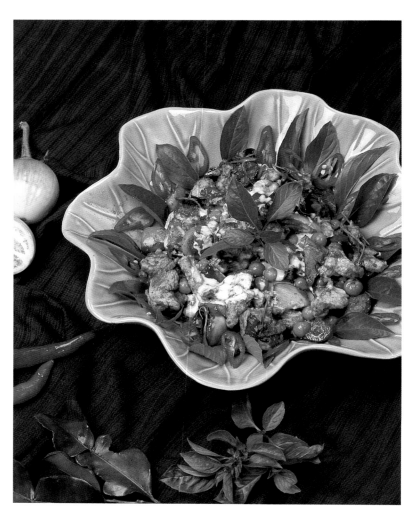

METHOD

Put the oil in a wok and when it is hot add the green curry paste and fry for 1-2 minutes. Then add the chicken and when the outside turns to white add the big egg plants, small egg plants and the kaffir lime leaves and stir-fry for 1 minute. Add the chicken stock and stir to combine and then add the sauce ingredients and stir-fry again.

Add the big, red chilli and sweet basil leaves followed by the thick coconut milk. Stir-fry to combine and turn off the heat. Serve with the remaining thick coconut milk poured over the top.

CHICKEN WITH GREEN PEPPERS
GAI PHAD PRIK SOD - ไก่ผัดพริกสด

This dish is not as spicy as the name might imply as the main ingredient is bell peppers not chilli peppers.

INGREDIENTS
Serves 4

300g (11/2 cups ,10 oz) chicken - thinly sliced
60mls (4 tablespoons) oil
7 cloves of garlic
1 small onion - cut into 8
3 green peppers - seeds removed and cut into strips
100g (11/4 cups, 3 oz) straw mushrooms - cut in 1/2
1 big, red chilli - sliced
1/2 teaspoon white peppercorns - crushed
250mls (1 cup, 8 fl oz) chicken stock or water
7 spring onions - cut into 2cm (1 inch) pieces

Sauce
30mls (2 tablespoons) oyster sauce
30mls (2 tablespoons) soy sauce
15mls (1 tablespoon) light soy sauce
1/4 teaspoon sweet soy sauce
1/2 teaspoon sugar

METHOD

Put the oil into a wok and add the garlic followed by the onion and fry until the garlic starts to turn brown. Add the chicken and fry until the outside turns to white and then add the green peppers and stir-fry for another minute.

Then add the sauce ingredients and stir-fry on high heat. Add the mushrooms, big, red chilli and white peppercorns and stir-fry again.

Add the stock and when it is boiling add the spring onions.

Stir-fry to combine and serve.

CHICKEN WITH CASHEW NUTS

GAI PHAD MED MAMUANG - ไก่ผัดเม็ดมะม่วง

This is a dish that is Chinese in origin but is now very popular with Thais too. Personally, I love cashew nuts and think that this dish tastes wonderful. It is one of the most popular dishes in my restaurant too and is very easy to make.

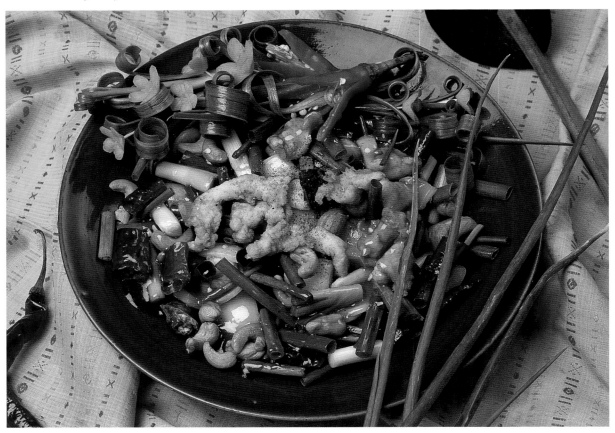

INGREDIENTS
Serves 4

300g (11/2 cups, 10 oz) chicken breast - thinly sliced

120g (2 cups, 4 oz) deep-fried cashew nuts - (if you have raw cashew nuts then fry them in 250mls (1 cup, 8 fl oz) oil, over a low heat until the cashew nuts are brown. Drain).

45mls (3 tablespoons) oil

8 cloves of garlic - crushed

2 small onions - sliced

2 big, red chillies - sliced

125mls (1/2 cup, 4 fl oz) chicken stock or water

4-8 spring onions - sliced

15mls (1 tablespoon) wine or 5mls (1 teaspoon) whisky

Sauce

30mls (2 tablespoons) oyster sauce

15mls (1 tablespoon) soy sauce

15mls (1 tablespoon) fish sauce

20g (1 tablespoons) palm sugar

METHOD

Put the oil into a wok and add the garlic and when it starts to turn brown add the chicken, onions and big, red chillies and stir-fry for about 3 minutes. Add the stock and stir to combine. Add the sauce ingredients and stir-fry to combine. Then add the cashew nuts and spring onions and stir-fry briefly. Add the wine or whisky and turn off the heat and serve.

BEEF WITH RED CURRY PASTE
PHAD PHET NEUA - ผัดเผ็ดเนื้อ

This dish is made special by the addition of fresh green peppercorns which give the dish a lovely peppery flavour. It is also a good way of using red curry paste for something other than a curry.

INGREDIENTS
Serves 4

300g (11/2 cups, 10oz) lean beef - thinly sliced
60mls (4 tablespoons) oil
100g (4 tablespoons) red curry paste (see p.105)
250mls (1 cup, 8 fl oz) thick coconut milk - keep 30mls (2 tablespoons) for garnish
3 big egg plants - cut in 4 quarters and then sliced
120g (11/4 cup, 4 oz) small egg plants
20g (1/4 cup, 1 oz) young, green peppercorns
50g (1 cup, 2 oz) lesser ginger - cut into strips
6 kaffir lime leaves - stems removed
1 big, red chilli - sliced
30g (1 cup, 1 oz) sweet basil leaves
Enough oil to deep-fry the basil

Sauce
30mls (2 tablespoons) fish sauce
15mls (1 tablespoon) soy sauce
1 teaspoon sugar
60mls (4 tablespoons) chicken stock or water

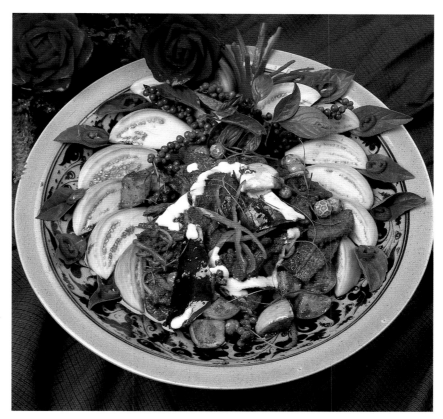

METHOD

Put the oil into a wok and when it is hot add the red curry paste and fry for 1-2 minutes. Then add half the thick coconut milk and the beef and stir-fry until the outside of the beef looks cooked (about 2 minutes). Then add the big egg plants, small eggplants and young, green peppercorns and stir-fry to combine. Add the lesser ginger and kaffir lime leaves and stir-fry again.

Then add the sauce ingredients and stir-fry for 1 minute. Add the remaining thick coconut milk and the big, red chilli and stir-fry to combine. Turn off the heat and transfer to a serving dish.
Deep fry the sweet basil leaves in very hot oil for 1 minute and drain. Then put them on top of the beef. Pour the remaining thick coconut milk over the top and serve.

PORK WITH GARLIC AND PEPPER

MUU PHAD GRATIUM PRIK THAI - หมูผัดกระเทียมพริกไทย

For people who love the taste of garlic this is an amazing dish.

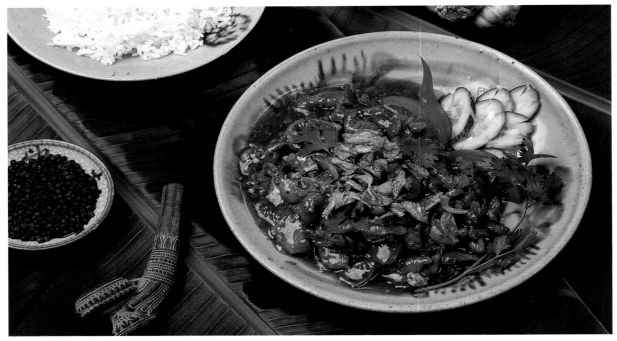

INGREDIENTS
Serves 4

450g (21/4 cups, 1lb) pork filet or tenderloin - thinly sliced
Enough oil to deep-fry

Marinade
15mls (1tablespoon) light soy sauce
15mls (1 tablespoon) soy sauce
1 teaspoon white peppercorns - crushed
1 teaspoon tapioca flour

120mls (1/2 cup, 4 fl oz) oil
50g (1/2 cup, 11/2 oz) garlic with skin on - chopped
60mls (4 tablespoons) chicken stock or water

Sauce
30mls (2 tablespoons) oyster sauce
15mls (1 tablespoon) light soy sauce
1/2 teaspoon sugar

METHOD

Put the pork into a bowl along with the light soy sauce, soy sauce, white peppercorns and tapioca flour. Mix together and leave to marinate for 10 minutes.

Meanwhile put the oil into a wok and when it is hot add the unpeeled garlic and cook on a high heat until the garlic starts to turn brown. Turn down the heat and keep stirring until the garlic is crispy (about 2-3 minutes). Drain the oil and put the garlic on some kitchen paper.

Put the oil for deep-frying into a wok and when it is hot add the marinated pork and fry for about 1 minute. Remove the pork from the oil.

Heat an empty wok and when it is hot add the fried pork and the sauce ingredients and stir-fry quickly. Add the stock and stir-fry to combine for about 2 minutes and then turn off the heat.

Put the fried pork on a plate and sprinkle the crispy garlic over the top.

LONG BEANS WITH PORK AND RED CURRY PASTE

PHAD PHED TUA SAI MUU - ผัดเผ็ดถั่วฝักยาวใส่หมู

INGREDIENTS

Serves 4

300g (11/2 cups, 10oz) pork - thinly sliced
400g (4 cups, 14 oz) long beans or string beans -
cut into 2cm (1 inch) pieces
60mls (4 tablespoons) oil
200g (1/2cup, 7 oz) red curry paste *(see p.105)*
15 kaffir lime leaves - stems removed from all and
5 shredded to use as a garnish
5 big, red chillies - sliced
30g (1 cup, 1 oz) sweet basil leaves

Sauce

60mls (4 tablespoons) fish sauce
20g (1 tablespoon) palm sugar
20g (2 tablespoons) sugar

METHOD

Put the oil in a wok and when it is hot, add the curry paste and stir-fry for 1-2 minutes. Then add the pork and fry until the outside turns white.

Then add the long beans, the kaffir lime leaf pieces and the big, red chillies. Stir-fry to combine for 2 minutes. Then add the sauce ingredients and stir-fry together.

Finally add the sweet basil leaves. Turn off the heat and serve garnished with the shredded kaffir lime leaves.

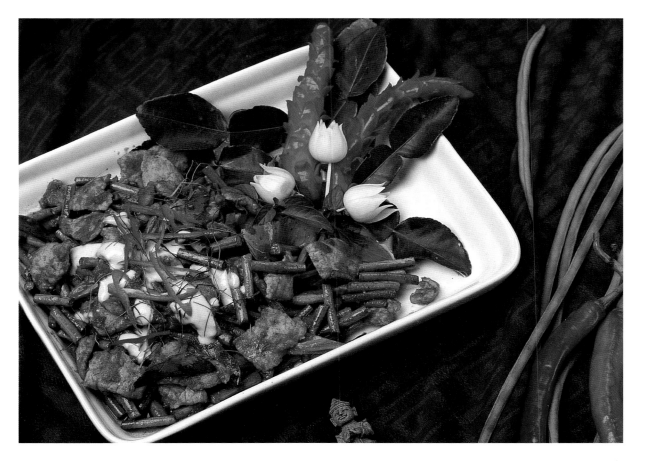

SPICY PORK WITH YOUNG GREEN PEPPERCORNS

PHAD PHET MUU - ผัดเผ็ดหมู

I like to make this dish really spicy and I like the combination of the spiciness from the curry paste mixed with the hotness from the young, green peppercorns.

INGREDIENTS
Serves 4

300g (11/2 cups, 10 oz) pork - thinly sliced
250mls (1 cup, 8 fl oz) thick coconut milk
50g (2 tablespoons) red curry paste *(see p.105)*
3 big egg plants - cut into bite sized pieces
30g (cup, 1 oz) young, green peppercorns
4 lesser ginger roots - thinly sliced
2 big, red chillies - thinly sliced
45mls (3 tablespoons) fish sauce
5 kaffir lime leaves - shredded, discarding the stem

METHOD

Put 90mls (6 tablespoons) of the thick coconut milk into a wok and when it is boiling, add the red curry paste and fry for 1-2 minutes. Add the pork and stir-fry until the outside turns white. Then add the rest of the thick coconut milk and bring to the boil. Add the big egg plants, young, green peppercorns, lesser ginger and half the red chillies. Stir to combine and add the fish sauce and shredded kaffir lime leaves. Simmer for another 2 minutes.

Turn off the heat and serve garnished with the rest of the red chillies.

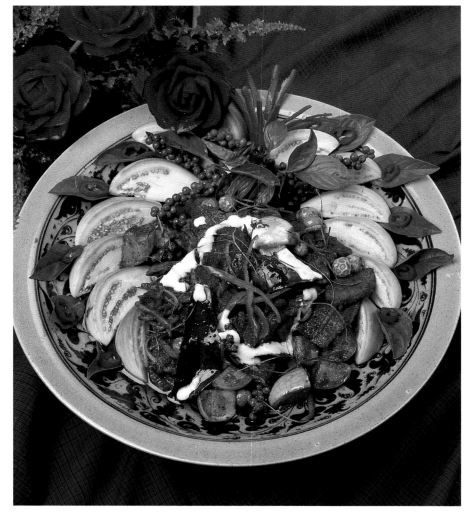

PUMPKIN WITH PORK
PHAD FUK THONG SAI MUU - ผัดฟักทองใส่หมู

If you like pumpkin you will enjoy this dish. It is really simple to make and in Thailand they normally use golden pumpkin.

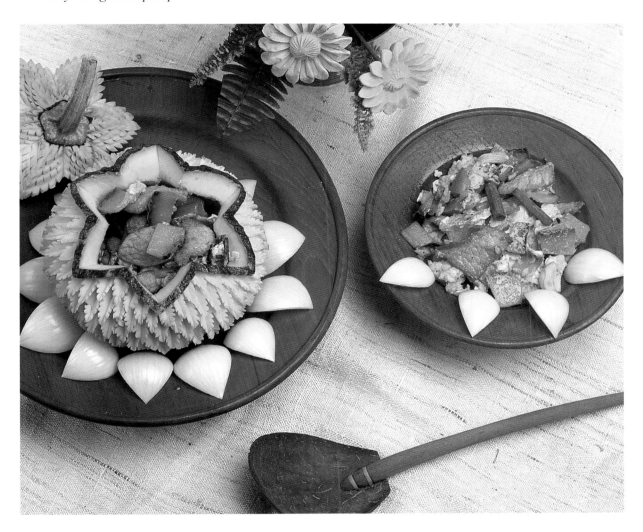

INGREDIENTS
Serves 4

500g (4 cups, 1lb 2 oz) pumpkin - thinly sliced
300g (11/2 cups, 10oz) pork - thinly sliced
90mls (6 tablespoons) oil
9 cloves of garlic - smashed
125mls (1/2 cup, 4 fl oz) chicken stock or water
60mls (4 tablespoons) fish sauce
2 eggs - beaten

METHOD

Put the oil into a wok and when it is hot add the garlic, pumpkin and chicken stock. Simmer for 2 minutes and then add the pork. Stir-fry to combine and simmer for 4 minutes. Add the fish sauce and stir, then add the eggs and stir-fry to cook the eggs and combine well. Serve.

CHICKEN WITH GINGER
GAI PHAD KING - ไก่ผัดขิง

Chicken and ginger go together excellently. If possible try to get young ginger which has a pink root.

INGREDIENTS
Serves 4

300g (11/2 cups, 10oz)
chicken breast - thinly
sliced
60mls (4 tablespoons) oil
6 cloves or garlic - chopped
1 small onion - cut in ½
and then sliced
60g (1 cup, 2 oz) ginger
shredded
2 big, red chillies - sliced
120mls (1/2 cup, 4 fl oz)
chicken stock or water
60g (1 cup, 2 oz) spring
onions - cut into 2cm
(1 inch) pieces
60g (1 cup,2 oz) eye
mushrooms cut bite-sized
pieces

Sauce
30mls (2 tablespoons)
fish sauce
45mls (3 tablespoons)
oyster sauce
30mls (2 tablespoons)
light soy sauce
15mls (1 tablespoons)
Soya bean paste

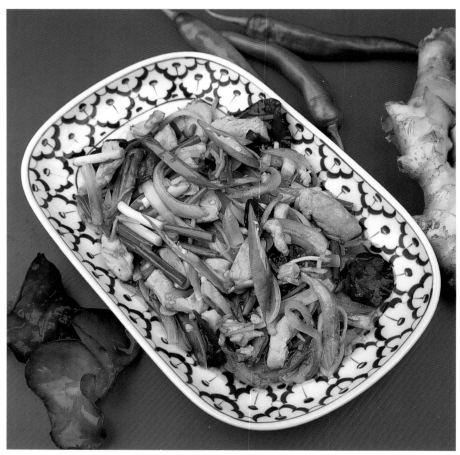

METHOD

Put the oil into a wok and when it is hot fry the garlic until it starts to turn brown. Then add the onion and the chicken and stir-fry until the outside of the chicken turns to white. Then add the ginger and mushrooms stir-fry to combine. Add the sauce ingredients and stir-fry again. Add the chillies and chicken stock and stir-fry for 1 minute. Add the spring onions and stir-fry to combine. Serve.

BEEF WITH BASIL LEAVES
PHAD KRAPOW NEUA - ผัดกระเพราเนื้อ

This dish is made using holy basil which has a slightly hot taste to it but you can use any sort of basil you like.

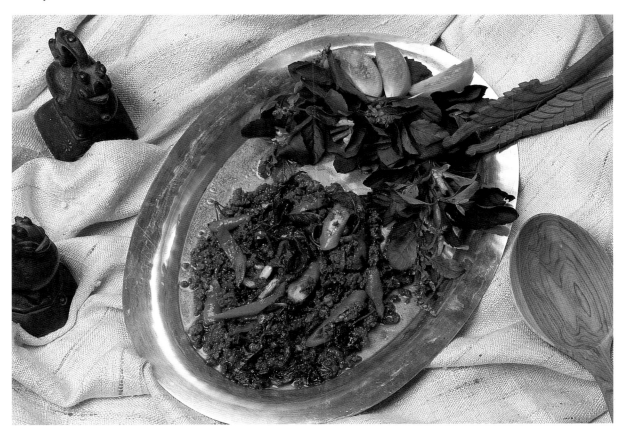

INGREDIENTS
Serves 4

500g (21/2 cups, 1lb 2 oz) minced beef
60mls (4 tablespoons) oil
15 cloves of garlic - smashed
30 small chillies - chopped
2 big, red chillies - sliced
250mls (1 cup, 8 fl oz) chicken stock or water
45g (11/2 cups, 11/2 oz) holy basil leaves

Sauce
90mls (6 tablespoons) oyster sauce
60mls (4 tablespoons) fish sauce
1/4 tablespoon sugar
10mls (2 teaspoons) sweet soy sauce

METHOD

Put the oil into a wok and when it is hot add the garlic and the small chillies and stir-fry until the garlic starts to turn brown. Add the beef and stir-fry until the outside is cooked (1-2 minutes). Add the sauce ingredients and stir-fry to combine. Add the big, red chillies and stir again. Then add the chicken stock and when it is boiling add the basil leaves. Cook for another 1 minute. Turn off the heat and serve.

CHICKEN WITH CHILLI JAM

GAI PHAD NAM PRIK POW - ไก่ผัดน้ำพริกเผา

Chilli jam is used often in Thai cooking. You can buy it ready made or make your own. This dish is also very good made with prawns.

INGREDIENTS
Serves 4

300g (11/2 cups, 10 oz) chicken - thinly sliced
60mls (4 tablespoons) oil
9 cloves of garlic - smashed
1 onion - cut into wedges
125mls (1/2 cup, 4 fl oz) chilli jam *(see p.49)*
250mls (1 cup, 8 fl oz) chicken stock or water
30mls (2 tablespoons) soy sauce
10g (1 tablespoon) sugar
8 spring onions - cut into 2cm (1 inch) pieces
3 big, red chillies - sliced

METHOD

Put the oil into a wok and when it is hot add the garlic and fry until the garlic starts to turn brown. Add the chicken and onion and stir-fry until the outside of the chicken turns white. Then add the chilli jam and fry for 2-3 minutes, stirring continuously. Add the stock and when it is boiling, add the soy sauce and sugar and stir-fry to combine. Add the spring onions and big red chillies.

Turn off the heat and serve.

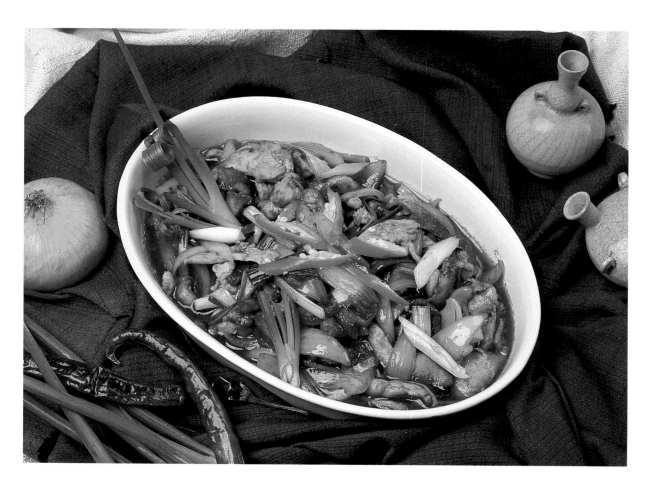

CHINESE LEAVES IN OYSTER SAUCE
PHAD PHAK KANA NAM MUN HOI - ผัดผักคะน้าน้ำมันหอย

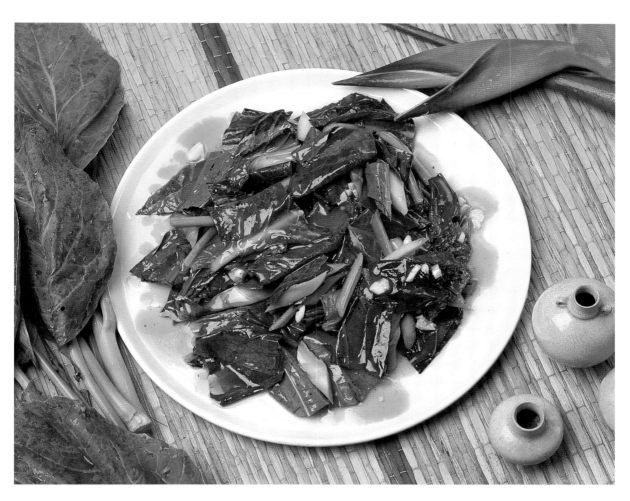

INGREDIENTS
Serves 4

400g (8 cups, 14oz) Chinese leaves or Chinese bokshoi
60mls (4 tablespoons) oil
9 cloves of garlic - smashed
1 teaspoon ground black peppercorns
120mls (1/2 cup, 4 fl oz) oyster sauce
15mls (1 tablespoon) soy sauce
250mls (1 cup, 4 fl oz) chicken stock or water

METHOD

Put the oil into a wok and when it is hot, add the garlic and the Chinese leaves. Stir-fry together for about 1 minute. Then add the oyster sauce, soy sauce and chicken stock. Stir-fry to combine.
Add the pepper and stir to mix well.

Turn off the heat and serve.

MIXED VEGETABLES
PHAD PHAK RUAM - ผัดผักรวม

This dish can be made using any selection of vegetables that you like. You need to put the vegetables that take the longest to cook in first.

INGREDIENTS
Serves 4

60mls (4 tablespoons) oil
5 cloves of garlic - chopped
1 onion - cut in 1/2 and sliced
50g 1/2 cup, 2 oz) carrot - cut in 1/2 lengthways and sliced
10 baby corn - each cut into 3 pieces
50g (1/2 cup, 2 oz) snow peas
100g (1 cup, 3 oz) cauliflower - cut into bite-sized pieces
100g (11/4 cup, 3 oz) straw mushrooms - cut in ½
120mls (1/2 cup, 4 fl oz) chicken stock or water

Sauce
60mls (4 tablespoons) oyster sauce
30mls (2 tablespoons) soy sauce
1/2 teaspoon sugar
1/2 teaspoon ground black peppercorns
15mls (1 tablespoon) sesame oil

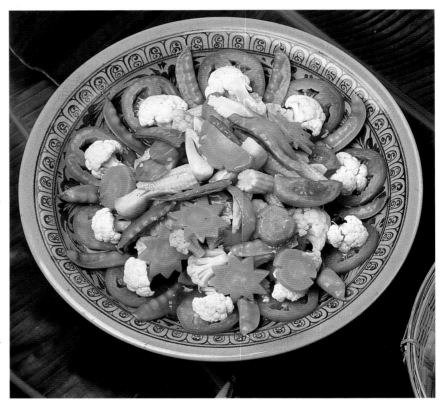

METHOD

Put the oil into a wok and when it is hot add the garlic, followed by all the vegetables except for the mushrooms. Stir-fry for about 2 minutes and then add the mushrooms. Stir-fry to combine and add the chicken stock and stir-fry to combine again. Then add the sauce ingredients. Stir-fry to combine and serve.

MORNING GLORY
PHAD PHAK BOONG - ผัดผักบุ้ง

This is a delicious dish and is often cooked as a show piece in some restaurants. It is normally cooked very fast and furiously over a high heat and then, in some establishments, a waiter will run over to the other side of the road while the cook stands with his back to the road. The cook will then throw the contents of his wok over his head, over the road and it is caught (or not!) on a plate by the waiter.

INGREDIENTS
Serves 4

700g (81/2 cups, 1 lb 6 oz) morning glory or spinach
60mls (4 tablespoons) oil
120mls (1/2 cup, 4 fl oz) chicken stock or water
9 cloves of garlic - chopped
10 small green and red chillies - smashed

Sauce

120mls (1/2 cup, 4 fl oz) soya bean paste
10g (1 tablespoon) sugar
75mls (5 tablespoons) oyster sauce
1 teaspoon ground black pepper

METHOD

Put all the ingredients except the oil into a bowl. Put the oil into a wok and when it is hot add all the ingredients. Stir-fry quickly for 2-3 minutes until the morning glory or spinach is cooked.

Serve.

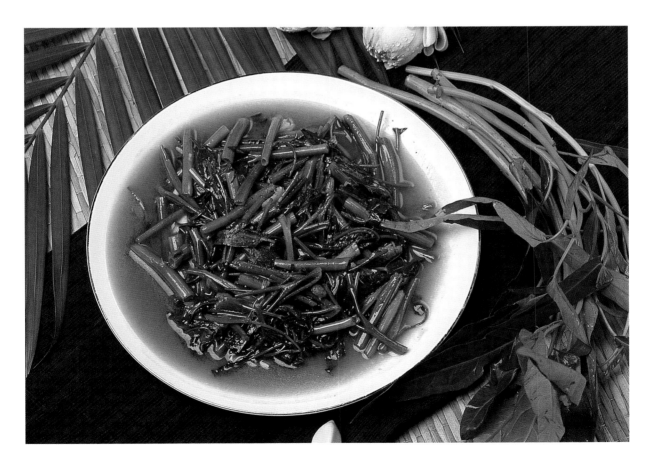

FRIED MIXED MUSHROOMS WITH BABY CORN

PHAD HED RUAM KHAO POD ORN - ผัดเห็ดรวมข้าวโพดอ่อน

You can use any selection of mushrooms that you like. This is a good dish for people who are vegetarian.

INGREDIENTS
Serves 2

45mls (3 tablespoons) oil
100g (13/4 cups, 31/2 oz)
Chinese mushrooms - cut in
half (if you are using dried
mushrooms, they need to be
soaked in water for at least 30
minutes before using)
100g (11/4 cups, 31/2 oz) straw
mushrooms - cut in half
3 cloves of garlic - chopped
1 onion - cut into bite-sized
pieces
6 baby corn - cut in half
lengthways and then cut in half
again
125mls (1/2 cup, 4 fl oz) chicken
stock or water
1 big, red chilli - sliced
4 spring onions - sliced
5g (1 teaspoon) tapioca flour -
dissolved in 45mls
(3 tablespoons) water
10g (1/2 cup, 1/2 oz) coriander -
chopped

Sauce
15mls (1 tablespoon) fish sauce
15mls (1 tablespoon) soy sauce
15mls (1 tablespoon) oyster
sauce

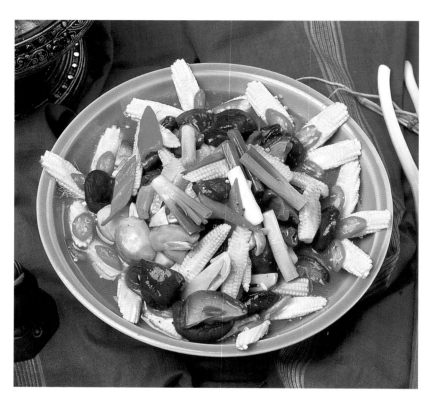

METHOD

Put the oil into a wok and fry the garlic over a high heat until it starts to turn brown. Add the onion and stir-fry and then add the Chinese mushrooms and straw mushrooms and stir - fry for about 1 minute. Add the babycorn and stir-fry again. Then add the chicken stock and stir to combine. Add the sliced chilli, spring onions and the sauce ingredients and stir-fry until all the vegetables are cooked. Then add the tapioca flour and stir-fry once more until the sauce is thick.

Serve garnished with the coriander.

SWEET AND SOUR VEGETABLES

PHAD PRIO WAN PHAK - ผัดเปรี้ยวหวานผัก

INGREDIENTS
Serves 4

45mls (3 tablespoons) oil
5 cloves of garlic - crushed
1 onion - cut into bite-sized
pieces
100g (11/4 cups, 31/2 oz)
cauliflower - cut into bite
sized pieces
1 medium carrot - peeled and
cut into 2cm (1 inch) lengths
1 cucumber - cut into 2cm
(1 inch) pieces
8 baby corn - cut in 1/2
lengthways
220g (11/2 cups, 71/2 oz)
pineapple - cut into bite
sized pieces
1 big, red chilli - seeds
removed and cut into thin
strips
2 tomatoes - cut into bite-
sized pieces
70g (1 cup, 21/2 oz) snow peas
60mls (1/4 cup, 4
tablespoons) chicken stock
or water

Sauce
15mls (1 tablespoon) lime
juice
30g (3 tablespoons) sugar
15mls (1 tablespoon) fish
sauce
15mls (1 tablespoon) oyster
sauce
15mls (1 tablespoon) soy
sauce
45mls (3 tablespoons)
tomato sauce

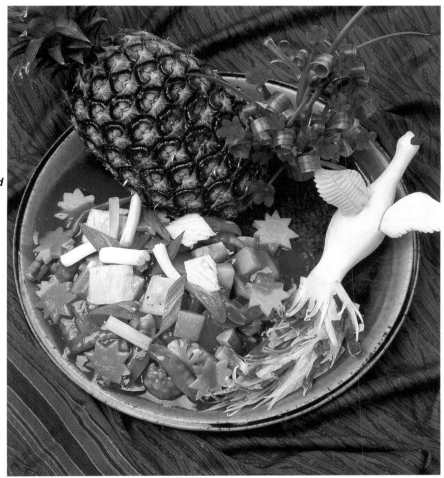

METHOD

Put the oil into a wok and fry the garlic over a high heat until it starts to turn brown. Add the onion and stir - fry. Add the cauliflower and carrot followed by the cucumber, baby corn and pineapple and stir-fry for 2 minutes. Add the chillies, tomatoes and peas and stir-fry for 1 minute until all the vegetables are cooked. Add the chicken stock and stir-fry briefly.

Add the sauce ingredients and stir to combine. Serve immediately.

PRAWNS WITH ASPARAGUS

GOONG PHAD NOR MAI FARANG - กุ้งผัดหน่อไม้ฝรั่ง

This is a lovely light dish and I think that the prawns and asparagus go together really well.

INGREDIENTS

Serves 4

250g (13/4 cups, 6 oz) prawns - washed, peeled and deveined and then boiled in water for 1 minute

500g (61/4 cups, 1 lb 2 oz) asparagus - cut into 1 inch pieces

60mls (4 tablespoons) oil

12 cloves of garlic - chopped

1/2 teaspoon sugar

10g (1 tablespoon) tapioca flour dissolved in 30mls (2 tablespoons) water

Sauce

45mls (3 tablespoons) light soy sauce

45mls (3 tablespoons) oyster sauce

500mls (2 cups, 16 fl oz) chicken stock

45mls (3 tablespoons) sesame oil

1/4 teaspoon pepper

METHOD

Put the oil into a wok and when it is hot add the garlic and fry until it starts to turn brown. Then add the asparagus and stir-fry for 2 minutes.

Add all the sauce ingredients and stir-fry to combine. Add the sugar and prawns and stir-fry for 1 minute.

Then over a high heat add the tapioca flour and stir-fry until the sauce is thick. Serve.

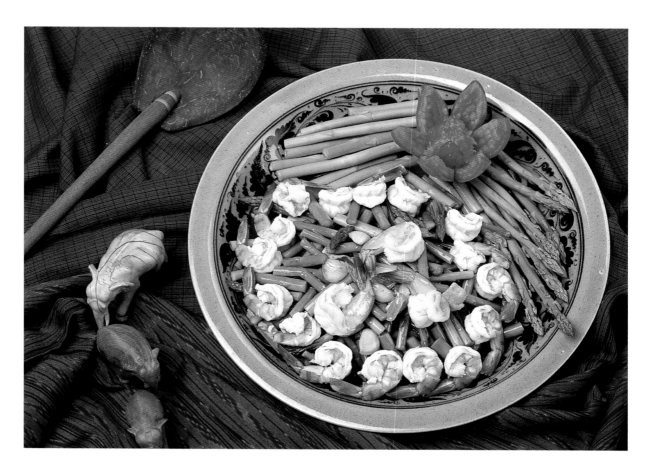

CRAB WITH YELLOW CURRY POWDER

POO PHAD PONG GAREE - ปูผัดผงกระหรี่

This is an unusual dish where the crab is fried with a slightly curried sauce.

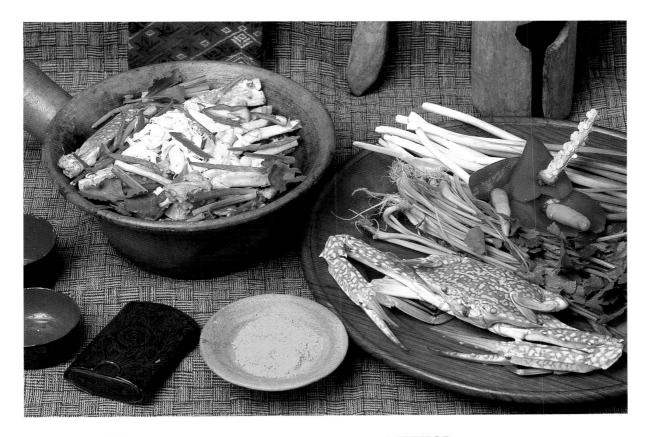

INGREDIENTS
Serves 4

2 crabs - each one cut into 4 pieces
250mls (1 cup, 8 fl oz) unsweetened, condensed milk
125mls (1/2 cup, 4 fl oz) chilli oil
1 teaspoon of chilli powder
1 egg
60mls (4 tablespoons) oil
1 big, red chilli - shredded
4 spring onions - roughly chopped
10g (1/4 cup, 1/2 oz) Chinese celery - roughly chopped

Sauce
15mls (1 tablespoon) soy sauce
15mls (1 tablespoon) light soy sauce
1/2 teaspoon sugar

METHOD

Boil some water and cook the crab for about 4-5 minutes. Drain.

Put the condensed milk, chilli oil, chilli powder and egg into a bowl and mix together well. Add the sauce ingredients and mix again.

Put the oil into a wok and when it is hot, add the above mixture. Keep stirring and when it is boiling, add the crab and stir-fry to combine.
Cook for 2 minutes. Turn off the heat and serve garnished with the big, red chilli, spring onions and Chinese celery.

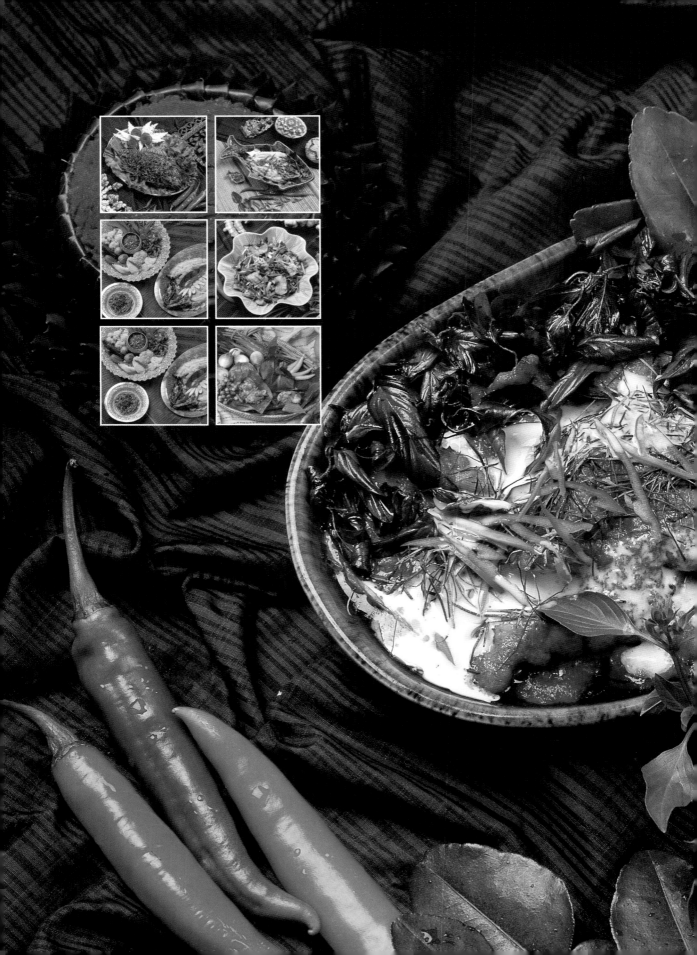

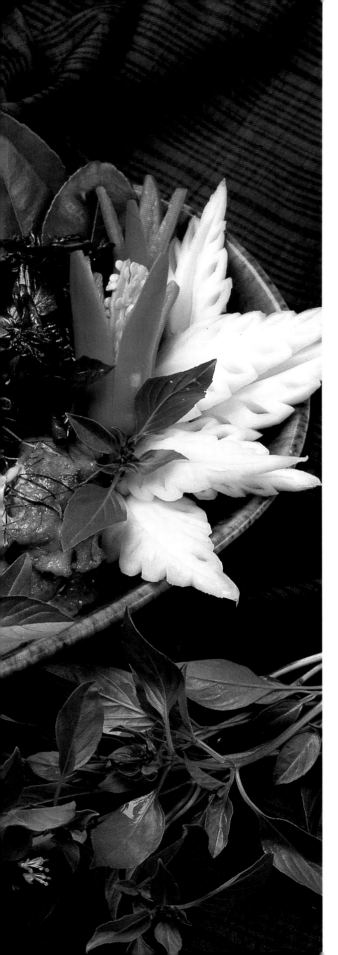

FISH DISHES

Thai people absolutely love fish and they will eat it as often as they can get it. They are not too fussy about what sort of fish they use for any particular dish and their main concern is that it is fresh. If you are not sure what sort of fish to use then tell your fishmonger what you are planning to do with the fish and he will be able to tell you what sort of fish he has that you can use.

In Thailand they often serve the whole fish, head and all, as they eat the eyes and the meat in the cheeks of the fish. However if you are put off by this then you can serve the fish without the head or you can just use fish fillets if you are not too sure about the bones.

STEAMED FISH WITH LIME SAUCE

PLAA CHON NEUNG MANOW - ปลาช่อนนึ่งมะนาว

This is a really tasty and healthy dish. The fresh taste of the lime combined with the spicy chillies makes this dish absolutely delicious. You can use less chillies if you do not want the sauce to be so spicy.

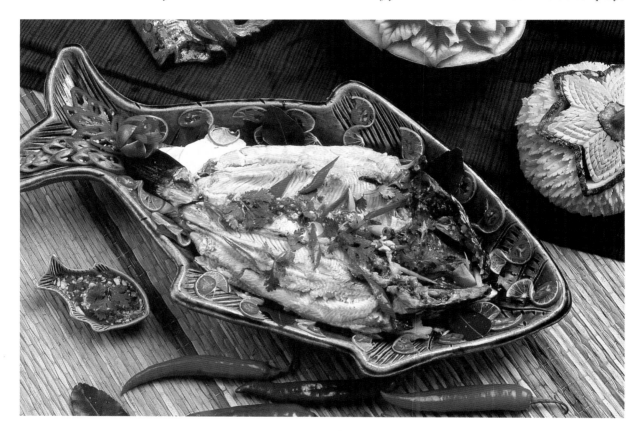

INGREDIENTS
Serves 2

2 fish fillets or one whole fish such as sole, sea bass, plaice or monkfish
1 lime - thinly sliced

Sauce
2 stalks of lemongrass - lower 1/3 only, chopped
20g (2 tablespoons) coriander root - chopped
50g (1/2 cup, 2oz) garlic - chopped
10g (1/4 cup, 1/2 oz) Chinese celery - chopped

1 big, red chilli - chopped
40 small red and green chillies - chopped
180mls (3/4 cup, 6 fl oz) fish sauce
125mls (1/2 cup, 4 fl oz) lime juice
45mls (3 tablespoons) chicken stock or water
40g (2 tablespoons) palm sugar
10g (1 tablespoon) sugar
1/2 teaspoon salt

METHOD

Put the fish onto a plate and put the slices of lime on top of the fish. Steam the fish until it is cooked (about 15 -20 minutes).

Put all the remaining ingredients into a blender and blend until nearly smooth. Pour the sauce over the fish and serve.

STEAMED FISH WITH CHILLI DIPPING SAUCE
PLAA CHON NEUNG NAM PRIK - ปลาช่อนนึ่งน้ำพริก

INGREDIENTS
Serves 2

1 whole fish such as sole, sea bass, plaice or monkfish - make diagonal slashes in the skin at 2cm (1 inch) intervals

50g (1/2 cup, 2oz) cauliflower - divided into florets
3 baby corn
3 long beans - sliced into 2cm (1 inch) pieces
80g (3/4 cup, 3oz) cucumber - cut into chunks
70g (1/2 cup, 21/2 oz) carrot - cut into chunks
1 big eggplant - cut into 4

4 kaffir lime leaves - chopped
10g (1 tablespoon) ginza - chopped
1/2 teaspoon ground, roasted sticky rice (see p.19)
15mls (1 tablespoon) chicken stock or water
5 shallots - chopped
5 eryngo leaves - chopped
2 spring onions - chopped

Sauce
90mls (6 tablespoons) fish sauce
60mls (4 tablespoons) lime juice
30mls (2 tablespoons) melted palm sugar
30mls (2 tablespoons) tamarind juice (see p.17)
10g (3 tablespoons) chilli powder

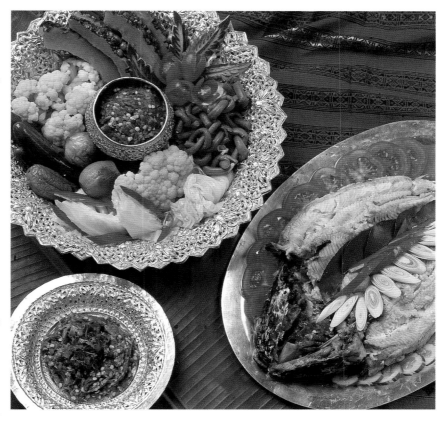

METHOD

Put the fish onto a plate and steam until it is cooked (about 15-20 minutes).

Boil some water and add the cauliflower, baby corn, long beans, cucumber, carrot and big egg plant and boil for 5 minutes. Drain.

Put the kaffir lime leaves, ginza, and sauce ingredients into a pan and bring to the boil, stirring continuously. Simmer for 2 minutes and then turn the heat off.

Add the roasted sticky rice and stock and stir to combine. Add the shallots, eryngo leaves and spring onions and mix together.

Serve the steamed fish with the chilli dipping sauce and boiled vegetables.

STEAMED FISH LUI SUAN

PLAA CHON LUI SUAN - ปลาช่อนลุยสวน

The name of this dish implies that the fish is very fresh and is still swimming around in the herb garden. Try to use fish that is really fresh.

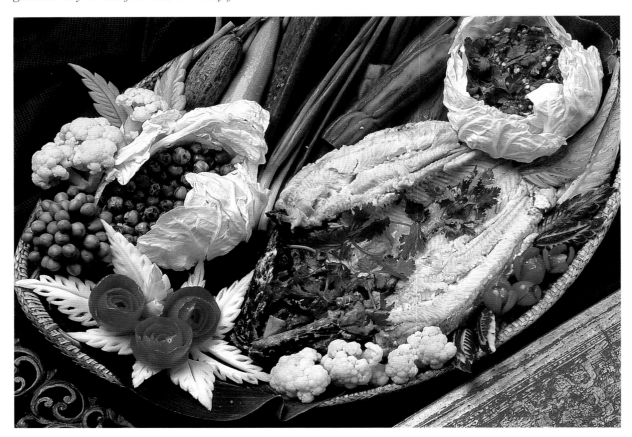

INGREDIENTS
Serves 2

1 whole fish such as sole, sea bass, plaice or monkfish - make diagonal slashes in the skin at 2cm (1 inch) intervals
1 stalk of lemongrass - lower 1/3 only, sliced
10 kaffir lime leaves
10 slices of ginza

50g (1/2 cup, 2oz) cauliflower - divided into florets
3 baby corn
3 long beans - sliced into 2cm (1 inch) pieces
80g (3/4 cup, 3oz) cucumber - cut into chunks
70g (1/2 cup, 21/2 oz) carrot - cut into chunks
1 big eggplant - cut into 4

70g (1/2 cup, 21/2 oz) young chilli dipping sauce *(see p.46)*

METHOD

Put the fish onto a plate along with the lemongrass, kaffir lime leaves and ginza. Steam for about 15-20 minutes, until cooked.

Boil some water and add the cauliflower, baby corn, long beans, cucumber, carrot and big egg plant and boil for 5 minutes. Drain.

Serve the steamed fish with the boiled vegetables and young chilli dipping sauce.

STEAMED FISH IN BANANA LEAVES
HOR NEUNG PLAA - ห่อนึ่งปลา

If you do not want to cook this dish using banana leaves or silver foil then it can be cooked by stir-frying it in a wok over a low heat. You will need to add a bit more water and then put a lid on the wok and cook for about 3 minutes so that the fish is cooked properly. Cod is a good fish to use for this dish.

INGREDIENTS
Serves 4

300g (2 cups, 10 oz) fresh water fish fillets - thinly sliced
60mls (4 tablespoons) oil
100g (4 tablespoons) red curry paste *(see p.105)*
2 big egg plants - cut into bite-sized pieces
20 small egg plants
4 long beans - cut into 1cm (1/2 inch) long pieces
60mls(4 tablespoons) chicken stock or water
30mls (2 tablespoons) fish sauce
8 eryngo leaves or coriander leaves - finely shredded
15g (1 tablespoon) roasted, ground sticky rice *(see p.19)*
1 teaspoon prickly ash - broken into small pieces
4 pepper leaves or cabbage leaves
4 kaffir lime leaves - finely shredded
Banana leaves or silver foil

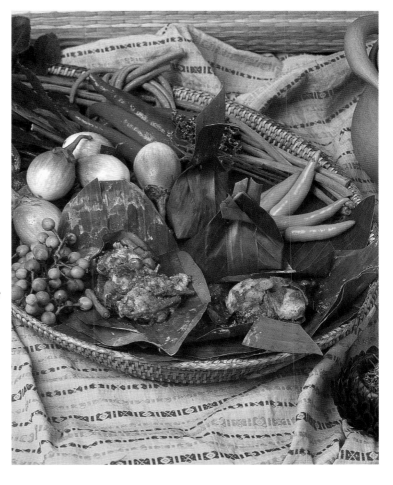

METHOD

Put the oil into a wok and add the red curry paste and fry for about 1 minute. Add the big egg plant, small egg plants and long beans and stir together. Then add the chicken stock, fish sauce, eryngo leaves and stir-fry. Add the fish and stir-fry and then add the roasted, ground sticky rice and prickly ash. Stir-fry briefly and remove from the heat.

Divide the mixture into 4 portions. Put the pepper leaf into the middle of the banana leaf and spoon one portion of the fish mixture onto it. Then sprinkle some of the shredded kaffir lime leaves on top. Fold the edges of the banana leaf up and secure with a tooth pick so that it makes a parcel. Repeat for the remaining 3 portions. Steam them for about 10 -15 minutes (or bake in the oven for about 20 minutes at 180°C or 360°F) until cooked. It can be eaten hot or cold by opening up the banana leaves and eating the fish mixture inside.

FRIED FISH WITH CHINESE CELERY

PLAA CHON PHAD KHUN CHAI - ปลาช่อนผัดคื่นฉ่าย

I love to eat fish and the flavours of the Chinese celery and ginger combine together excellently in this dish.

INGREDIENTS
Serves 4

300g (2 cups, 10oz) fish fillets (any sort of fresh water fish) - thinly sliced
Enough wheat flour to coat the fish
Enough oil to deep fry the fish
120mls (1/2 cup, 4 fl oz) oil
9 cloves of garlic - smashed
100g (11/2 cups, 31/2 oz) spring onion - cut into 2cm (1 inch) pieces
150g (21/2 cups, 5½1/2oz) Chinese celery - cut into 2cm (1 inch) pieces
60g (1 cup, 2 oz) ginger - cut into strips
2 big, red chillies - thinly sliced
250mls (1 cup, 8 fl oz) chicken stock or water
1/2 teaspoon pepper
1/2 teaspoon sugar

Sauce
30mls (2 tablespoons) soya bean paste
30mls (2 tablespoons) light soy sauce
30mls (2 tablespoons) soy sauce
125mls (1/2cup, 8 fl oz) oyster sauce

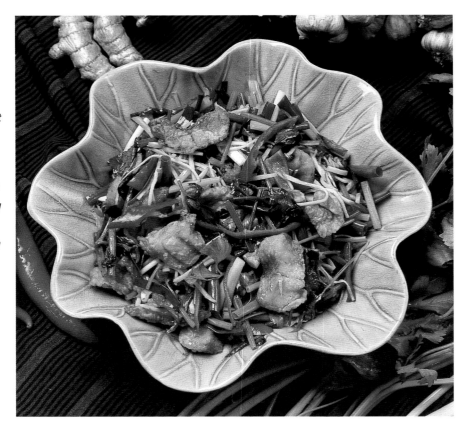

METHOD

Coat the fish in the flour and shake off any excess flour. Heat the oil in a wok and when it is hot add the fish. Fry the fish until it turns a golden brown colour (about 3 minutes). Drain.

Put the oil into a wok and when it is hot, add the garlic and fry until it starts to turn golden brown. Then add the fish, followed by the spring onion, Chinese celery, ginger, big red chillies and the sauce ingredients. Stir-fry to mix the ingredients together well.

Then add the chicken stock and stir-fry over a high heat for 2 minutes.

Add the pepper and sugar and mix together.

Turn off the heat and serve.

FRIED FISH WITH RED CURRY SAUCE
CHOO CHEE PLAA - อู่ฉี่ปลา

This is one of my favourite dishes. The sauce is like a thick version of red curry coconut sauce which I think goes together excellently with the fried fish.

INGREDIENTS
Serves 4

300g (2 cups, 10oz) fish filets such as red snapper, plaice or halibut - thinly sliced
Enough flour to coat the fish
Enough oil to deep fry the fish

500mls (2 cups, 16 fl oz) thick coconut milk (reserve 30mls, 2 tablespoons for garnish)
100g (4 tablespoons) red curry paste (see p.105)
40g (2 tablespoons) palm sugar
30mls (2 tablespoons) fish sauce
6 kaffir lime leaves - stems removed and shredded. Keep some for garnish.
1 big, red chilli - cut in 1/2 lengthways and shredded. Keep some for garnish.
15g (1/2cup, 1/2 oz) sweet basil leaves. Keep some for garnish.

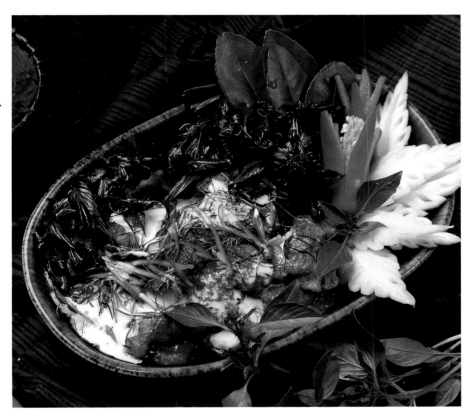

METHOD

Cover the fish in the flour and shake off any excess flour. Heat the oil in a wok and when it is hot add the fish. Fry the fish until it turns a golden brown colour (about 3 minutes). Drain and put on a serving dish.

Put half the thick coconut milk into a wok and fry for 3-5 minutes until the coconut oil starts to separate out. Add the red curry paste and fry for 1-2 minutes.

Once the paste is cooked add the other half of the coconut milk and stir for 1 minute. Add the palm sugar along the side of the wok and stir for another minute. Add the fish sauce and stir together. Add the kaffir lime leaves, big red chilli and basil leaves. Stir to combine. Turn off the heat and pour the sauce over the fried fish. Garnish with the remaining kaffir lime leaves, big red chilli and basil leaves. Pour the remaining thick coconut milk over the top and serve.

FRIED FISH WITH CHILLI AND BASIL
PLAA NIN LAAD PRIK BAI HORAPA - ปลานิลราดพริกใบโหระพา

This is a recipe that I devised myself and I think that the fresh taste of the sweet basil combined with the fried fish is amazing. If you do not want to use a whole fish or do not want to deep fry the fish then you can use fish fillets pan-fried in a little oil or grilled.

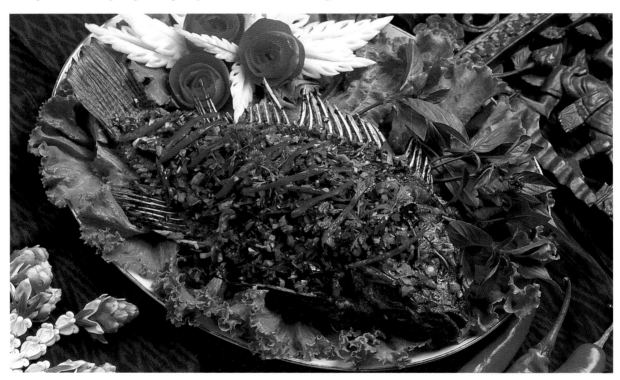

INGREDIENTS
Serves 2

300g (10 oz) whole fish (cod, haddock, plaice, halibut, red mullet) - scales and fins removed
Enough oil to deep fry the fish

Sauce
30mls (2 tablespoons) oil
6 cloves of garlic - crushed
1 onion - chopped
5 medium, red chillies - thinly sliced
1 big, red chilli - sliced
1 big, green chilli - sliced
15mls (1 tablespoon) fish sauce
15mls (1 tablespoon) soy sauce
60mls (1/4 cup, 4 tablespoons) chicken stock or water
20g (3/4 cup, 3/4 oz) sweet basil leaves
10g (1/2 cup, 1/2 oz) coriander - chopped

METHOD

Deep fry the fish in very hot oil until it is crispy on both sides.

To make the sauce, put the oil into a wok and add the garlic, onion and chillies and fry until the garlic starts to turn brown. Then add the fish sauce, soy sauce and chicken stock and fry for 1 minute. Add the basil leaves and stir - fry well to combine.

Turn off the heat and pour the sauce over the fish. Garnish with the coriander.

CURRY PASTES

That curry pastes are usually made up of a combination of fresh and dried ingredients. If some of the ingredients are difficult to obtain then it is a good idea to make the pastes in big quantities so that you do not have to get all the ingredients together too often.

When you are making a paste any dried ingredients need to be made into a powder form before they can be added to the fresh ingredients otherwise they will not be pounded properly. If possible it is best to use the dried ingredients in their natural form (eg. coriander seeds as opposed to coriander powder) and then make them into a powder yourself as the flavour is better. To do this you will need to put the dried ingredients into a wok (do not use any oil) and roast them until they become a brown colour. The different ingredients must be roasted separately as some of the ingredients will burn before the others are brown. eg. cumin seeds will go brown much faster than coriander seeds.

Once all the dried ingredients have been roasted then they can be put into a mortar and pounded into a powder using a pestle. You can also use a coffee grinder to grind the seeds.

Once you have prepared the dried ingredients you then need to prepare all the fresh ingredients. If you are going to use a pestle and mortar to make the paste it is a good idea to chop the ingredients finely as this will mean less pounding later on. Once all the ingredients have been prepared you can put them into a mortar and pound for about 10 minutes, using a pestle, until the paste is smooth. If there are too many lumps in the paste then they will float on the top of the curry so try to get the paste fairly smooth.

If you are using a liquidizer the ingredients can be roughly chopped. You may find that if you use a liquidizer the paste is a bit dry and you will need to add some water to get the paste to combine. If you are making a paste for a recipe where the paste is going to be fried it is best not to use too much water so just add the water a tablespoon at a time. If the paste is going to be fried and there is too much water then when you fry the paste it will spit. If the paste is too watery then you can reduce it by putting it into a wok and boiling it until all the water has evaporated before it is fried. If the paste is not going to be fried then you can add 250mls (1 cup, 8 fl oz) water to the paste when it is being liquidized.

Once you have made the paste it can be stored in the refrigerator for about 1 week. If not it can be frozen and it will last for about 6 months. If you are going to freeze it you might like to freeze it in an ice cube tray so that you can just take out as many cubes as you want to use.

However, if you want to make the paste in a big quantity, the best way to store it so that it lasts for a long time is to fry it in oil. To do this you will need about 250mls (1 cup, 8 fl oz) oil to 1kg (2½ cups, 2lbs 3oz) curry paste. Our recipes for 4 people use about 100g (4 tablespoons) of curry paste so the above mentioned quantity would be enough paste for about 10 curries for 4 people. Put the oil into a wok and when it is hot add the curry paste and fry it over a low heat stirring occasionally. You need to fry the curry paste until there is an aroma released and the paste will change colour slightly. If you have made the paste in a liquidizer it may take a little longer to fry than paste that has been made using a pestle and mortar as the extra water that has been added needs to evaporate.

Once the paste is ready it can be stored in a jar along with a tight fitting lid. You should store the paste along with the oil that it was fried in as the oil will help the curry paste keep its colour and its flavour. It can be stored in a jar for about one month but if you keep the jar in the refrigerator it will last for a few months. You will probably use the curry paste before it goes off.

GREEN CURRY PASTE

NAM PRIK GAENG KHEO WAN - น้ำพริกแกงเขียวหวาน

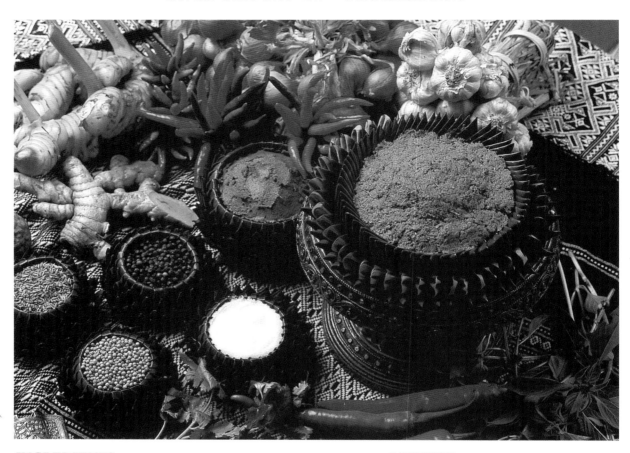

INGREDIENTS
Dried
1 teaspoon coriander seeds - roasted until brown
1/2 teaspoon cumin seeds - roasted until brown
1/2 teaspoon black peppercorns
1/2 teaspoon salt

Fresh
5g (1 teaspoon) ginza - skin removed, chopped
15g (3 tablespoons) lemongrass - lower 1/3 only, chopped
5g (1 teaspoon) kaffir lime peel - chopped
20g (2 tablespoons) coriander root - chopped
10g (2 tablespoons) shallots - chopped
5g (1 tablespoon) garlic - crushed
5g (1 teaspoon) shrimp paste
5g (1 teaspoon) tumeric - skin removed, chopped
20 small, green chillies
30g (1cup, 1oz) sweet basil leaves

METHOD

Put the coriander seeds, cumin seeds and black peppercorns into a mortar and grind them into a powder using a pestle. Then add all the remaining ingredients and pound using a pestle for about 10 minutes until the paste is smooth. All the ingredients for the paste can also be put into a blender and liquidized. If the paste is too dry to liquidize then you may need to add a bit of water.

This recipe will make about 100-130g (4-5 tablespoons) of curry paste.

RED CURRY PASTE

NAM PRIK GAENG PHED - น้ำพริกแกงเผ็ด

INGREDIENTS

Dried

1 tablespoon coriander seeds - roasted until brown
2 cardamom pods - roasted until brown
1/2 teaspoon black peppercorns
1/2 teaspoon salt
10 big, red, dried chillies - seeds removed and soaked in water for at least 10 minutes and then finely chopped

Fresh

5g (1 teaspoon) ginza - skin removed, chopped
5g (2 teaspoons) lemongrass - lower 1/3 only, chopped
5g (1 teaspoon) kaffir lime peel - chopped
10g (1 tablespoon) coriander root - chopped
15g (3 tablespoons) shallots - chopped
15g (3 tablespoons) garlic - crushed
5g (1 teaspoon) shrimp paste
10 small, red chillies

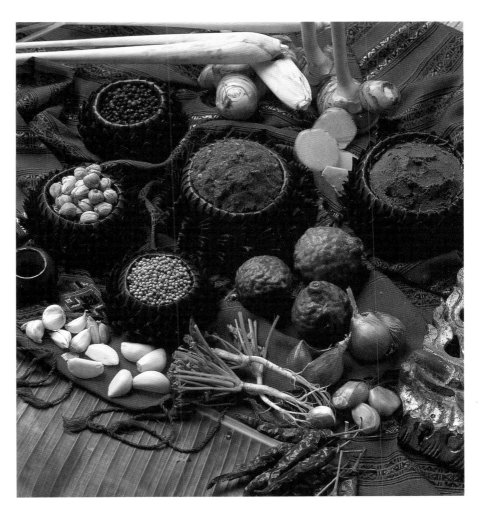

METHOD

Put the coriander seeds, cardamom pods and black peppercorns into a mortar and grind them into a powder using a pestle. Then add the rest of the ingredients and pound using a pestle for about 10 minutes until the paste is smooth. All the ingredients for the paste can also be put into a blender and liquidized. If the paste is too dry to liquidize then you may need to add a bit of water.

This recipe will make about 100-130g (4-5 tablespoons) of curry paste.

PANAENG CURRY PASTE

NAM PRIK PANAENG - น้ำพริกแพนง

INGREDIENTS

Dried

2 teaspoons coriander seeds - roasted until brown

1/2 teaspoon cumin seeds - roasted until brown

3 pieces of mace - roasted until brown

3 long, green peppers - roasted until brown

2 cardamom pods - roasted until brown

1/2 teaspoon black peppercorns

1/2 teaspoon salt

12 big, red, dried chillies - seeds removed and soaked in water for at least 10 minutes and then finely chopped

Fresh

10g (2 teaspoons) ginza - skin removed, chopped

10g (2 tablespoons) lemongrass - lower 1/3 only, chopped

5g (1 teaspoon) kaffir lime peel - chopped

10g (1 tablespoon) coriander root - chopped

15g (3 tablespoons) shallots - chopped

10g (2 tablespoons) garlic - crushed

5g (1 teaspoon) shrimp paste

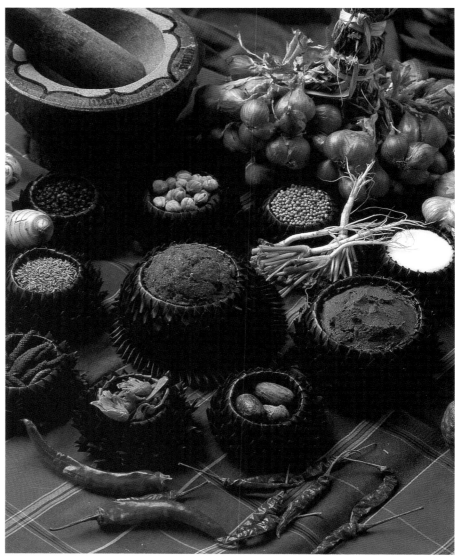

METHOD

Put the coriander seeds, cumin seeds, mace, long green peppers, cardamom pods and black peppercorns into a mortar and grind them into a powder using a pestle. Then add the rest of the ingredients and pound using a pestle for about 10 minutes until the paste is smooth. All the ingredients for the paste can also be put into a blender and liquidized. If the paste is too dry to liquidize then you may need to add a bit of water.

This recipe will make about 100-130g (4-5 tablespoons) of curry paste.

YELLOW CURRY PASTE
NAM PRIK GAENG GAREE - น้ำพริกแกงกะหรี่

INGREDIENTS

Dried

1/2 teaspoon salt
12 big, red, dried chillies - seeds removed and soaked in water for at least 10 minutes and then finely chopped

Fresh

10g (1 tablespoon) ginza - skin removed, chopped
20g (4 tablespoons) lemongrass - lower 1/3 only, chopped
20g (4 tablespoons) garlic - crushed
5g (1 teaspoon) shrimp paste

METHOD

Put all the ingredients for the paste into a mortar and pound using a pestle for about 10 minutes until the paste is smooth. All the ingredients for the paste can also be put into a blender and liquidized. If the paste is too dry to liquidize then you may need to add a bit of water.

This will make about 100-130g (4-5 tablespoons) of yellow curry paste.

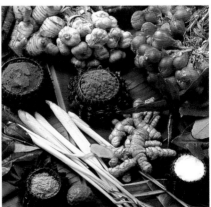

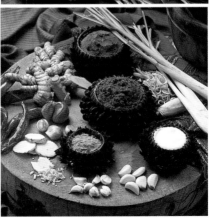

CHIANG MAI CURRY PASTE
NAM PRIK GAENG HANGLAY - น้ำพริกแกงฮังเล

INGREDIENTS

Dried

1/2 teaspoon salt
3 big, red, dried chillies - seeds removed and soaked in water for at least 10 minutes and then finely chopped

Fresh

20g (2 tablespoons) ginza - skin removed, chopped
10g (2 tablespoons) lemongrass - lower 1/3 only, chopped
10g (2 tablespoons) shallots - chopped
5g (1 tablespoon) garlic - crushed
5g (1 teaspoon) shrimp paste
5g (1 teaspoon) tumeric - skin removed, chopped

METHOD

Put all the ingredients for the paste into a mortar and pound using a pestle for about 10 minutes until the paste is smooth. All the ingredients for the paste can also be put into a blender and liquidized. If the paste is too dry to liquidize then you may need to add a bit of water.

This recipe will make about 80-100g (3-4 tablespoons) of curry paste.

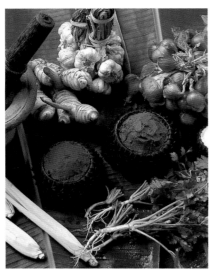

NORTHERN STYLE CURRY PASTE
NAM PRIK GAENG OHM - น้ำพริกแกงอ่อม

INGREDIENTS

Dried

1/2 teaspoon salt

5 big, red, dried chillies - seeds removed and soaked in water for at least 10 minutes and then finely chopped

Fresh

20g (2 tablespoons) ginza - skin removed and chopped

5g (1 tablespoon) lemongrass - lower 1/3 only, chopped

10g (1 tablespoon) coriander root - chopped

20g (4 tablespoons) shallots - chopped

10g (2 tablespoons) garlic - crushed

15g (1 tablespoon) shrimp paste

METHOD

Put all the ingredients for the paste into a mortar and pound using a pestle for about 10 minutes until the paste is smooth. All the ingredients for the paste can also be put into and liquidized. If the paste is too dry to liquidize then you may need to add a bit of water.

This recipe will make about 100-130g (4-5 tablespoons) of curry paste.

MIXED VEGETABLE CURRY PASTE
NAM PRIK GAENG CARE - น้ำพริกแกงแค

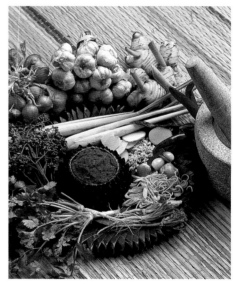

INGREDIENTS

Dried

1/2 teaspoon salt

7 big, red, dried chillies - seeds removed and soaked in water for at least 10 minutes and then finely chopped

Fresh

10g (2 tablespoons) lemongrass - lower 1/3 only, chopped

5g (1 tablespoon) coriander root - chooped

15g (3 tablespoons) shallots - chopped

10g (2 tablespoons) garlic - crushed

15g (1 tablespoon) shrimp paste

METHOD

Put all the ingredients for the paste into a mortar and pound using a pestle for about 10 minutes until the paste is smooth. All the ingredients for the paste can also be put into and liquidized. If the paste is too dry to liquidize then you may need to add a bit of water.

This recipe will make about 100-130g (4-5 tablespoons) of curry paste.

MUSSAMAN CURRY PASTE
NAM PRIK GAENG MUSSAMAN - น้ำพริกแกงมัสมั่น

INGREDIENTS

75mls (5 tablespoons) oil
15g (3 tablespoons) garlic - crushed
5g (1 tablespoon) shallots - chopped
4 big, red chillies - seeds removed and soaked in water for at least 10 minutes and finely chopped

Put the oil into a wok and when it is hot, add all the above ingredients. Fry on a low heat for 2-3 minutes, until they go a slightly brown colour. Drain the oil and set aside.

Dried
2 tablespoons coriander seeds - roasted until brown
1 tablespoon cumin seeds - roasted until brown
1 tablespoon star anise - roasted until brown
1 stick of cinnamon - roasted until brown
5 cloves
1/2 teaspoon salt

Fresh
5g (1 teaspoon) ginza - skin removed, chopped
5g (1 tablespoon) lemongrass - lower 1/3 only, chopped
1/2 teaspoon kaffir lime peel - chopped

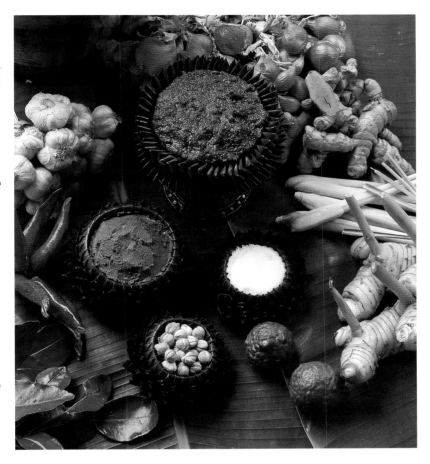

METHOD

Put the coriander seeds, cumin seeds, star anise, cinnamon and cloves into a mortar and grind them into a powder. Then add the rest of the ingredients and pound using a pestle for about 10 minutes until the paste is smooth. All the ingredients for the paste can also be put into a blender and liquidized. If the paste is too dry to liquidize then you may need to add a bit of water.

This recipe will make about 100-130g (4-5 tablespoons) of curry paste.

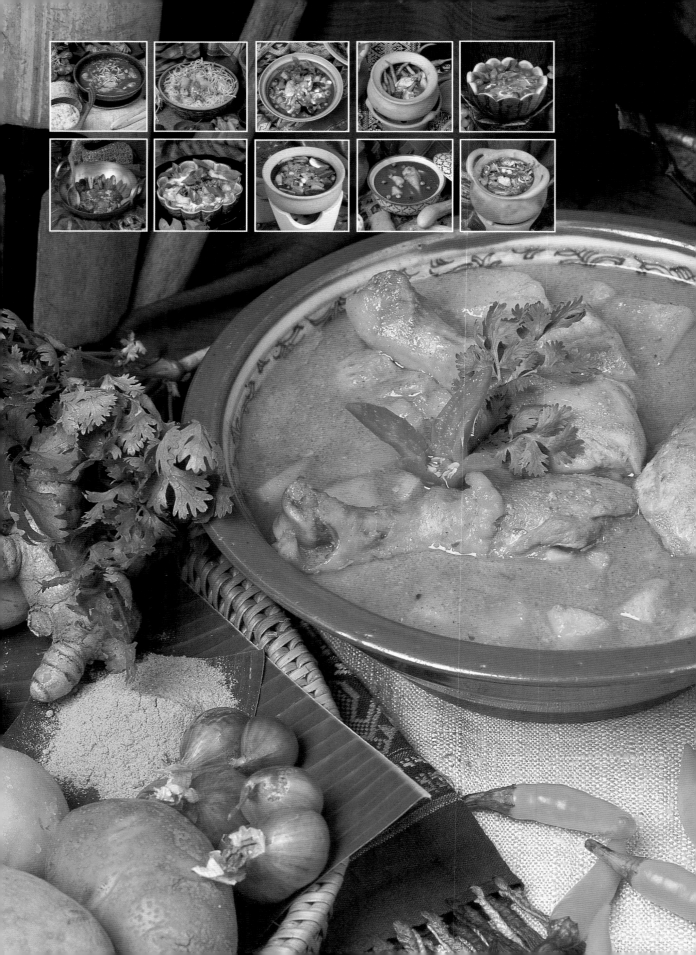

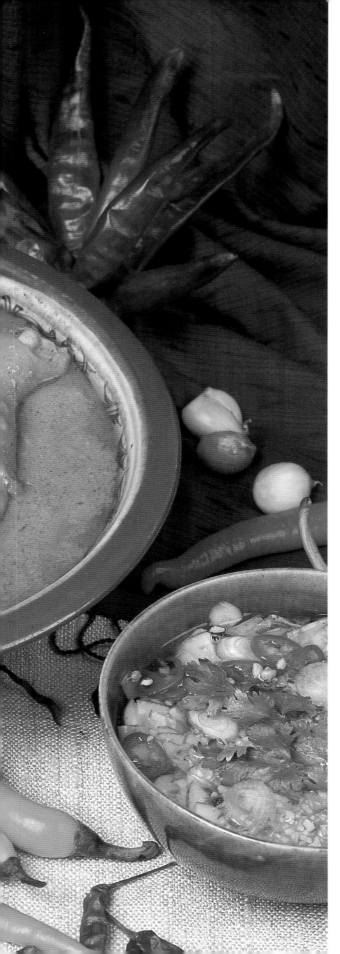

CURRIES

Curries are very popular in Thailand and are a part of every meal. There are basically two different sorts of curries. One is made with coconut milk and the other is made with water. Curries from central and southern Thailand are normally made using coconut milk and are richer than the curries from the north and north-east which are made from water. Coconuts are very plentiful in the south which is why they use more coconut milk.

COCONUT MILK CURRIES

In Thailand fresh coconut milk is used to make the curries but abroad it may not be so easy to find. If you cannot get fresh coconut milk then you can use tinned, creamed or powdered coconut milk instead. Sometimes if you are not using fresh coconut milk, the oil will not separate out from the coconut milk. If it looks as if the coconut milk is going to burn and no oil has appeared then you will need to add 15-30mls (1-2 tablespoons) of oil and then you can add the curry paste and follow the recipe as normal. The main difference between the curries is that different pastes are used to change the taste and colours of the curries.

Traditionally Thai people like their curries to have a film of oil on the top as they think that it adds to the colour. However, coconut oil is very high in cholesterol so if you want you can spoon off any excess oil that is on the top before it is served. In our recipes we use 500mls (2 cups, 16 fl oz) coconut milk for 4 people. If you like your curries to have a bit more sauce then you can add an extra 250mls (1cup, 8 fl oz) thick coconut milk.

If you do not want to use coconut milk at all then you can also make the curries using cows milk or soya milk. It will make the curry have a thinner consistency and a slightly different taste but it is more healthy.

WATER BASED CURRIES

These are very simple to make as plain water or stock is used. Some of the pastes are fried in oil but some of the pastes do not need to be fried and can just be cooked along with the water or stock. Each recipe will tell you which method needs to be used.

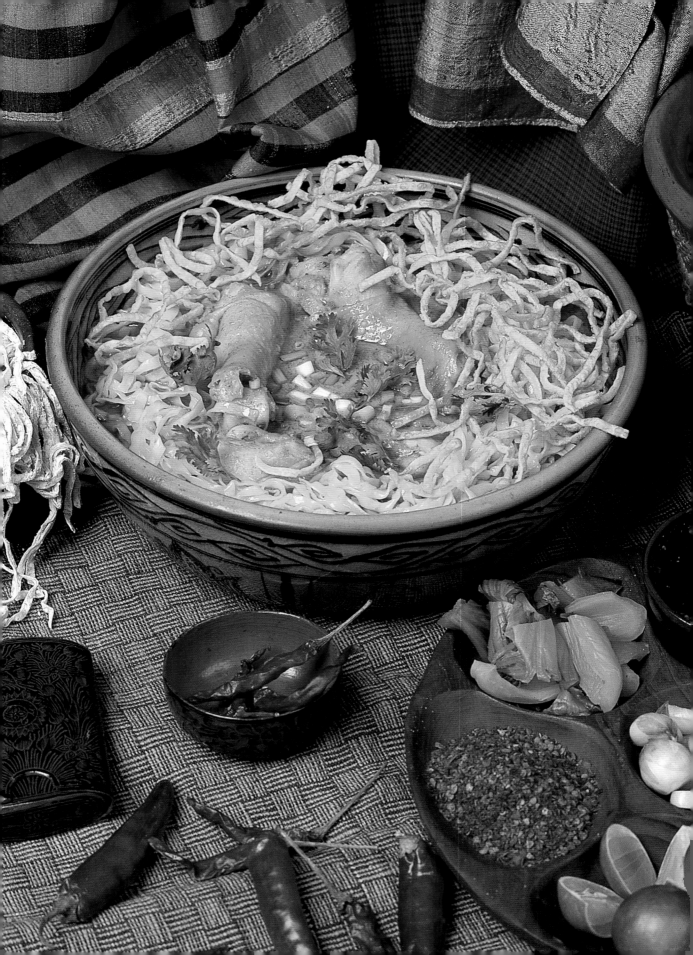

CHIANG MAI NOODLE CURRY WITH CHICKEN
KHAO SOI GAI - ข้าวซอยไก่

This dish is specific to Chiang Mai. It has quite a lot of different parts to it but it is worth it in the end. It is an amazing dish that impresses all who come to Chiang Mai.

INGREDIENTS

Serves 4

500g (5 cups, 1 lb 2oz) fresh egg noodles
Enough oil to deep-fry 100g (1 cup, 3½ oz) egg noodles
8 chicken legs
1 litre (4 cups, 32 fl oz) thick coconut milk
1 litre (4 cups, 32 fl oz) thin coconut milk
250mls (1 cup, 8 fl oz) chicken stock or water
60g (3 tablespoons) palm sugar
20g (2 tablespoons) sugar
125mls (½ cup, 4 fl oz) soy sauce
125mls (½ cup, 4 fl oz) fish sauce

Paste
Dried

1 teaspoon curry powder
½ teaspoon salt
15 big, red, dried chillies - seeds removed and soaked in water for 10 minutes and then finely chopped

Fresh

30g (2 tablespoons) ginza - skin removed, chopped
30g (6 tablespoons) lemongrass - lower 1/3 only, chopped
50g (5 tablespoons, 2 oz) coriander root - chopped
60g (6 tablespoons) shallots - chopped
15g (3 tablespoons) garlic - crushed
30g (3 tablespoons) ginger - chopped
15g (1 tablespoon) shrimp paste
250mls (1 cup, 8 fl oz) water

Accompaniments

180mls (¾ cup, 6 fl oz) oil
80g (½ cup, 3 oz) chilli powder

Pickled cabbage or cucumber
10 shallots - cut into quarters
2 limes - cut into wedges
30mls (2 tablespoons) sweet soy sauce

METHOD

Put all the ingredients for the paste into a blender and blend until smooth.

Put 250mls (1 cup, 8 fl oz) of thick coconut milk into a wok and fry for 3-5 minutes, stirring continuously, until the coconut oil begins to separate out. Add the paste and fry for 1-2 minutes until it is cooked and then add the chicken legs, chicken stock, remaining thick coconut milk and half the thin coconut milk. Bring to the boil and then add the palm sugar along the side of the wok until it melts followed by the sugar, soy sauce and fish sauce and simmer on a low heat for about 30 minutes or until the chicken is tender. Add the remaining thin coconut milk as needed, while simmering. If it get too dry you can also add some more chicken stock.

Meanwhile put the oil for frying the egg noodles into a wok and when it is hot add 100g (1 cup, 3½ oz) of egg noodles and fry until they are crispy (30 seconds). Drain and set aside.

For the accompaniments, put the oil into a wok and when it is hot add the chilli powder. Stir together and remove from the heat. Leave to cool.

When you are ready to eat put the egg noodles into some boiling water for 2 minutes and drain and put into a serving dish. Add the chicken legs and curry sauce and serve garnished with the crispy egg noodles, coriander leaves and spring onions.

Serve along with the 5 accompaniments which are added to taste.

NORTHERN STYLE CURRY WITH PORK
GAENG OHM MUU - แกงอ่อมหมู

This curry is a typical northern curry and is one of the most popular. Although it is made using water the final curry has a thick gravy-like consistency and reminds me of a Thai equivalent to steak and kidney.

INGREDIENTS
Serves 4

300g (11/2 cups, 10 oz) pork tenderloin - thinly sliced

30mls (2 tablespoons) oil

100g (4 tablespoons) gaeng ohm *(see p.108)* **or red curry paste** *(see p.105)*

500mls (2 cups, 16 fl oz) chicken stock or water

1 stalk of lemongrass - lower 1/3 only, sliced

50g (1/2 cup, 2 oz) young ginza - peeled and sliced

6 kaffir lime leaves - stems removed

30mls (2 tablespoons) fish sauce

15mls (1 tablespoon) soy sauce

1/4 teaspoon salt

5 eryngo leaves - roughly chopped

1 spring onion - sliced

10g (1/2 cup, 1/2 oz) coriander leaves

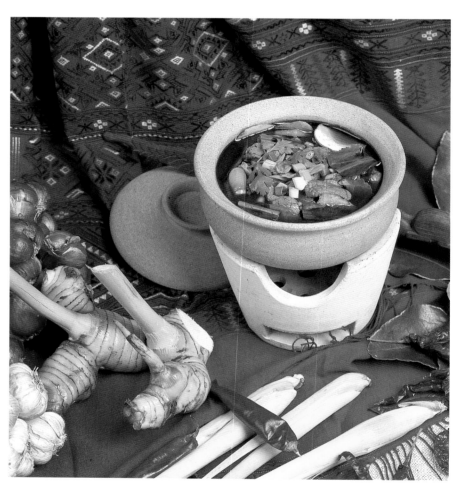

METHOD

Put the oil into a wok and when it is hot add the curry paste and fry for about 1-2 minutes. Then add the pork and stir-fry for another 2 minutes. Add the chicken stock, lemongrass, young ginza and kaffir lime leaves and bring to the boil. When it is boiling add the fish sauce, soy sauce and salt and let it simmer for about 20 minutes, until the pork is tender.

Serve garnished with the eryngo leaves, spring onion and coriander.

PICKLED BAMBOO SHOOT CURRY WITH CHICKEN

GAENG NOR MAI DORNG GAI - แกงหน่อไม้ดองไก่

I like the sour taste of the pickled bamboo shoots in this curry and it is also very good made with catfish or pork.

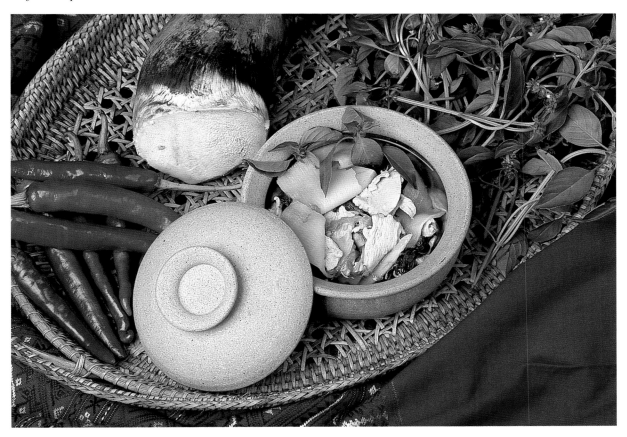

INGREDIENTS

Serves 4

300g (11/2 cups, 10oz) chicken - thinly sliced

150g (1 cup, 5 oz) pickled bamboo shoots - sliced

250mls (1 cup, 8 fl oz) chicken stock or water

15mls (1 tablespoon) fish sauce

15mls (1 tablespoon) lime juice

15g (1/2 cup, 1/2 oz) lemon basil

Paste

3 big green chillies - roasted

6 shallots - roasted

10g (2 tablespoons) garlic - roasted

5g (1 teaspoon) shrimp paste

250mls (1 cup, 8 fl oz) chicken stock or water

METHOD

Put all the ingredients for the paste into a blender and blend until smooth. Put the paste into a pan along with the chicken stock and bring to the boil. Simmer for 2 minutes and then add the chicken and cook for 3 minutes. Add the bamboo shoots, fish sauce and lime juice and simmer for another 2-3 minutes. Add the lemon basil and serve.

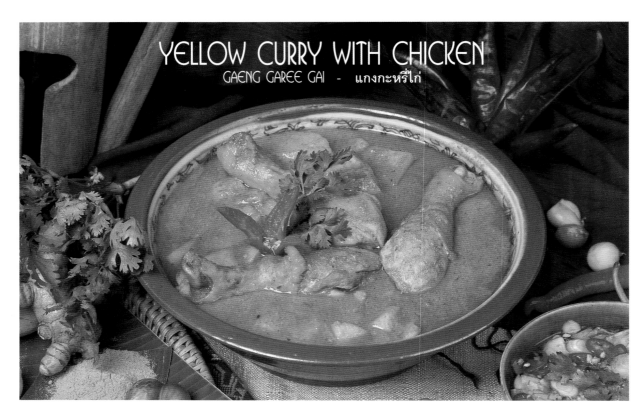

YELLOW CURRY WITH CHICKEN
GAENG GAREE GAI - แกงกะหรี่ไก่

This curry is quite similar to Indian curries and has curry powder in it. It is a creamy curry which has potatoes in it making it popular with travelers in Thailand who are missing their native food. If you like you can make this curry using chicken legs instead of chicken breast.

INGREDIENTS
Serves 4

300g (11/2 cups, 10oz) chicken breast - thinly sliced
250mls (1 cup, 8 fl oz) thick coconut milk
250mls (1 cup, 8 fl oz) thin coconut milk
1 teaspoon yellow or normal curry powder
100g (4 tablespoons) yellow curry paste *(see p.107)*
2 medium potatoes - peeled and cut into small cubes and then boiled in water for 5 minutes. (Sweet potato, taro root or pumpkin can be used instead of the potato).
40g (2 tablespoons) palm sugar
45mls (3 tablespoons) soy sauce

Sauce
90mls (6 tablespoons) sugar syrup
30mls (2 tablespoons) vinegar
4 tablespoons cucumber - thinly sliced
20g (11/2 tablespoons) ground, roasted peanuts
1 shallot - thinly sliced
1 tablespoon coriander leaves - chopped
A few slices of big, red chilli

METHOD

Put the thick coconut milk into a wok and fry for 3-5 miniutes, stirring continuously, until the coconut oil begins to separate out. Then add the yellow curry paste and the yellow curry powder and fry for 1-2 minutes. Once the paste is cooked add the chicken and potato and cook until the outside of the chicken turns white. Then and the thin coconut milk and bring to the boil. Add the palm sugar along the side of the wok until it melts and then add the soy sauce. Simmer for about 5 minutes until the chicken and potato are cooked.

Mix the ingredients for the sauce together and serve with the yellow curry.

MIXED VEGETABLE CURRY WITH CHICKEN

GAENG CARE GAI - แกงแคไก่

This dish reminds me of my childhood when my mother would often cook this dish for me and it is a northern curry. It has an unusual texture due to the inclusion of ground, roasted sticky rice and can be made using whatever selection of vegetables you have available. In Thailand it is often made with frog.

INGREDIENTS
Serves 4

300g (11/2 cups, 10oz) chicken - thinly sliced
60mls (4 tablespoons) oil
100g (4 tablespoons) gaeng care curry paste *(see p.108)* **or red curry paste** *(see p.105)*
1 big eggplant - cut into 1cm (1/2 inch) pieces
20g (1/4 cup, 1 oz) small green eggplants
30g (1/4 cup, 1 oz) long green aubergine or eggplant
2 long beans - cut into 2 cm (1 inch) pieces
20g (1 cup, 1 oz) cotton buds - optional
500mls (2 cups, 16 fl oz) chicken stock or water
1/4 teaspoon prickly ash
30mls (2 tablespoons) fish sauce
7 eryngo leaves - roughly chopped
4 pepper leaves - roughly chopped
30g (1 cup, 1 oz) acacia leaves - roughly chopped
1 big, red chilli - sliced
1/4 teaspoon salt
10g (1 tablespoon) ground, roasted sticky rice *(see p.19)*

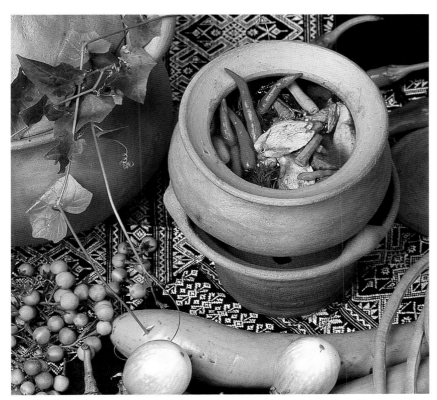

METHOD

Put the oil into a wok and fry the curry paste for 1-2 minutes. Add the chicken and fry it until it turns white. Add big eggplants, small eggplants, long green aubergine, long beans and cotton buds. Stir-fry to combine. Add half the chicken stock and the prickly ash and simmer for 2 minutes. Then add the rest of the chicken stock and the fish sauce followed by the eryngo leaves, pepper leaves, acacia leaves and the big, red chilli. Bring it to the boil and add the salt and roasted sticky rice powder. Simmer for another 2 minutes and turn off the heat and serve.

JUNGLE CURRY WITH PORK
GAENG PAH MUU - แกงป่าหมู

This curry is quite similar to red curry but it is made using water instead of coconut milk and it has more vegetables in.

INGREDIENTS
Serves 4

300g (11/2 cups, 10oz) pork - thinly sliced
60mls (4 tablespoons) oil
100g (4 tablespoons) red curry paste (see p.105)
1 big eggplant - cut into 1cm (1/2 inch) pieces
20g (1/4 cup, 1oz) small eggplants
50g (1/2 cup, 2 oz) lesser ginger - sliced into thin strips
2 long beans - cut into 2cm (1 inch) pieces
10g (1/4 cup,1/2 oz) young, green peppercorns
2 baby corn - each cut into 3 pieces
500mls (2 cups, 16 fl oz) chicken stock or water
30mls (2 tablespoons) fish sauce
1/4 teaspoon salt
5 kaffir lime leaves - stems removed
1 big, red chilli - sliced
15g (1/2 cup, 1/2 oz) holy basil

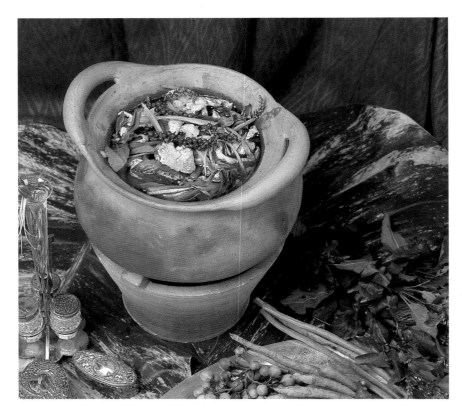

METHOD

Put the oil in a wok and fry the curry paste for 1-2 minutes. Add the pork and stir-fry until it turns white (about 2 minutes).

Add the big eggplants, small eggplants, lesser ginger, long beans, young green peppercorns, baby corn and half the chicken stock.
Bring to the boil, while stirring and simmer for 2 minutes.

Then add the rest of the chicken stock and bring back to the boil.
Add the fish sauce and salt, followed by the kaffir lime leaves and the big, red chilli.
Bring to the boil once again and add the holy basil leaves. Turn off the heat and serve.

GREEN CURRY WITH CHICKEN
GAENG KHEO WAN GAI - แกงเขียวหวานไก่

This is one of the most popular dishes that we teach. Ready-made versions are now widely available in supermarkets but nothing can beat our home-made green curry and it is a wonderful dinner party dish. You can make the sauce as thick and creamy as you like. This curry is one of the most spicy.

INGREDIENTS
Serves 4

300g (11/2 cup, 10 oz) chicken breast - thinly sliced
250mls (1 cup, 8 fl oz) of thick coconut milk - keep 30mls (2 tablespoons) set aside to use as a garnish
250mls (1 cup, 8 fl oz) thin coconut milk
100g (4 tablespoons) green curry paste *(see p.104)*
3 big egg plants - cut into 1cm (1/2 inch) pieces
50g (1/2 cup, 2oz) small egg plants
40g (2 tablespoons) palm sugar - optional
30mls (2 tablespoons) fish sauce
2 kaffir lime leaves - torn into pieces discarding the stem
30g (1 cup, 1 oz) sweet basil leaves
1 big, green chilli - sliced
1 big, red chilli - sliced

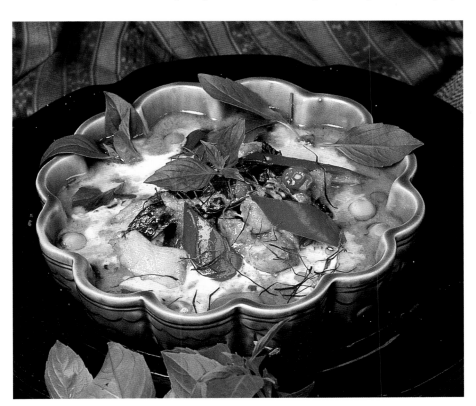

METHOD

Put the thick coconut milk into a wok and fry for 3-5 minutes, stirring continuously, until the coconut oil begins to separate out. Then add the green curry paste and fry for 1-2 minutes. Once the paste is cooked add the chicken and cook until the outside of the chicken turns white. Then add the thin coconut milk and when it is boiling add the big and small egg plants. Simmer for about 4 minutes until the egg plants are slightly soft. Then add the palm sugar along the edge of the wok so that it melts and add the fish sauce, kaffir lime leaves and half of the basil leaves.

Turn off the heat and serve garnished with the big, green chillies, big, red chillies, the remaining basil leaves and remaining thick coconut milk.

PANAENG CURRY WITH PORK
PANAENG MUU - พะแนงหมู

Panaeng curry is slightly different from the other coconut milk curries in that it has a thicker sauce. The paste is made using an amazing array of dried spices which give the curry its unique flavour.

INGREDIENTS
Serves 4

300g (11/2 cups, 10oz) pork fillet or tenderloin - thinly sliced
500mls (2 cups, 16 fl oz) thick coconut milk - keep 30mls (2 tablespoons) set aside to use as a garnish
100g (4 tablespoons) panaeng (see p.106) or red curry paste (see p.105)
40g (2 tablespoons) palm sugar
30-45mls (2-3 tablespoons) fish sauce
7 kaffir lime leaves - 3 torn into pieces discarding the stem and 4 shredded
15g (1/2 cup, 1/2 oz) sweet basil leaves
1 big, red chillies - sliced

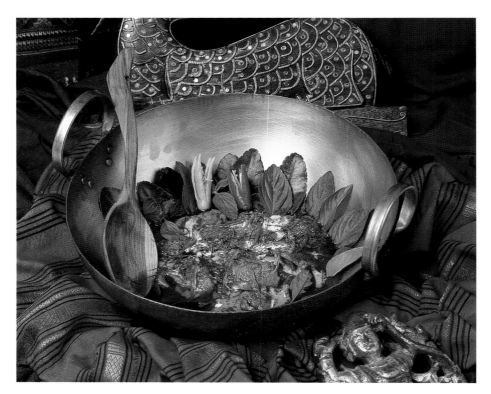

METHOD

Put half of the thick coconut milk into a wok and fry for 3-5 minutes, stirring continuously, until the coconut oil begins to separate out. Then add the panaeng curry paste and fry for 1-2 minutes. Once the paste is cooked add the pork and cook until the outside of the pork is cooked. Then add the rest of the thick coconut milk and bring to the boil. Simmer and add the palm sugar along the side of the wok until it melts and then and add the fish sauce and kaffir lime leaf pieces. Stir to combine and then add half the basil leaves.

Turn off the heat and serve garnished with the shredded kaffir lime leaves, red chillies, remaining basil leaves and remaining coconut milk.

RED CURRY WITH FISH
GAENG PHED PLAA - แกงเผ็ดปลา

Red curry is not as hot as green curry despite its colour. It is made using coconut milk and is also often made with chicken or beef.

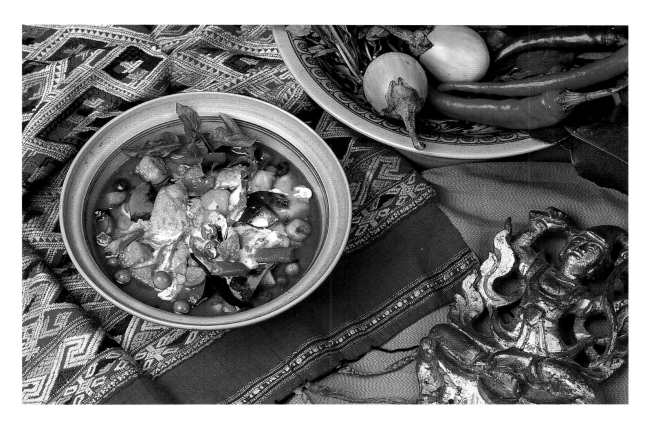

INGREDIENTS
Serves 4

300g (11/2 cups, 10 oz) fish fillets - thinly sliced
45mls (3 tablespoons) oil
100g (4 tablespoons) red curry paste *(see p.105)*
250mls (1 cup, 8 fl oz) thick coconut milk - keep 30mls
(2 tablespoons) set aside to use as a garnish
250mls (1 cup, 8 fl oz) thin coconut milk
2 big egg plants - cut into 1cm (1/2 inch) pieces
100g (1 cup, 31/2 oz) bamboo shoots - cut into bite-sized pieces
30mls (2 tablespoons) fish sauce
3 kaffir lime leaves - 2 torn into pieces discarding the stem and 1 shredded
30g (1 cup, 1 oz) sweet basil leaves
2 big, red chillies - sliced

METHOD

Put the oil into a wok and when it is hot add the curry paste and fry for 1-2 minutes. Once the paste is cooked add the thick coconut milk and when it is boiling, add the egg plants and bamboo shoots followed by the thin coconut milk. Simmer for about 4 minutes until the egg plants are slightly soft. Then add the fish sauce and kaffir lime leaf pieces. Add the fish and cook for about 2 minutes until the fish is cooked. Add half of the basil leaves.

Turn off the heat and serve garnished with the shredded kaffir lime leaf, big, red chillies and basil leaves and remaining thick coconut milk.

RED CURRY WITH ROAST DUCK

GAENG PHED PED YANG - แกงเผ็ดเป็ดย่าง

This version of red curry is very popular in my restaurant as it makes a change to the normal curries. It is quite rich due to the duck but pineapple is added to counter this richness. If you are used to eating Thai curries I think you will definitely enjoy this as it is a good variation.

INGREDIENTS
Serves 4

240g (2 cups, 8 oz) roast duck - thinly sliced
100g (4 tablespoons) red curry paste *(see p.105)*
250mls (1 cup, 8 fl oz) thick coconut milk - keep 30mls
(2 tablespoons) set aside to use as a garnish
250mls (1 cup, 8 fl oz) thin coconut milk
3 kaffir lime leaves - 2 torn into pieces discarding the stem and 1 shredded
40g (1/2 cup, 11/2 oz) young, green peppercorns
4 big egg plants - cut into 1cm (1/2 inch) pieces
50g (1/2 cup, 2oz) small egg plants
150g (1 cup, 5oz) pineapple - cut into bite-sized pieces
6 cherry tomatoes
10 grapes
30g (1 cup, 1 oz) sweet basil leaves (keep some for garnish)
1 big, red chilli - sliced (keep some for garnish)

Sauce
30mls (2 tablespoons) fish sauce
30mls (2 tablespoons) soy sauce
10g (1 tablespoon) sugar
20g (1 tablespoon) palm sugar

METHOD

Put the thick coconut milk into a wok and fry for 3-5 minutes, stirring continuously, until the coconut oil begins to separate out. Then add the red curry paste and fry for 1-2 minutes. Once the paste is cooked add the thin coconut milk and when it is boiling, add the kaffir lime leaves, young, green peppercorns, big egg plants, small egg plants, pineapple and cherry tomatoes and simmer for 3 minutes. Then add the grapes, sweet basil leaves, big, red chilli, sauce ingredients and duck and simmer for another 3 minutes. Then turn off the heat and serve garnished with the remaining basil leaves, big, red chilli and thick coconut milk.

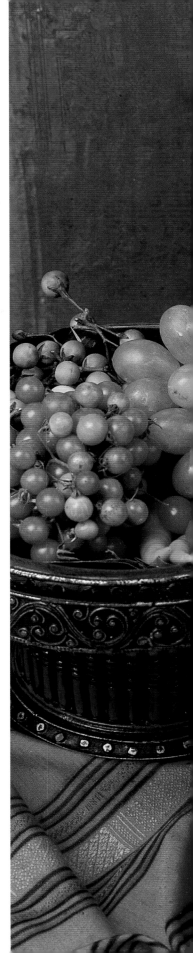

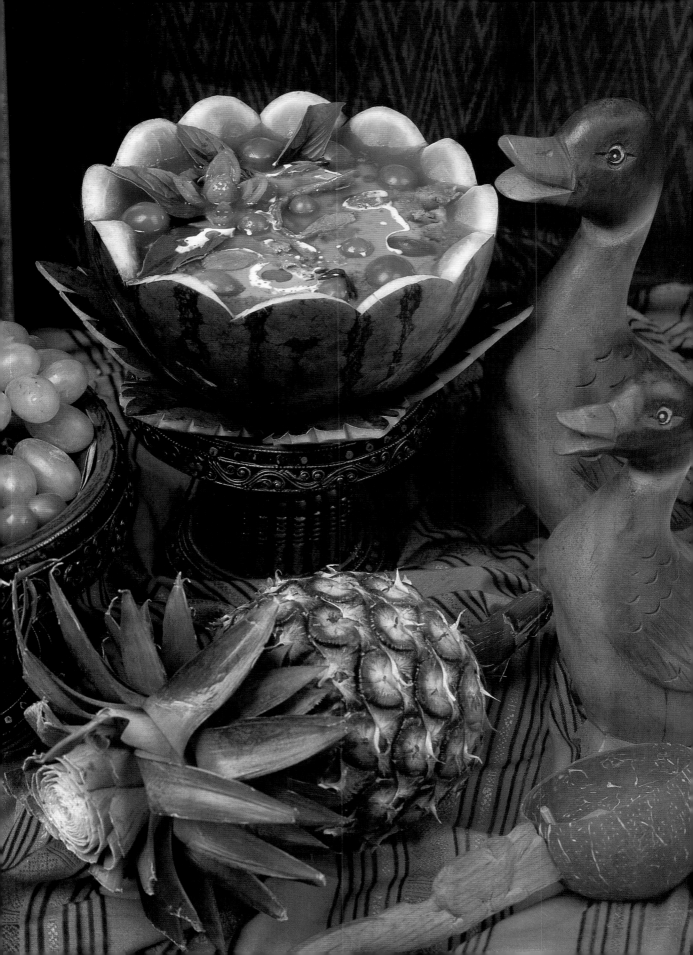

CHIANG MAI CURRY WITH PORK
GAENG HANGLAY MUU - แกงฮังเลหมู

This dish is used on ceremonial occasions in the north and is often prepared in big quantities at weddings, new house ceremonies, temple ceremonies and funerals. The sauce becomes quite thick if the dish is simmered for an hour or so and many people are surprised to learn than there is no coconut milk in this dish. If you want you can simmer it in a cool oven, an aga is especially good.

INGREDIENTS
Serves 4

500g (21/2 cups, 1 lb 2 oz) pork - cut into 2cm (1 inch) pieces
30mls (2 tablespoons) fish sauce
40g (2 tablespoons) palm sugar
5g (1 teaspoon) gaeng hanglay or normal curry powder (gaeng hanglay curry powder is made up of cumin powder, tumeric powder, coriander powder and mace powder in equal quantities)
60mls (4 tablespoons) oil
80g (3 tablespoons) gaeng hanglay curry paste (see p.107) or red curry paste (see p.105)
500mls (2 cups, 16 fl oz) water
50g (3 tablespoons) peanuts - roasted until brown
30g (1/2 cup, 1 oz) ginger - skin removed and cut into strips
45mls (3 tablespoons) tamarind juice (see p.17)

METHOD

Put the pork into a bowl along with the paste, fish sauce, palm sugar and gaeng hanglay curry powder and mix well. Leave for 20 minutes or overnight.

Put the oil into a wok and fry the pork and marinade until the outside of the pork is cooked. Then add the water and bring to the boil. Add the peanuts, ginger and tamarind juice and simmer for 15 minutes until the sauce is thick. It may be necessary to add some more water.

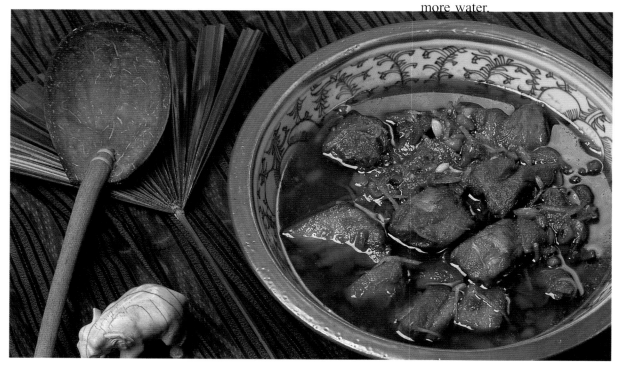

MUSSAMAN CURRY WITH BEEF
GAENG MUSSAMAN NEUA - แกงมัสมั่นเนื้อ

This curry reflects the Muslim influence in Thai cooking. Mussaman curry paste is quite different from the normal pastes used in Thai curries.

INGREDIENTS
Serves 4

300g (11/2 cups, 10oz) beef - thinly sliced
250mls (1 cup, 8 fl oz) thick coconut milk
250mls (1 cup, 8 fl oz) thin coconut milk
4 tablespoons of mussaman curry paste *(see p.109)*
10g (1 teaspoon) palm sugar
5 cardamom pods
5 bay leaves
2 medium potatoes - peeled and cut into bite-sized pieces (sweet potato, taro root or pumpkin can be used instead of the potato)
45mls (3 tablespoons) fish sauce
75mls (5 tablespoons) tamarind juice *(see p.17)*

Sauce
45mls (3 tablespoons) sugar syrup *(see p.49)*
15mls (1 tablespoon) vinegar
2 tablespoons cucumber - thinly sliced
10g (2 teaspoons) ground, roasted peanuts
1/2 shallot - thinly sliced
A few slices of big, red chilli

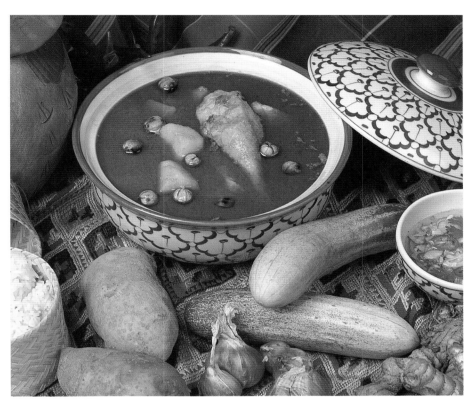

METHOD

Put the thick coconut milk into a wok and fry for 2-3 minutes, stirring continuously, until the coconut oil begins to separate out. Add the mussaman curry paste and fry for 1-2 minutes.

Once the paste is cooked add the beef and potato and cook until the outside of the beef is cooked (2-3 minutes). Then add the thin coconut milk and when it is boiling add the palm sugar along the side of the wok until it melts and then add the cardomom pods, bay leaves, fish sauce and tamarind juice. Simmer for about 20 minutes until the beef and potato are cooked.

Mix all the ingredients for the sauce together and serve as an accompaniment to the mussaman curry.

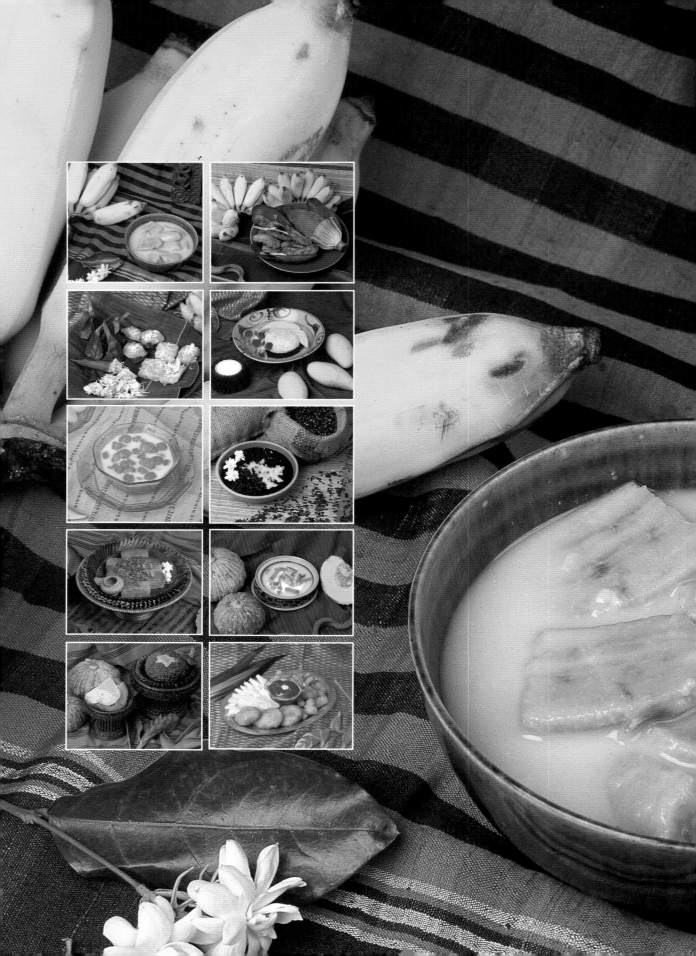

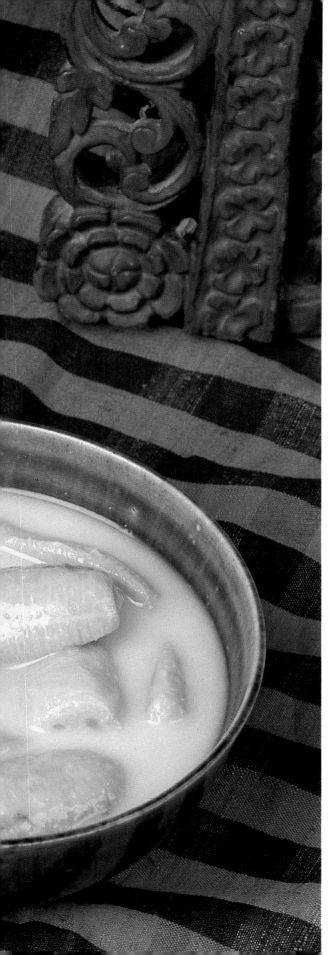

DESSERTS

Most Thai desserts are very sweet and are made of a combination of rice, coconut milk and sugar. Some foreigners find that they are too sweet but you can always put in less sugar if you are making them yourself. It can be quite difficult to get Thai desserts in restaurants as many places will opt for ice-cream and fresh fruit instead. Thai people love to eat fresh fruit and they will cut a selection of fruits into bite sized pieces and put them on a plate in the centre of the table and everyone will help themselves. This is only a small selection of Thai desserts but I have tried to choose desserts that I think will appeal to a western palate.

FRIED BANANAS
KLUAY KHEK - กล้วยแขก

Often when you walk along the streets in Thailand you will see street vendors with large woks full of hot oil deep-frying various different foods such as bananas, sweet potatoes and pumpkin. They are normally eaten as a snack and are best eaten while they are still hot.

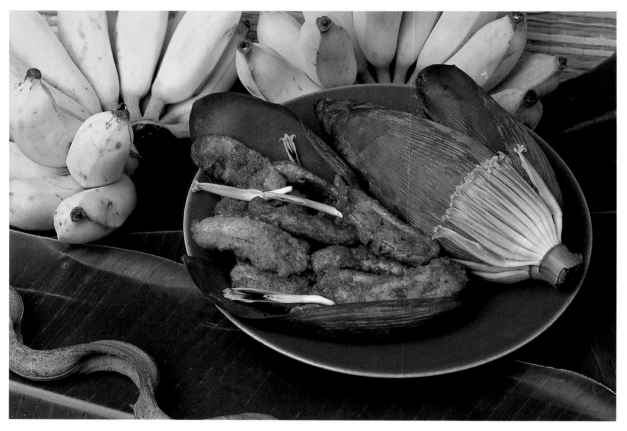

INGREDIENTS
Serves 4

4 small bananas - each sliced lengthways into 3 pieces
Enough oil to deep-fry - about 500mls (2 cups, 16fl oz)
300g (3 cups, 10oz) rice flour
300g (11/2 cups, 10oz) sugar
150g (3 cups, 5oz) grated coconut
250mls (1 cup, 8 fl oz) water
40g (2 tablespoons) palm sugar
½ teaspoon salt
5g (3 tablespoons) sesame seeds

METHOD

Put the rice flour, sugar, grated coconut, water, palm sugar and salt into a bowl and mix together using your hand. When it is well combined add the sesame seeds and mix again.

Dip the bananas into the mixture and make sure they are thoroughly coated. Put the oil into a wok and when it is hot add the banana and fry until they start to turn golden brown. They will keep on cooking once they are removed from the oil so do not over-fry them. Put them on some draining paper and then serve.

PUMPKIN IN COCONUT MILK
BUAD FUK THONG -บวดฟักทอง

Pumpkins are used quite a lot in Thai desserts and this dessert is an unusual way of serving pumpkin.

INGREDIENTS
Serves 4

200g (2 cups, 7oz) pumpkin - cut into bite-sized
chunks but leave the skin on
750mls (3 cups, 24 fl oz) water
1 teaspoon bicarbonate of soda
250mls (1 cup, 8 fl oz) thick coconut milk
250mls (1 cup, 8 fl oz) thin coconut milk
2 pandanus leaves
40g (4 tablespoons) sugar
40g (2 tablespoons) palm sugar
1/4 teaspoon salt

METHOD

Dissolve the bicarbonate of soda in the water and add the pumpkin. Leave to soak for about 10 minutes and then drain the water out.

Put the thin coconut milk into a pan along with the pandanus leaves, sugar and palm sugar and bring to the boil. Add the pumpkin and leave to simmer until the pumpkin is soft (about 10 minutes).

Add the thick coconut milk and salt and bring back to the boil and then turn off the heat and serve.

If the coconut milk is not thick enough then add 1 teaspoon of corn flour dissolved in 30mls (2 tablespoons) of water and bring back to the boil. Turn off the heat and serve either hot or cold.

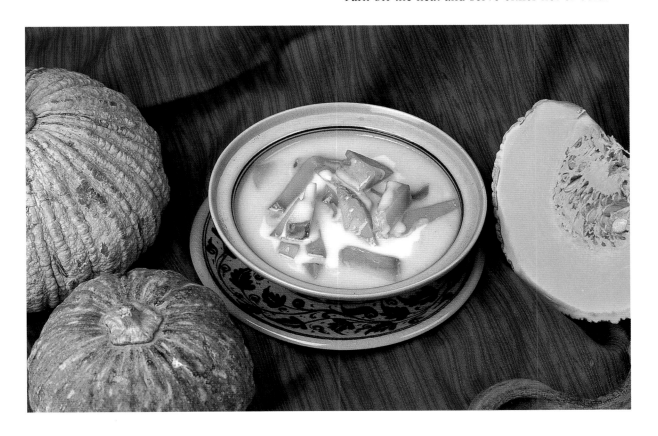

THAI CUSTARD
SANKAYA - สังขยา

I think Thai custard is wonderful and Thais will often dip pieces of bread into it but you can eat it on its own.

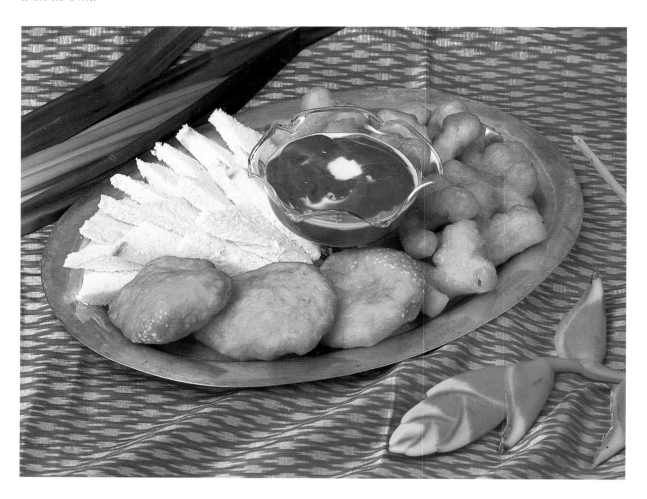

INGREDIENTS
Serves 4

200g (7oz) pandanus leaves - thinly sliced or 4 drops of pandanus extract

500mls (2 cups, 16 fl oz) water

500mls (2 cups, 16 fl oz) unsweetened, evaporated milk

250g (1 cup, 81/2 oz) sugar

15g (3 tablespoons) corn flour

1 egg

METHOD

Put the pandanus leaves into a blender along with the water and blend until smooth. Strain through some muslin into a bowl. Add the unsweetened, evaporated milk, sugar, corn flour and egg and put the entire mixture in a blender and blend until smooth.

Pour the custard mixture into a pan and cook over a very low heat, stirring continuously. Cook for 20 minutes and leave to cool before serving.

THAI CUSTARD IN A PUMPKIN
SANKAYA FUK THONG - สังขยาฟักทอง

The outside of the pumpkin is sometimes beautifully carved which makes this dessert look absolutely stunning. The richness of the custard is counterbalanced by the pumpkin. I think that this dish is quite rich but my wife absolutely loves it and thinks that it is one of the most delicious Thai desserts that there is. It is definitely worth trying and is an excellent dish for a dinner party.

INGREDIENTS
Serves 4

1 small pumpkin
4 ducks eggs
120g (6 tablespoons) palm sugar
250mls (1 cup, 8 fl oz) thick coconut milk

METHOD

Cut a square in the top of the pumpkin where the stem is. Keep, to use as a lid. Remove all the seeds and some of the pulp from the centre.

Put the eggs into a bowl and lightly whisk. Add the palm sugar and thick coconut milk and mix all the ingredients together until well blended. Pour the custard mixture into the pumpkin and steam for about 20 -25 minutes until the custard is set. The lid should also be steamed.

Serve once the pumpkin has cooled.

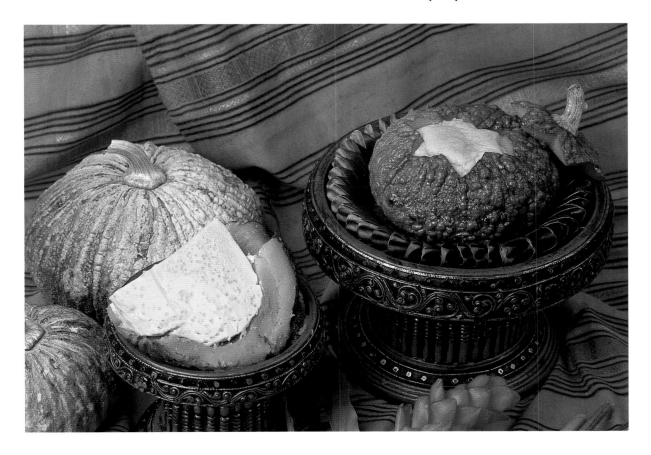

BANANAS IN COCONUT MILK
KLUAY BUAD CHEE - กล้วยบวดชี

Bananas are often used in desserts and this dish is really easy to make and has a lovely creamy sauce.

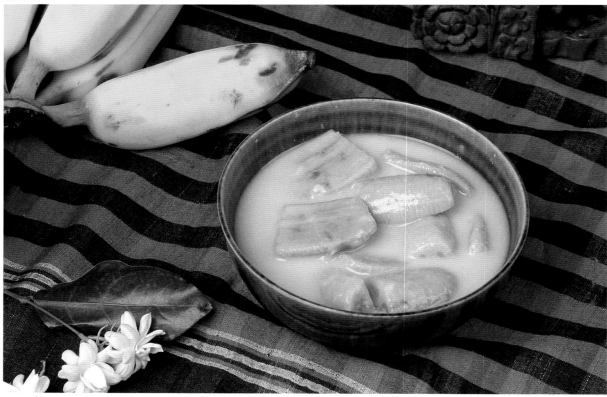

INGREDIENTS
Serves 4

8 small bananas (or pumpkin, sweet potato, or taro)
500mls (2 cups, 16 fl oz) thick coconut milk
500mls (2 cups, 16 fl oz) thin coconut milk
2 pandanus leaves or 2 drops of pandanus extract
40g (2 tablespoons) firm palm sugar
40g (4 tablespoons) sugar
Pinch of salt to taste

METHOD

Steam the bananas in their skins for about 5 minutes (or boil for 2 minutes) until the skins starts to break. Once the skin breaks remove the bananas and peel. Cut each banana into about 4 pieces.

Put the thin coconut milk into a pan along with the pandanus leaf and bring to the boil. When it is boiling add the banana pieces followed by the firm palm sugar, sugar and salt. Bring to the boil and add the thick coconut milk. Boil gently in all for about 3 minutes. If you want the sauce to be thicker then add 5g (1 teaspoon) of tapioca flour to the coconut milk. Do not boil for too long or the oil will start to separate out from the coconut milk and the bananas will be too soft. The bananas should be slightly hard. It can be eaten hot or cold.

WATER CHESTNUTS WITH SUGAR SYRUP AND COCONUT MILK
TAB TIM GROB - ทับทิมกรอบ

This is one of the most unusual desserts that we have and the crunchy water chestnuts make it a really refreshing dessert when combined with the sweet sugar syrup and ice.

INGREDIENTS

Serves 4

130g (1 cup, 41/2 oz) water chestnuts - peeled and cut into quarters
Chunks of melon - optional
125mls (1/2 cup, 4 fl oz) water
1/2 teaspoon red food colouring

30g (1/4 cup, 1 oz) tapioca flour
1000mls (4 cups, 32 fl oz) water

Sugar Syrup
130g (1/2 cup, 41/2 oz) sugar
125mls (1/2 cup, 4 fl oz) water

125mls (1/2 cup, 4 fl oz) thick coconut milk
Ice - crushed

METHOD

Put the water chestnuts into the water along with the red food colouring. Leave to soak for 20 minutes.

Meanwhile put the water and sugar for the sugar syrup into a pan and dissolve the sugar over a low heat. Once the sugar has dissolved bring the water to the boil and boil for 2 minutes.

Put the 1000mls of water into a pan and bring it to the boil. Drain the water chestnuts and roll each one in the tapioca flour. Once the water is boiling drop the water chestnuts into the water and leave for about 2 minutes until they float. Then remove them and put them into a bowl of cold water. If you are not going to serve the water chestnuts straight away then remove them from the water and store them in a bowl in the refrigerator.

To serve, put the water chestnuts into individual bowls and spoon over some of the sugar syrup and thick coconut milk. Add some crushed ice and serve.

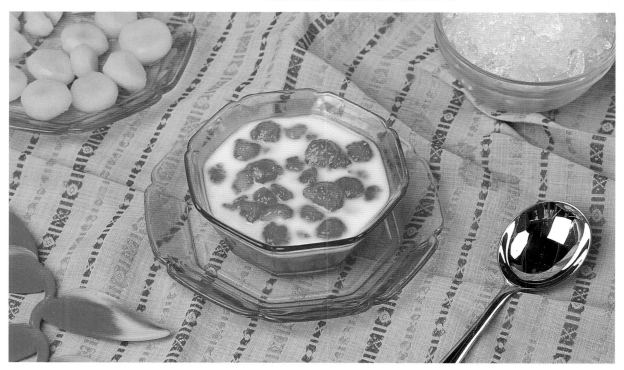

BLACK STICKY RICE PUDDING
KHAO NEOW DAM PIAK - ข้าวเหนียวดำเปียก

I still remember when I was a young boy using buffaloes to plough the rice fields with my father and I noticed that the leaves on the rice were black. This was my first introduction to black rice as everything about this rice is black. Many people think that colour is added to the rice but infact it is naturally black. This pudding will be appreciated by anybody who likes rice pudding.

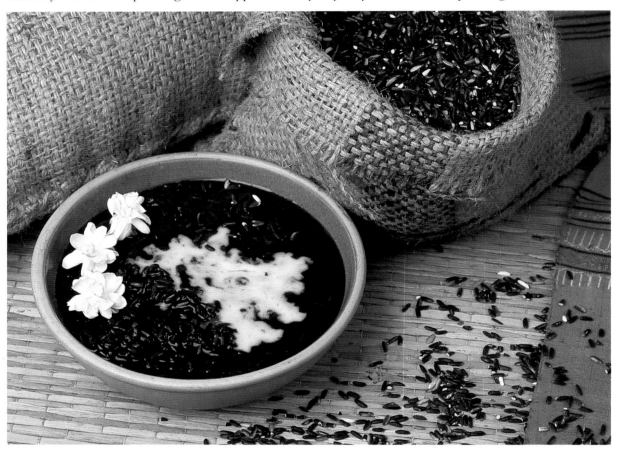

INGREDIENTS
Serves 2

130g (½ cup, 41/2 oz) black sticky rice (white sticky rice can also be used)
750mls (3 cups, 24 fl oz) water
250mls (1 cup, 8 fl oz) thick coconut milk - reserve 60mls (1/4 cup, 4 tablespoons) for garnish
70g (1/4cup, 21/2 oz) sugar

METHOD

Put the black sticky rice into a pan along with the water and bring to the boil.

Simmer for 30 minutes until the rice is cooked, stirring occasionally.

Once the rice is cooked, add the coconut milk and sugar and simmer for 3-5 minutes.

Serve with the remaining thick coconut milk spooned on top. It can be eaten either hot or cold.

STEAMED BANANA CAKE

KHANOM KLUAY - ขนมกล้วย

This is a really simple cake to make and in Thailand it is sometimes steamed in little banana leaf boats or in little bowls. If you cannot obtain grated coconut then you can use unsweetend dessicated coconut but it needs to be soaked in water for about 10 minutes before using.

INGREDIENTS

Serves 6

10 small bananas (or 5 large bananas) - mashed
120g (1 cup, 4 oz) rice flour
30g (1/4 cup, 1oz) tapioca flour
130g (1/1/2 cup, 41/2 oz) sugar
1/2 teaspoon salt
125mls (1/2 cup, 4 fl oz) thick coconut milk
100g (3 cups, 1/2 oz) grated coconut

METHOD

Put the bananas into a bowl along with the rice flour, tapioca flour, sugar, salt, coconut milk and 3/4 of the grated coconut. Mix well until all the ingredients are thoroughly combined. Put the mixture into a steaming or baking tin (8"x 8" or 20cm x 20cm) and sprinkle the rest of the grated coconut on the top.

Steam for 30 minutes or bake in the oven (180°C or 360°F) for 30 minutes. Once it is cooked turn the cake out of the tin and serve hot or cold.

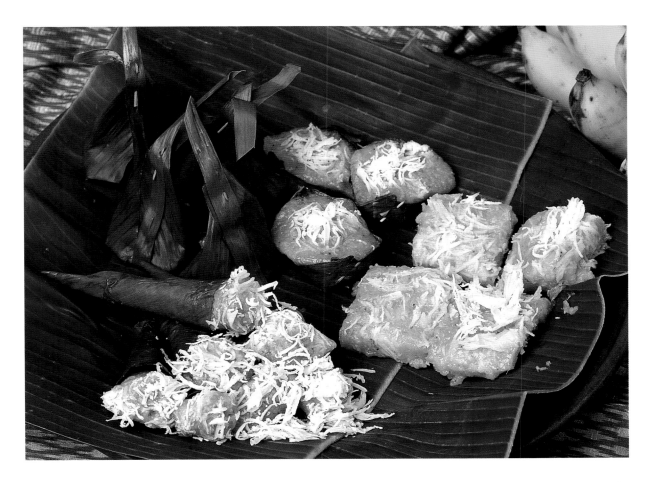

MANGO WITH STICKY RICE
KHAO NEOW MAMUANG - ข้าวเหนียวมะม่วง

This is one of the most popular Thai desserts and many foreigners who come to Thailand regularly make sure that they come in the mango season so that they can have this dessert every day! The sweet sticky rice can be made in advance but should be eaten the same day that it is made.

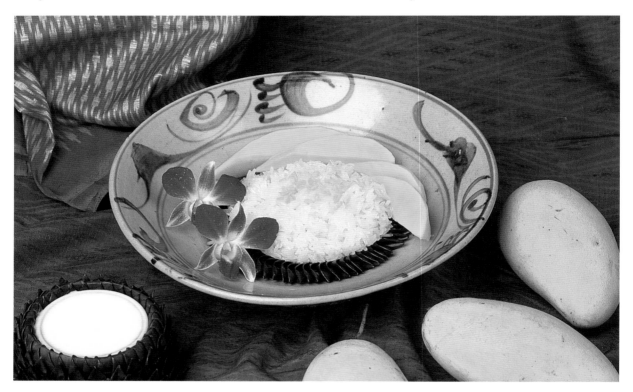

INGREDIENTS

Serves 6

2 mangoes
600g (4 cups, 1 lb 5oz) sticky rice - soaked in
water for at least 3 hours or overnight
500mls (2 cups, 16 fl oz) thick coconut milk
200g (1 cup, 81/2 oz) sugar
1/2 teaspoon salt
5g (1 tablespoon) of sesame seeds - roasted

Sauce
120mls (1/2 cup, 4 fl oz) thin coconut milk
30g (2 tablespoons) sugar
pinch of salt

METHOD

Steam the soaked sticky rice for 15-20 minutes until it is cooked. Mix the thick coconut milk, sugar and salt together. Once the rice is cooked put it in a bowl and while it is still hot add the coconut milk, sugar and salt mixture and combine thoroughly. Leave to rest for about 30-50 minutes so that the rice has time to absorb the coconut milk. Mix the sauce ingredients together and set aside.

When you are ready to serve the dessert, divide the sticky rice into 6 portions and put into separate bowls. Peel the mangoes and slice thinly. Put the mango slices on top of the sticky rice. Then pour the thin coconut milk sauce over the mangoes and sprinkle the sesame seeds on top and serve.

BAKED MUNG BEAN CAKE
KHANOM MOH GAENG - ขนมหม้อแกง

The first time I had this cake I was not sure what it would taste like but the combination of mung beans and crispy fried shallots is really good.

INGREDIENTS

250g (1 cup, 81/2 oz) dried mung bean
1 litre (4 cups, 32 fl oz) water
250mls (1 cup, 8 fl oz) thick coconut milk
200g (1/2 cup, 7 oz) palm sugar
1/2 teaspoon salt
3 eggs
3 shallots - thinly sliced and fried in
30mls (2 tablespoons) oil until brown and crispy

METHOD

Cover the mung beans with some water and soak for 4 hours or overnight.

Drain the mung beans and put into a pan with the 1litre (4 cups, 32 fl oz) water. Simmer for 30 minutes or until soft. Stir occasionally.

Put the thick coconut milk, palm sugar and salt into a bowl and mix together.

Add the eggs and mix well. Strain the mixture into another bowl and add the mung beans. Mix well.

Pour the mixture into a baking tray (8" x 8" or 20cm x 20cm) and bake in the oven (180°C or 360°F) for 40 minutes. Sprinkle the shallots on top and cook for another 5 minutes. Allow to cool and cut into squares to serve.

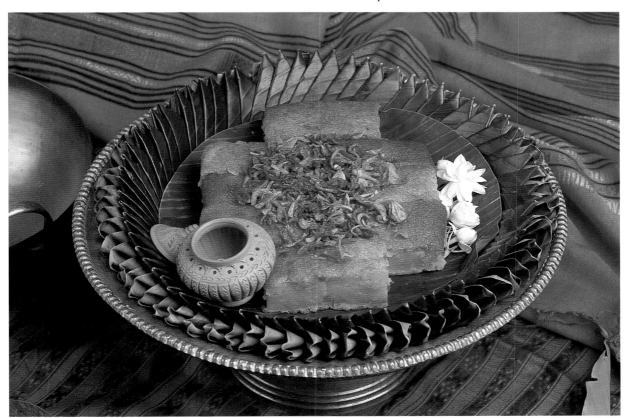

INDEX